Neuropsychiatric

DISORDERS

Neuropsychiatric
DISORDERS

Gareth W Roberts, PhD

Senior Lecturer in Neuroanatomy

Department of Anatomy and Cell Biology

St Mary's Hospital Medical School

London, UK

P Nigel Leigh, PhD, FRCP

Head of University Department of Neurology

Institute of Psychiatry and King's College School of Medicine and Dentistry

London, UK

Daniel R Weinberger, MD

Chief, Clinical Brain Disorders Branch

National Institute of Mental Health

Division of Intramural Research Programs

NIMH Neuropsychiatric Research Hospital

Washington, DC, USA

with a contribution by

Robert H Perry, FRCP, FRCPath

Consultant Neuropathologist and Reader in Neurochemical Pathology

Newcastle General Hospital

Newcastle upon Tyne, UK

Foreword by

Stanley B Prusiner, MD

Professor of Neurology

University of California

San Francisco, USA

WOLFE

London St. Louis Baltimore Boston Chicago Philadelphia Sydney Toronto

For full details of all Mosby Europe Limited titles please write to
Mosby Europe Limited, Brook House, 2–16 Torrington Place,
London WC1E 7LT, England.

Publisher:	Fiona Foley
Project Manager:	Robert Whittle
Design:	Mark Willey
	Jim Evoy
Illustration:	Mark Willey
	Maurice Murphy
Index:	Nina Boyd
Production:	Susan Bishop

British Library Cataloguing in Publication Data:
Library of Congress Cataloging in Publication Data:
Catalogue records for this title are available

ISBN 1-56375-510-6
Text set in Garamond; captions set in Gill
Originated in Hong Kong by Mandarin Offset Ltd
Printed in Singapore
Produced by Imago Productions, Singapore

Foreword

The costs to society of neuropsychiatric disorders are extraordinarily expensive both in terms of human suffering and economic resources. Dementing illnesses are among the most prevalent of these disorders and are thought to be the fourth leading cause of death in many developed nations following heart disease, cancer and stroke. Dementia takes its toll not only in the patients who are afflicted with an illness that robs them of the qualities that made them humans but also in non-affected family members who are forced to devote their lives caring for their impaired loved ones. The most common dementia is Alzheimer's disease — not only is the cause of this disease unknown but there are no effective treatments or methods of prevention.

The incidence of many neuropsychiatric disorders increases with age. Demographic studies predict staggering increases in the number of patients afflicted with neuropsychiatric disorders since improved medical care, which effectively treats many acute illnesses, often results in greater longevity. This medical paradox can only be remedied by first elucidating the causes of illnesses such as Alzheimer's disease and then developing effective therapies. As medical scientists have deepened their understanding of this murky and once seemingly impenetrable morass of vague, poorly defined illnesses, several new nosological entities have emerged in the last decade — AIDS dementia complex, cortical Lewy body disease, and prion disease — to produce their additional burden of complexity.

The development and application of new research tools emerging from microelectronics, scanning and confocal microscopy, image analysis and reconstruction, immunology and molecular biology, have produced a deluge of new information on the anatomy, physiology and chemistry of the brain. The advent of this new neuroscience is an enormously exciting avenue but applying all this new information to the improved care of patients is a daunting task.

Some of the benefits of this new neuroscience derive from the influx of skilled scientific and technical staff working with clinicians to investigate the etiology and pathogenesis of disease. As invariably occurs, this cross-fertilization among such disciplines as neurology, psychiatry, genetics, neuroanatomy, neuroimaging and neuropathology has produced a cornucopia of insights into the biology of the brain and its relationship to disease. The progeny of this union is the phoenix of neuropsychiatry newly risen from the arid slough of 'syndrome-ology'.

This emergent and rapidly expanding field which is so interdisciplinary has produced many clinicians who believe that their training in neuroscience has been inadequate to permit them to capture and appreciate the full meaning of so many stellar advances. From the point of view of the scientist, neuropsychiatric diseases have risen from vague entities to be avoided at all costs to areas of investigation which are considered by many to be among the most challenging and rewarding. The rapid progress of scientific investigation means that the classic phenomenology of psychiatry and neurology must be remolded to accommodate new concepts of disease and that accepted concepts of pathophysiology must be reassessed in the light of recent findings.

The process of communicating and disseminating so much new information presents problems, which are particularly acute for those who are beginning to study neuropsychiatric disease, and for those who try to relate their knowledge of the pathophysiology of one disease to another.

This volume so beautifully illustrated and clearly written by Gareth Roberts, Nigel Leigh and Daniel Weinberger addresses many of these problems. By distilling a torrent of data the authors have tried to capture the essence of the various disease processes. The etiology, clinicopathology, and physiology are presented concisely but accurately while illustrations augment the presentation of important concepts. Their refreshing approach has been to describe the trunks rather than the branches of individual trees of knowledge. The latter task is reserved for more comprehensive texts.

The last ten years of the twentieth century have been called the 'Decade of the Brain'. This designation highlights the challenges for clinicians and biomedical scientists in trying to unravel the causes of many dreaded, neuropsychiatric disorders that have resisted investigation for so long. It is the hope of the authors that this volume will be helpful to both clinicians and scientists as they try to find new ways to ameliorate the tragic burdens cast by many neuropsychiatric illnesses.

Stanley B Prusiner *San Francisco*

Preface

Over the last decade, great advances have been made in understanding the biology of neuropsychiatric disorders. In addition, neuroscience has come of age, giving birth to many courses and publications which are designed to integrate the study of anatomy, physiology and the functions of the brain. As teachers, we are asked to provide overviews on the biology of these disorders to scientists and clinicians at various stages of their training. However, these requests often create a formidable problem in presenting the mass of information in a way which is accessible, balanced, and which integrates natural history, clinical features and basic science. Because we could not find a book which seems to combine these aspects adequately, we decided to write our own text, and hence this volume was conceived.

We have gathered up-to-date information on many aspects of the major neuropsychiatric and neurodegenerative disorders, and combined a succinct text with key illustrations, culminating in a series of chapters that we hope will provide a useful starting point for an audience interested in the causes, symptoms, pathology and biology of these disorders. We did not aim for exhaustive detail, but rather to place before the reader balanced accounts of the most important topics, and to provide an entry to more detailed study through key references to more detailed reading.

The work of assembling the text and illustrations generated many new ideas and collaborations, and we received helpful advice from many colleagues, both in basic and clinical neuroscience. Many friends and colleagues have responded to our requests for illustrations, and we thank them for their unstinted help.

This project might have remained a fanciful notion but for the drive and enthusiasm of our publishers. Our vague concepts were transformed by the application of 'Gower Power' personified by publisher Fiona Foley, who with a velvet hand in a velvet glove ensured the project's completion; Robert Whittle, project manager and editor provided guidance, and a bottomless coffee pot; and Mark Willey (artist) whose ability to metamorphose scribbled sketches into meaningful illustrations was little short of awesome. Working with you was a pleasure!

Any errors or omissions are our own. We hope that the book will prove to be a useful introduction for those working at the interface between clinical and basic neuroscience, be they undergraduate or postgraduate students, neurologists or psychiatrists in training, or more senior colleagues who will find the text and illustration useful for teaching. We hope also that the book illustrates the excitement and intellectual challenges posed by the study of these complex disorders.

Acknowledgement

Dr Robert Perry would like to thank Mr AE Oakley for photographic assistance in the preparation of the coronal maps in chapter 1.

Contents

1 A Guide to the Cortical Regions

Brodmann's areas are often used to localize function and/or damage in the cerebral cortex. However, MRI and CT scans, which detect regions of damage, are generally presented as coronal slices. An integration of these two systems of describing regions of interest within the brain is desirable. The first such synthesis is presented here.

This *Guide to the Cortical Regions* shows a series of 33 coronal slices at standard intervals through the brain – slice number 1 at the anterior pole of the cerebrum, through to slice number 33 at the posterior pole – to demonstrate Brodmann's areas of the cortex. The angle of these coronal slices is indicated on the diagrammatic lateral view of the brain below. The Brodmann's areas are coloured consistently throughout; the colours are keyed below. All the diagrams are approximately life size. Brodmann areas in primary sensory cortex (3, 1, 2, 5) have been demonstrated in the coronal plane as Brodmann area 3.

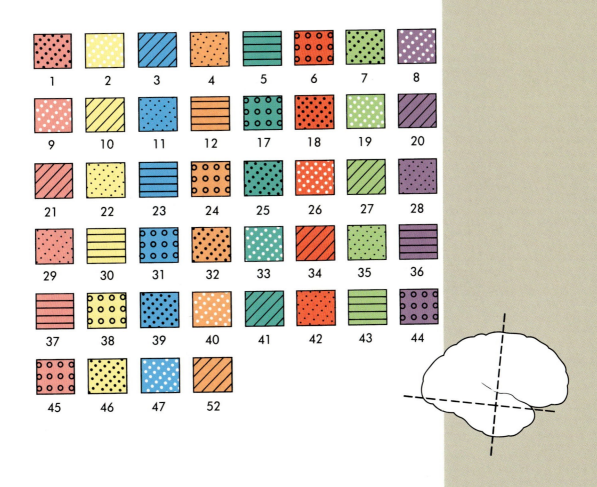

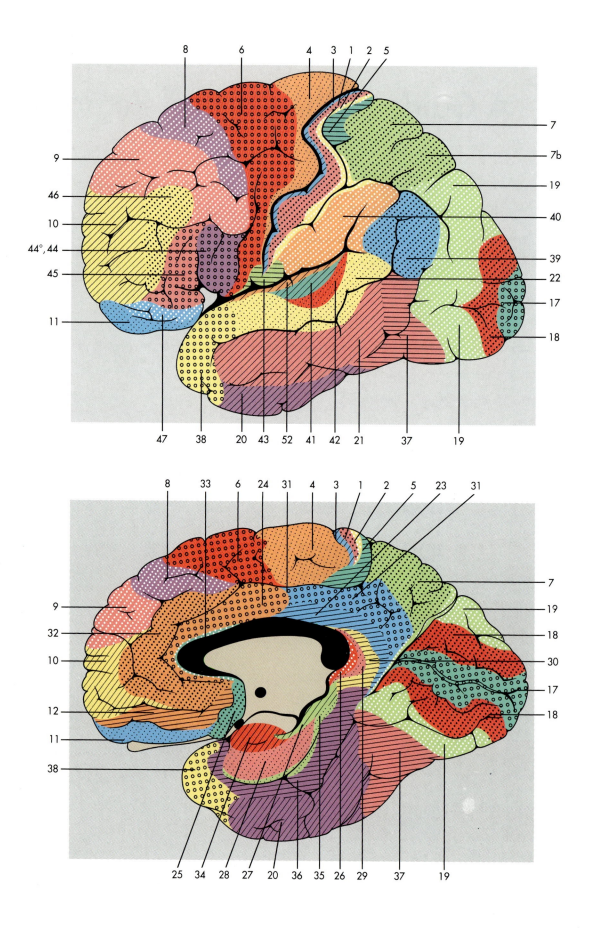

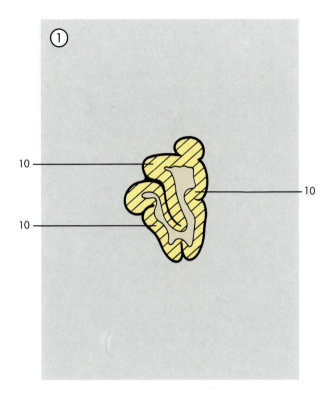

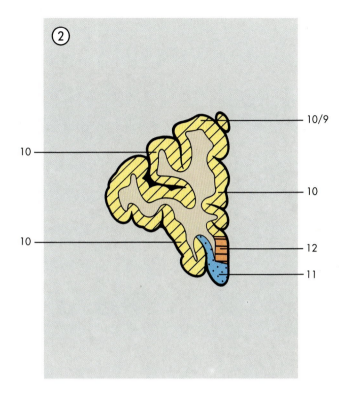

①

10 —

10 —

10 —

②

10 —

10 —

— 10/9

— 10

— 12

— 11

③

9 —

10 —

10 —

— 9

— 10/32

— 10

— 12

— 11

④

9 —

10/46 —

10/45/47 —

olfactory bulb

— 9

— 32

— 12

— 11

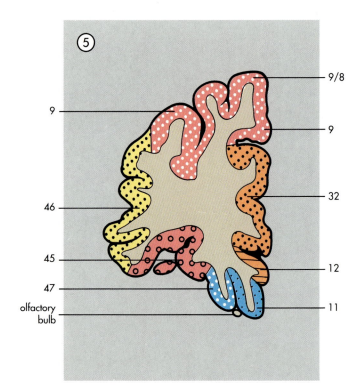

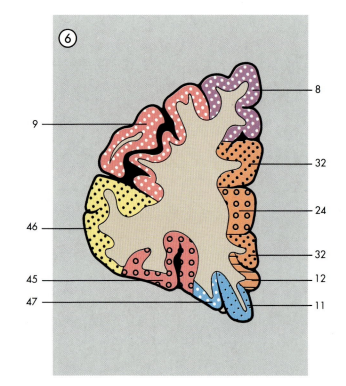

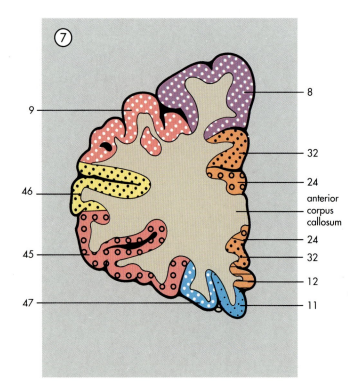

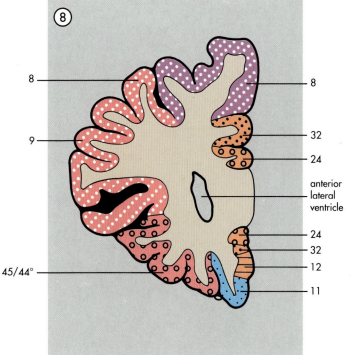

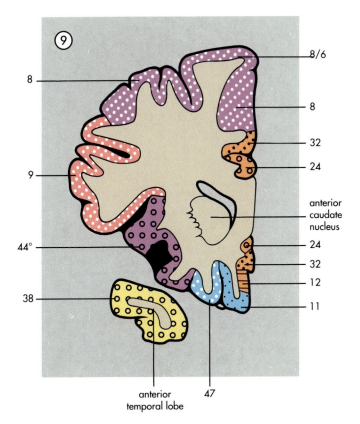

⑨

8/6

8

32

24

anterior caudate nucleus

24

32

12

11

8

9

44°

38

anterior temporal lobe

47

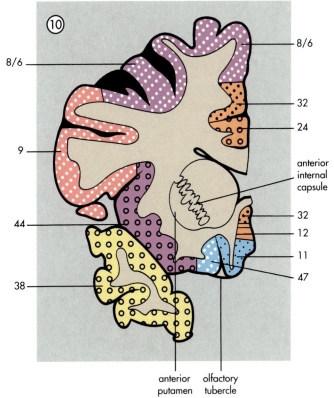

⑩

8/6

8/6

9

44

38

8/6

32

24

anterior internal capsule

32

12

11

47

anterior putamen

olfactory tubercle

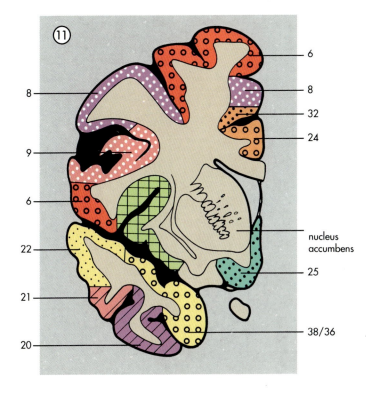

⑪

8

9

6

22

21

20

6

8

32

24

nucleus accumbens

25

38/36

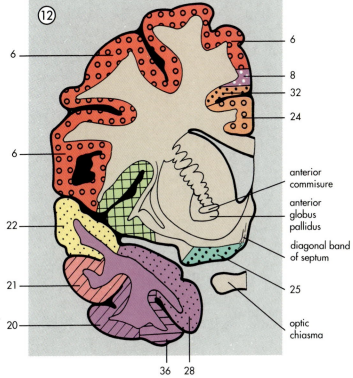

⑫

6

6

6

22

21

20

6

8

32

24

anterior commisure

anterior globus pallidus

diagonal band of septum

25

optic chiasma

36   28

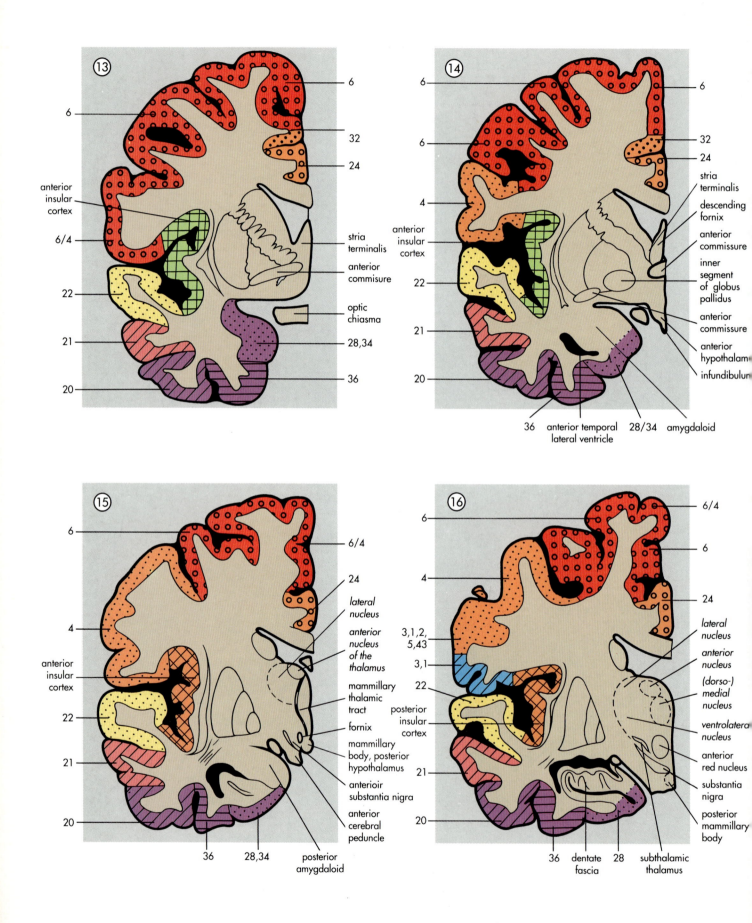

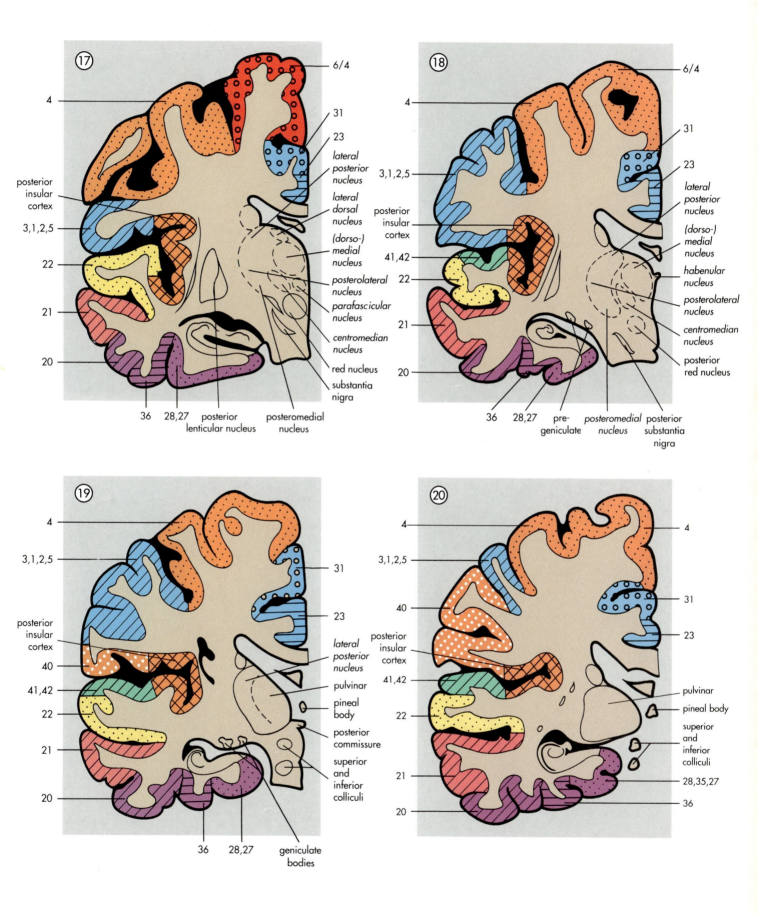

⑰

4

6/4

31

23

lateral posterior nucleus

lateral dorsal nucleus

(dorso-) medial nucleus

posterolateral nucleus

parafascicular nucleus

centromedian nucleus

red nucleus

substantia nigra

posterior insular cortex

3,1,2,5

22

21

20

36   28,27   posterior lenticular nucleus   posteromedial nucleus

⑱

4

6/4

31

23

lateral posterior nucleus

(dorso-) medial nucleus

habenular nucleus

posterolateral nucleus

centromedian nucleus

posterior red nucleus

3,1,2,5

posterior insular cortex

41,42

22

21

20

36   28,27   pre-geniculate   *posteromedial nucleus*   posterior substantia nigra

⑲

4

3,1,2,5

posterior insular cortex

40

41,42

22

21

20

31

23

lateral posterior nucleus

pulvinar

pineal body

posterior commissure

superior and inferior colliculi

36   28,27   geniculate bodies

⑳

4

3,1,2,5

40

posterior insular cortex

41,42

22

21

20

4

31

23

pulvinar

pineal body

superior and inferior colliculi

28,35,27

36

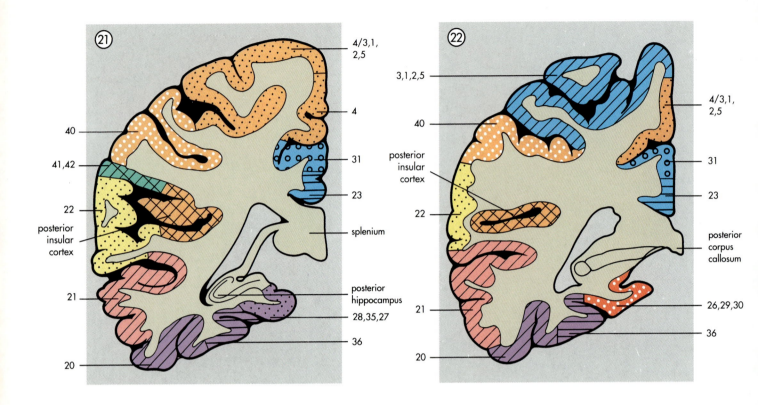

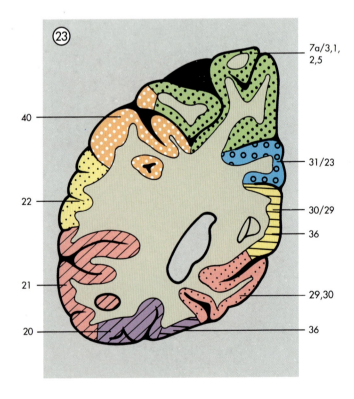

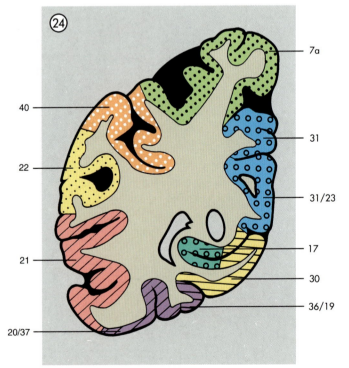

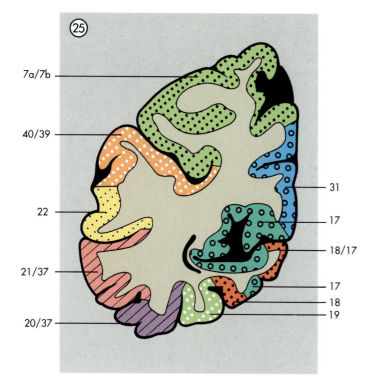

(25)

7a/7b

40/39

22

21/37

20/37

31

17

18/17

17
18
19

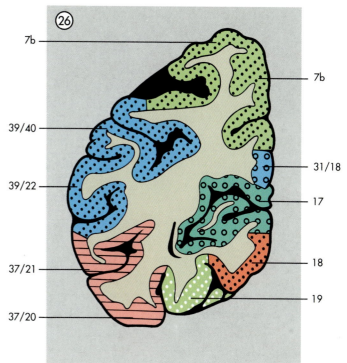

(26)

7b

39/40

39/22

37/21

37/20

7b

31/18

17

18

19

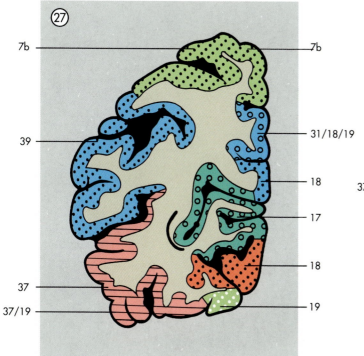

(27)

7b

39

37

37/19

7b

31/18/19

18

17

18

19

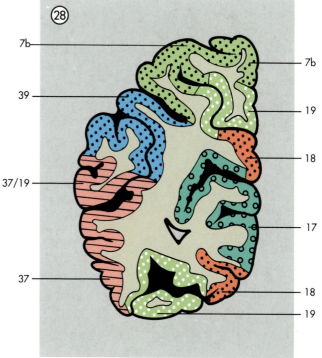

(28)

7b

39

37/19

37

7b

19

18

17

18

19

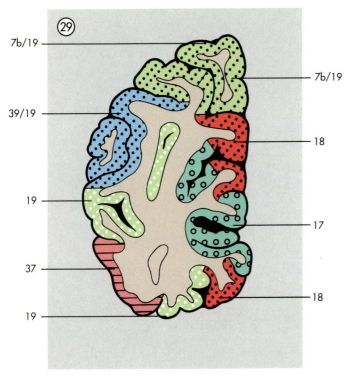

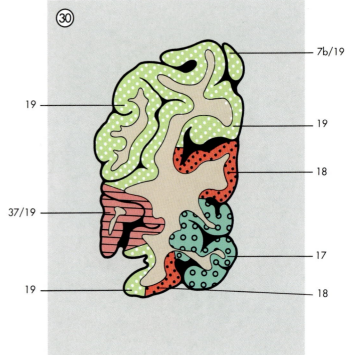

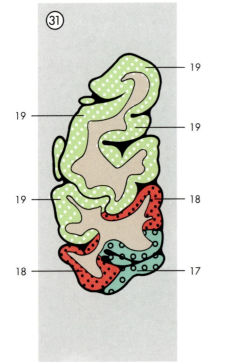

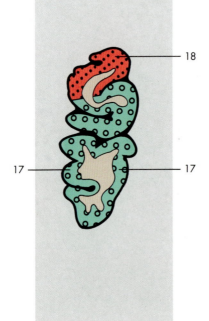

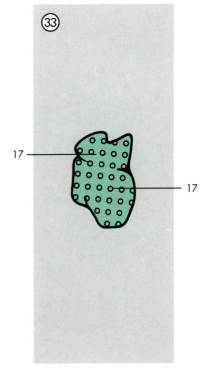

SECTION 1

Dementias

Dementia is the most disabling psychiatric disorder of adulthood. It is very common and incidence rates rise dramatically with age, from 0.5 per cent of the population at age 40 up to 20 per cent of those aged 80 and over.

As a consequence of increased longevity and improvements in therapy (e.g. for hypertension and head trauma), the number of cases has increased and continues to increase dramatically. It is estimated that there are 1 500 000 persons in the USA requiring constant medical care and a further 3 000 000 who cope in the community with support. Dementia is now the fourth commonest cause of death in the USA. Its clinical manifestations may be widespread and diverse, so that dementia can seldom be omitted from consideration in diagnosing mental illness, especially in old age.

A work group under the auspices of the US Department of Health and Human Services proposed the following criteria for dementia:

Dementia is the decline of memory and other cognitive functions in comparison with the patient's previous level of function as determined by a history of decline in performance and by abnormalities noted from clinical examination and neuropsychological tests. A diagnosis of dementia cannot be made when consciousness is impaired by delirium, drowsiness, stupor or coma or when other clinical abnormalities prevent adequate evaluation of mental status. Dementia is a diagnosis based on behaviour and cannot be determined by CT and MRI scans, EEG or other laboratory instruments although specific causes of dementia may be identified by these means.

Diagnosing Dementia When establishing the presence of a dementia and determining a differential diagnosis as to the probable cause, it is important to differentiate between acute and chronic states of dementia (Fig. 1); to determine whether the dementia can be treated; and to establish a prognosis so that appropriate counselling and support can be provided.

Establishing the existence of a dementia and uncovering its aetiology is based largely on clinical findings supported by appropriate imaging and laboratory investigations. Given that the patient's cognitive function is often poor, an informant (usually a close relative) may be required to ensure that a thorough clinical assessment and detailed history is obtained.

a. Causes of Acute Organic Disorders

Hypoxia

heart failure, myocardial infarction
respiratory disorders

Infections

general: bronchopneumonia, urinary tract, topical infections
cerebral: meningitis, encephalitis

Metabolic disorders

electrolyte disturbance
uraemia
hepatic encephalopathy
porphyria
hypoglycaemia

Vitamin deficiencies

thiamine (Wernicke's encephalopathy)
vitamin B_{12}
nitotinic acid (pellagra)

Endocrine diseases

myxoedema, thyrotoxicosis
parathyroid disorder
diabetes mellitus
Cushing's disease, Addison's disease
hypopituitarism

Trauma

head injury

Epilepsy

psychomotor seizure
post-ictal state
non-convulsive seizures

Space-occupying lesions

tumours: primary, metastatic
subdural haematoma
cerebral abscess

Vascular disorders

transient ischaemic attacks
multi-infarct dementia
cerebral embolism
hypertensive encephalopathy
subarachnoid haemorrhage
disseminated lupus erythematosis
transient global amnesia

Toxic disorders

drugs: alcohol, barbiturates, amphetamines, LSD, opiates,
    cannabis, cocaine, salicylates, phenacetin, tricyclic
    antidepressants, MAOIs, lithium, benzhexol, L-Dopa,
    isoniazid, cycloserine, steroids, digoxin
industrial metals: lead, mercury, manganese

b. Causes of Chronic Organic Disorders

Degenerative disorders

presenile dementia: Alzheimer's disease, Pick's disease, Prion
    disease, Cortical Lewy body disease, Huntington's chorea
senile dementia

Vascular disorders

multi-infarct dementia
subarachnoid haemorrhage
cerebral haemorrhage
cerebral embolism
disseminated lupus erythematosis

Space-occupying lesions

tumours
subdural haematoma

Infections

encephalitis
general paresis

Trauma

post-traumatic dementia
subdural haematoma

Toxic and metabolic disorders

myxoedema, hypoglycaemia, hypopituitarism
vitamin deficiency: thiamine (Korsakoff's psychosis), nicotinic
    acid (pellagra), vitamin B_{12} and folic acid
chronic alcoholic dementia
heavy metals

Anoxia

post-cardiac arrest
carbon monoxide poisoning
epilepsy

Other disorders affecting the CNS

multiple sclerosis
Parkinson's disease
normal-pressure hydrocephalus

Fig. 1 (a) Causes of acute organic disorders; (b) causes of chronic organic disorders.

Clinical History A full history should be obtained. This should also include an account of the patient's pre-morbid intellectual attainments, personality, and social functioning, in addition to current behaviour patterns and competence. Such information is often best obtained from an informant other than the patient. Although a basic procedure, this process is often executed inadequately. As a result the process of differential diagnosis is considerably more difficult.

The mental state should be assessed systematically. Such examinations should comprise an objective examination of cognitive functions (see below) and also an assessment of appearance, demeanour, mood, speech, thought content, and any perceptual disturbance.

The quality and reliability of any such assessment are dramatically improved by using one of the many standardized structured or semi-structured diagnostic interview schedules currently in wide use.

The Cambridge Mental Disorders of the Elderly Examination (CAMDEX) is a structured interview covering details of present state, past history, and family history. Information is obtained from both the patient and an informant. The Hachinski Ischaemia Score and a dementia score (Blessed *et al*, 1966) are incorporated. Cognitive function is assessed by brief neuropsychological tests which include the Mini Mental State Examination. Clinical observations during the interview and a brief physical examination form part of the assessment along with the results of any investigations. The procedure takes about 80 minutes to administer and is very reliable.

The Diagnostic Interview Schedule (DIS) is a procedure devised by the US National Institute of Mental Health. It can be used to generate a range of psychiatric diagnosis based on DSM III criteria. The schedule has been used to determine the prevalence rates of various psychiatric disorders among elderly community residents. However, the DIS was devised for a general population sample and it provides insufficient information for a conclusive diagnosis of dementia. For example, no enquiries are conducted into the history of onset or mode of progression of cognitive symptoms. As a consequence, the schedule can only establish the presence of severe cognitive impairment based on performance on the Mini Mental State Examination. However the procedure is a useful screen and a diagnosis of dementia can be confirmed by conventional clinical methods.

The Geriatric Mental State (GMS) is derived from the Present State Examination and adapted by the inclusion of items relating to organic mental disorder and additional questions concerning cognitive function. A computerized diagnosis based on the procedure (AGECAT) has been developed. This is similar to the CATEGO ID of the Present State Examination. The GMS is effective in the discrimination of organic brain syndromes from functional psychiatric disorders but cannot provide a differential diagnosis between Alzheimer's disease, cerebrovascular disease, and confusional states.

The Comprehensive Assessment and Referral Evaluation (CARE) is a long, semi-structured interview covering psychiatric symptoms, physical disability and performance in the activities of daily living, along with information about nutritional status and economic and social aspects of illness. It incorporates most of the GMS and has been widely used in community surveys. Assessment with CARE can be valuable in determining the degree of social support required by a patient. An abbreviated form, the SHORT-CARE is also available.

Assessment of dementia should also include an estimate of the severity of the disorder. This is often given as a global rating in terms of mild, moderate, or severe dementia. Such a rating is usually adequate for assessing prognosis and for counselling relatives. Global ratings correlate reasonably well with objective measures of cognitive performance, degree of cerebral atrophy seen on CT and MRI scans, and the hypometabolism seen with PET and SPECT.

Physical Examination   A physical examination will include blood pressure, neurological examination, examination of sight and hearing (important for cognitive assessment), and examination of gait.

Laboratory Investigations and Imaging   Laboratory investigations will include a full blood count, glucose, urea and electrolyte profile, and tests of thyroid and liver function. Serological tests for syphilis and HIV are also appropriate to determine the presence of infectious agents and (in the light of a family history) serum DNA should be assessed for genetic lesions (β-APP or Prion gene). EEG, although diagnostic only in cases of seizure disorders, is useful in ruling out non-convulsive status epilepticus which can present with cognitive and psychiatric symptoms as its only manifestations.

Imaging techniques (CT and MRI, PET and SPECT) are useful adjuncts to other procedures. However, in many cases the overlap that exists between measures of cortical atrophy or reduced metabolism in demented and normal elderly individuals means that the findings must be integrated with the results of clinical observation before a final diagnosis of dementia is made. The result of the imaging alone should not be permitted to override the clear clinical observations indicating dementia.

Main Causes of Dementia   Over 80 per cent of patients with dementia suffer from a limited number of conditions, associated with characteristic types of pathology and different aetiologies (Fig. 2).

Prognosis and Treatment   In most cases the presence of dementia is due to a progressive neuro-degenerative pathological process. In view of this, the prognosis is universally poor. At present the scope for therapeutic intervention is very limited with the exception of cerebrovascular disease.

Main Causes of Dementia	
Aetiology	**% of cases**
Alzheimer's disease	45
Cerebrovascular disease	15
Cortical Lewy body disease	10
Head trauma	3
Parkinson's disease	3
Motor neuron disease	2
Others	5
AIDS dementia	>1 (?)
Prion disease	>1 (?)
Unknown	15

Fig. 2 Main identifiable causes of dementia.

2 Alzheimer's Disease

INTRODUCTION

Alzheimer's disease (AD) is the fourth major cause of death in the developed world after heart disease, cancer, and stroke. It is largely a disease of the elderly, and afflicts an estimated 10 per cent of the population over 65 and 40 per cent of those over 85. AD is thought to affect over 4 million people at a cost of more than $35 billion a year in the USA.

Typically, AD begins with memory problems and becomes progressively worse until the patient is eventually bedridden and doubly incontinent. The progression from memory loss to global cognitive decline is inexorable, although the rate of decline varies from person to person.

The neuropathological characteristics of AD include extensive neuronal loss and formation of neurofibrillary tangles and amyloid plaques in the cortex.

Both genetic and environmental triggers of AD have now been identified. At present no effective treatment exists and clinical investigation and intervention is targeted towards differential diagnosis and management of the social and behavioural consequences of the progressive dementia.

DEFINITION

AD is a progressive neurodegenerative disorder characterized by marked intellectual decline sufficient to interfere with normal social functioning but occurring in the absence of clouding of consciousness. The intellectual decline is due to degeneration of the organization of the cortical architecture; this degeneration is caused by loss of synaptic connectivity due to amyloid plaque and neurofibrillary tangle formation.

EPIDEMIOLOGY

Over the last decade, several large studies in different countries have examined the epidemiology of AD in an attempt to discern relevant risk factors. A meta-analysis of recent case control studies (Eurodem study – see recommended reading) has identified several factors of aetiological importance. Case control studies have led to identification of possible risk factors associated with presence of disease (Fig. 2.1). The measure of risk usually used is relative risk or odd's ratios.

The relative risk indicates how much more likely exposed people are to develop the disease compared to unexposed people. The baseline figure of risk for a population is 1 and larger numbers indicate a proportionately higher risk for people exposed to a particular factor or a population subgroup. There can be difficulties with the definition of a baseline (relative risk = 1) if there is no negative exposure, since variability in the definitions of baseline exposure can lead to large differences in attributable risk. Exposure in different populations is likely to vary and each country will have different patterns of morbidity and mortality, i.e. survival effects. The pooling of data from many studies and appropriate statistical techniques (meta-analysis) means that, despite these limitations, we now have a much better idea of the risk factors which are related to AD and thus to the possible causes of AD (Fig. 2.2).

Risk Factors in AD	
Factor	**Relative Risk**
Family history of AD	3.5
Family history of Down's syndrome	2.7
Previous head trauma males females	2.67 0.85
Family history of Parkinson's disease	2.14
Depression	1.82
Maternal age (40+)	1.7
Epilepsy	1.6
Encephalitis/meningitis	1.6
Herpes zoster/simplex	1.15
General anaesthesis	1.0
Alcohol	1.0
Immune disorders, oesteoarthritis, poliomyelitis, thyroid disease, headaches, smoking, solvent exposure, head injury, blood transfusion	<1.0

Fig. 2.1 Risk factors in AD. (Data from the Eurodem Risk Factors Group, 1991.)

Risks Examined

Age

AD is a disease of old age. As is expected, increasing age is the best defined risk factor in AD. At 45 years, the population prevalence is less than 0.01 per cent; this rises to 2 per cent between 65 and 70, 5 per cent between 70 and 80, and over 20 per cent at 85. An early age of onset (< 65 years) is strongly associated with a positive family history.

Family history

Apart from age, family history of dementia in first-degree relatives is the most persistent positive association. In unselected population samples a high proportion of patients with AD have first- or second-degree relatives with either dementia or serious memory problems. Approximately 25 per cent of AD cases are thought to be familial (although not necessarily genetic). Of these familial cases some 10 per cent (2.5 per cent of all AD cases) have an autosomal dominant pattern of inheritance.

Genetics

A proportion of these families in the UK, USA, France, and Japan have been shown to have point mutations in the amyloid precursor protein (APP) gene on chromosome 21 (see page 2.18). These mutations are tightly linked to AD in these families. However, calculations indicate that these mutations account for less than 0.01 per cent of all AD cases. It is important to point out that these mutations in the APP gene probably cause AD in these families, and that this finding was a landmark scientific achievement in our understanding of AD.

Down's syndrome

People with Down's syndrome (trisomy 21) invariably develop the characteristic pathological changes of AD as they reach the age of 30–40. This is an age of onset some 30 years younger than that seen in the general population. The extent and type of the dementia present in these patients is difficult to determine because of the presence of the mental handicap which is typical of Down's syndrome.

Down's syndrome is caused by the extra copy (or partial copy) of chromosome 21 being over-expressed during fetal development. The additional copy of chromosome causes an over-expression (150 per cent of normal) of the genes on chromosome 21 during adult life. Appearance of AD pathology in older Down's syndrome sufferers is thought to be due to the over-expression of the APP gene during ageing. Thus the AD seen in Down's syndrome can be regarded as another example of a genetic lesion.

Maternal age

The risks associated with maternal age are particularly associated with the youngest and oldest mothers (those under 20 and over 40). This group of mothers also has increased risks of premature births, poor maternal fitness, and Down's syndrome babies. Only a tiny proportion of births, typically less than 1 per cent in most countries, are to women over 40.

Head injury

Descriptive reviews of case control studies often report the finding of head injury as a risk factor, although the proportion of cases which show this factor is usually small (2–15 per cent). Single studies have produced weak evidence that head injury is a risk factor. However, the status of a previous history of head trauma as a risk factor for AD is supported by the epidemiological meta-analysis. The factor is more marked in males and in cases where no family history is reported.

Repetitive head injury is known to cause a dementing syndrome in boxers (dementia pugilistica or punch-drunk syndrome – see Chapter 6) which shows the same molecular pathology as AD. Head injury has been found to be associated with other neurological disorders, and this may well be due to recall bias. Head injury is very common – about 5 per cent of the population will suffer a head injury with loss of consciousness sometime in their lives. Calculations indicate that head injury might be directly responsible for about 2.5 per cent of AD cases (Fig. 2.2).

Psychiatric history

Establishing and quantifying degrees of psychiatric history in a large group of people is an inexact science. The quality of this type of information collected varies considerably between studies. Overall, the odd's ratio is of a similar order to that seen for head injury, but there are important differences in the parameters of the risks due to head injury and psychiatric history. With psychiatric history, the risk for women is higher than that for men. This finding is attributable largely to symptoms of depression; since depression in women is relatively common this positive association could be of importance. The depression may be a prodromal manifestation of the dementia, but it may be that the two disorders share common underlying processes such

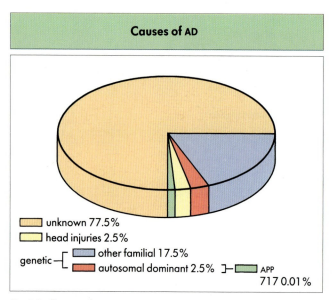

Causes of AD

unknown 77.5%
head injuries 2.5%
genetic — other familial 17.5%
autosomal dominant 2.5% — APP 717 0.01%

Fig. 2.2 Causes of AD.

as neurotransmitter disturbance. Alternatively later dementia could be related to the methods used to treat earlier episodes of depression.

Other diseases

Arthritis, headaches, blood transfusions, and thyroid disorders are weak associations and could be accounted for by bias or difficulties in assessing exposure. Headaches may not be reported by those who are demented and so informants would reply in the negative to questions about these. Blood transfusions may well be related to the likelihood of control selection and survival. All such associations are marginal and at present must be regarded as having doubtful significance.

Occupational exposure to chemicals

No clear associations have been shown. However, because of the difficulties in assessing the degree of exposure retrospectively, the ability of case control studies to test hypotheses concerning such exposures is very limited.

Smoking and alcohol

Exposure to both tobacco and alcohol have been shown to be negatively associated with AD. This association and the conclusion that smoking and drinking might prevent the onset of AD cannot be taken at face value. There are difficulties with both of these exposures in that the exposure itself is likely to bias the diagnostic process. Alcohol is related to a dementia syndrome and those with high intake are unlikely to be in an AD case series. Smoking is related to vascular disease, and this is likely to weight an individual to the vascular dementias. In addition to the problems of diagnostic bias, heavy alcohol and tobacco consumption reduce life expectancy, ensuring that many consumers do not live to be old enough to develop AD.

Other factors

In addition to those factors described above, cases have been made for an association between brain aluminium content, infective agents, myocardial infarction, and HLA types. The case for aluminium as a causative factor rests primarily on the phenomenon of dialysis encephalopathy and reports of increased aluminium levels in the brains of patients with AD. However, the brains of such patients rarely show significant plaque and tangle formation, which are the pathological hallmarks of AD. The increased levels of brain aluminium in AD are thought to be an epiphenomenon. Thus, direct evidence linking raised levels of aluminium in the central nervous system with an Alzheimer-like disease process is virtually non-existent. The epidemiological data linking intake of aluminium either in drinking water or prophylactically (e.g. antacid preparations) to the incidence of AD is weak.

To date no reliable evidence has ever been presented to show that AD is due to an infectious agent; this is in contrast to Prion disease.

DIAGNOSIS

The clinical criteria proposed for AD are:
- the disorder has an insidious onset;
- it is progressive;
- dementia occurs in the absence of other systemic or brain diseases which would account for the progressive cognitive deficit and personality change.

Absolute diagnostic accuracy requires neuropathological examination. However, skilled psychiatric, neurological, and psychological examinations together with CT, MRI, or PET imaging and laboratory investigations offer 80–90 per cent diagnostic accuracy. In view of this, rigid operational criteria such as those that appear in the *Diagnostic and Statistical Manual of Mental Disorders* (DSM III-R) appear premature in the light of present clinical experience. An interim solution to this problem can be found in the adoption of the categories: 'definite', 'probable', and 'possible' AD, as proposed by the Task Force on Alzheimer's disease (Fig. 2.3, see also further reading).

A diagnosis of *definite* AD requires confirmation by histopathology.

Probable AD can be diagnosed if there is a typical insidious onset with progression, and other possible causes can be excluded.

A diagnosis of *possible* AD may be made if the presentation or course is somewhat aberrant, or in the presence of other significant disease where AD is considered the most likely cause of the progressive dementia.

The NINCDS/ARDA Task Force definition of dementia rests heavily on documenting cognitive impairment. However, whilst evidence of cognitive impairment is essential for diagnosing dementia, changes in mood, behaviour, and personality are also often present. Such changes are not likely to be mere epiphenomena or secondary to the cognitive deficit; these symptoms are probably additional manifestations of the underlying degeneration of the brain.

Understanding the dementia of AD requires familiarity with the range of features which may be present. A good description of the typical progression in AD may be obtained from Sjögren's classic description (1952), and Slater and Roth's account (1977).

Early and Late Onset Forms of AD

AD is often described as having two forms, an early and late form. The difference between the two relates entirely to age of onset.

The early onset form, occurring before the age of 65, is often familial and, in onset before 55 years, often autosomal dominant. This is the form of AD originally described by Alzheimer in 1907. The late onset form of AD (onset over 65) is also called 'senile dementia' and 'senile dementia of the Alzheimer type'. The earlier onset is described as having a faster clinical course and being more aggressive. Neuropathological examination shows that atrophy, cell loss, tangle formation, and neurochemical deficit, can be more marked in the early onset cases (see page 2.5).

However, these differences are marginal and difficult to define, and the distinction of onset before or after the age of 65 is arbitrary. At present there is no sound evidence for concluding that the early and late onset forms of AD relate to differences in the underlying pathological processes.

CLINICAL FEATURES

The onset of AD is insidious and therefore difficult to judge, particularly in older patients. The disease may become manifest in patients after intervening medical conditions, trauma, or social upheaval (e.g. unemployment, moving home, bereavement). The diagnosis of dementia requires evidence of progressive change in two or more areas of cognition, one of which is usually memory; others may include language, mathematical ability, praxis, abstraction, visuo-spatial perception, and personality. A requirement for the DSM III criteria is that the above changes impair the ability of the individual to engage in a job or social activity.

Clinical Course

AD is progressive and this advancement has been described as having three stages by Roth.

First stage
- Memory impairment
- Disorientation in time and place
- Restlessness and anxiety

In the first stage (Fig. 2.4b), impairment of memory for recent events is usually the prominent feature. A patient will forget such things as what he had to eat that day or the details of recent conversations. Spatial perception and topographical memory decline, and disorientation, especially in time and place, is common, though the degree may vary during the course of the day. Examples would include forgetting the way to local shops or the way home, and uncertainty over the date of the month or time of day. Impaired concentration and fatigue may be noticed, alongside restlessness and anxiety. These latter features often occur at night and cause considerable difficulties for carers. Such symptoms are often targets for pharmacological treatment. Depression, when it occurs, is fleeting and variable, and does not

Diagnosis of AD – Clinical

Definite

Diagnosis of definite AD requires the clinical criteria for probable AD and histopathological evidence obtained from biopsy or autopsy.

Probable

A presence of dementia established by clinical examination and documented by the Mini-Mental Test, Blessed Dementia Scale, or some similar examination, and confirmed by neuropsychological tests. Patients should have: deficits in two or more areas of cognition, progressive worsening of memory and other cognitive functions, no disturbance of consciousness, onset between ages 40 and 90, most often after age 65, and absence of systemic disorders or other brain diseases that in and of themselves could account for the progressive deficits in memory and cognition.

The diagnosis is supported by: progressive deterioration of specific cognitive function such as language (aphasia), motor skills (apraxia), and perception (agnosia); impaired activities of daily living and altered patterns to behaviour; family history of similar disorders, particularly if confirmed neuropathologically; and laboratory reslts of: normal lumbar puncture as evaluated by standard techniques, normal pattern of non-specific changes in EEG, such as increased slow-wave activity; and evidence of cerebral atrophy on CT with progression documented by serial observation. Clinical features consistent with the diagnosis (after exclusion of causes of dementia other than AD) include: plateaux

in the course of progression of the illness, associated symptoms of depression, insomnia, incontinence, delusions, illusions, hallucinations, catastrophic verbal, emotional, or physical outbursts, sexual disorders, and weight loss, other neurological abnormalities in some patients, especially with more advanced disease and including motor signs such as increased muscle tone, myoclonus, or gait disorder; seizures in advanced disease; and CT normal for age.

Features that make the diagnosis of probable AD uncertain or unlikely include: sudden, apoplectic onset; focal neurological findings such as hemiparesis, sensory loss, visual field deficits, and inco-ordination early in the course of the illness; and seizures or gait disturbances at the onset or very early in the course of the illness.

Possible

Clinical diagnosis of possible AD: may be made on the basis of the dementia syndrome, in the absence of other neurological, psychiatric, or systemic disorders sufficient to cause dementia, and in the presence of variations in the onset, in the presentation, or in the clinical course; may be made in the presence of a second systemic or brain disorder sufficient to produce dementia, which is not considered to be the cause of the dementia; and can be used in research studies when a single, gradually progressive severe cognitive deficit is identified in the absence of other identifiable cause.

Fig. 2.3 Diagnosis of AD on clinical grounds. (CERAD criteria – see recommended reading.)

occur without other features of dementia. At this stage, exaggerations in or alterations to lifelong personality traits may appear, though they are rarely seen in the absence of obvious manifestations of memory or intellectual deficits.

Focal neurological deficits rarely occur early in AD. They tend to be more prominent in early onset cases. Generally the appearance of focal neurological deficits in patients over 65 or an unusual course of illness (e.g. stepwise decline in functioning) are indications that further neurological or imaging investigations are appropriate in order to exclude treatable diseases (e.g. hypertension or neoplasia).

Second stage
- Dysphasia, apraxia, agnosia
- Blunting of emotions and apathy
- Neurological signs

In the second stage of AD (Fig. 2.4c), all aspects of memory fail progressively and expressive dysphasia appears in association with parietal lobe deficits such as dyspraxia and agnosia. Epileptic fits occur in 5–10 per cent of cases. Blunting of emotions and apathy begin to take over the mood state. Judgement and

the capacity for abstract thought and calculation have also disappeared by this stage. Sourander and Sjögren have described a Klüver–Bucy syndrome as a common feature, but most studies have reported, at most, isolated features of this syndrome in AD. A degree of Parkinsonism may occur in about two-thirds of patients, but Parkinson-like features such as increased muscle tone and akinesia are only conspicuous in a small proportion of AD patients. Hemiparesis with extensor plantar responses, and a psychotic syndrome with hallucinations and delusions may be seen towards the end of the second stage or later.

Third stage
- Global cognitive decline
- Loss of personality
- Incontinence

In the third and final stage (Fig. 2.4d), there is gross disturbance of all intellectual functions. There are marked focal neurological deficits, and an increase in muscle tone appears with accompanying slow, wide-based and unsteady gait. There is gross emotional disinhibition, and the former personality becomes submerged. Patients cannot recognize relatives or even

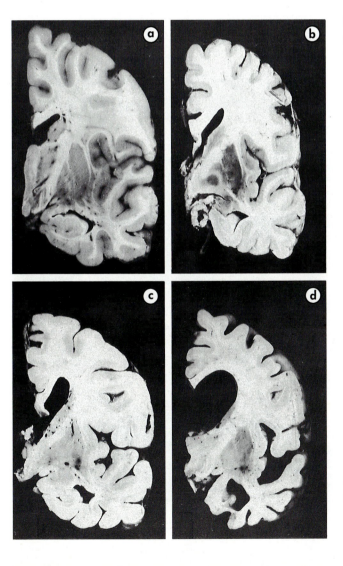

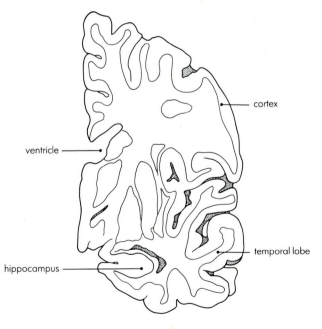

Fig. 2.4 Coronal brain slices in (a) normal elderly; (b) stage I AD (with slight cortical atrophy and ventricular enlargement). (Courtesy of Dr CJ Bruton, London.)

Coronal brain slices in (c) stage II AD (moderate atrophy of temporal lobe and ventricular enlargement); (d) stage III AD (severe cortical atrophy, particularly in the temporal lobe, and ventricular enlargement). (Courtesy of Dr CJ Bruton, London.)

deficits become more pronounced and progress from an increase in muscle tone with an accompanying slow, wide-based, and unsteady gait through spasticity and myoclonus. Patients become bedridden and invariably doubly incontinent. A vegetative state is reached, in which patients can survive for several years. There is progressive wasting despite a voracious appetite and death is usually caused by pneumonia.

Cognitive Deficits in AD

When approaching the task of formally assessing cognitive deficits in AD, two basic points should be noted:

(i) cognitive functions (e.g. memory) are made up of several separate components (e.g. short-term and long-term memory); and

(ii) that the extent and nature of cognitive deficits that arise from a diffuse neurodegenerative process and the deficits that result from diffuse brain damage may be different from those caused by multiple but localized brain lesions.

Studies of spatial function, language, and memory have established that the cognitive deficits seen in dementia are not the same as those in patients with circumscribed focal lesions. Thus, the view that the cognitive deficits and dementia in AD represent a collection of the symptoms associated with focal brain damage is probably inaccurate.

Memory

Memory is a composite of at least two different processes:

(i) learning and storing new information; and

(ii) recall of previously acquired information.

The process of learning and storing new information is the first casualty of the dementing process. This deficit grows as the disease progresses, and eventually the process of recall and retrieval of memories from the patient's remote past becomes impossible. The learning deficit of demented patients is similar to the amnesia of patients who have focal damage to the hippocampus or the midline structures or the diencephalon (e.g. Korsakoff patients). While the similarities are important it is useful to note several marked differences.

Patients with an amnesic syndrome have circumscribed memory deficits and, perhaps more importantly, their memory deficit is their primary clinical symptom – it far outweighs any other types of cognitive deficit that may be present. Patients with AD show deficits in memory, but these occur within the clinical picture of a general loss of cognitive function. An example is the name-finding deficit (impaired retrieval from semantic memory). This is typical of AD patients, and is often supposed to be a reflection of their memory deficit. However, it is extremely rare in patients suffering from amnesic disorders.

A further illustration of the two conditions is seen in the relative sparing of remote memory in severely affected amnesic patients when compared to patients with AD, in whom progressive impairment of remote memory is a characteristic feature.

Impairments in memory function of healthy elderly people are seen when their performance is compared with that of young or middle-aged people. The term benign senescent forgetfulness is used to refer to mild memory impairments in the absence of other signs of cognitive decline. It is very difficult to differentiate between senescent forgetfulness and senile forms of memory loss. Forgetfulness is not an inevitable consequence of ageing and it

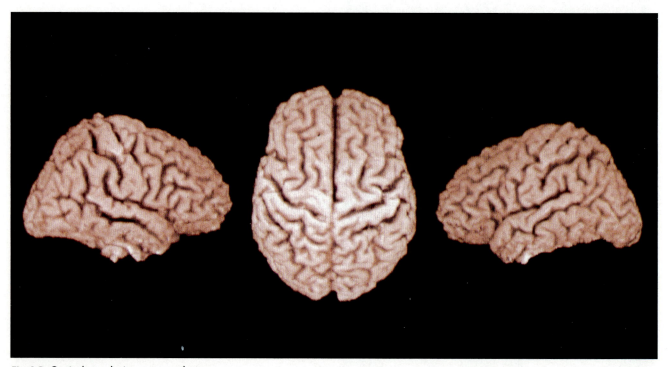

Fig. 2.5 Cortical atrophy in AD, as seen by MRI.

remains an open question as to whether its presence can be regarded as pathological.

Language

Language involves both the comprehension and use of speech and the ability to read and write. Patients with established AD invariably show deficits in many aspects of language function, including structure (phonology, syntax) and meaning (semantics). Despite the accumulating evidence of such deficits, many diagnostic protocols of moderate AD (including DSM-III-R) regard language impairment as a useful but non-essential feature.

During the early stages of AD, articulation, phrase length, and grammar show very little evidence of being affected. Detailed examination can reveal that the content of speech is shallow, with patients having naming problems and relying on stock phrases, although neologisms and phonemic substitution are rare. From an early stage, generative naming (where the patient provides lists of names when asked) is impaired, whereas nominal aphasia (examiner asks, 'What is this I'm holding?'), though common, is less often seen. Perseverative and semantic errors are common. In general, the ability to read is well preserved. However, comprehension of the written text and aural comprehension can be very poor.

As the disease progresses, patients confabulate and show disorders of written language. They begin to lose their knowledge of meaning and reference despite the relative preservation of other structural features of language. Although patients may be able to correct morphological and syntactic errors (e.g. 'He found Ed car'), even mildly demented patients experience great difficulty in correcting semantic errors (e.g. 'She lost Ed's temper').

Eventually, all aspects of language deteriorate, albeit at different rates. Structural features, simple phrases, and reading aloud showing the most resistance to deterioration.

Language deficit in AD differs from that seen in aphasia following a focal lesion in a manner analogous to that already discussed for amnesic syndromes. Patients with AD have a pattern of a broad range of moderate deficits in many aspects of language function compared to the pattern of severe but circumscribed language deficits seen in typical aphasias. This difference in the pattern of language deficits has led to the suggestion that the use of the term aphasia to describe the language deficits in AD is misleading.

Visuo-spatial function

Visuo-spatial function is impaired in AD, and the use of graded tests can help define abnormalities in patients with mild degrees of dementia. As the disease progresses, such tests reveal marked deficits in the patient's ability to copy simple drawings, to differentiate left from right, and to orientate objects in space. It is possible that such marked disturbances in visuo-spatial function have useful prognostic indications, since it has been reported that poor performance on such tests is associated with high mortality at six-month follow-up. Among low scorers, 26 per cent had died at follow-up, compared with only 4 per cent of high scorers, even though members of the former group were significantly younger.

SCANNING PROCEDURES AND IMAGING

Imaging procedures such as CT and MRI are useful aids for excluding other causes of dementia (such as space-occupying lesions, infarcts, lobar atrophy, or infection). However they have little diagnostic specificity in themselves. Whilst younger patients (those under 60) with AD may show marked cortical atrophy or ventricular enlargement on CT or MRI (Fig. 2.5), scans of older patients with AD often show no more atrophy and ventricular dilatation than that seen in a healthy person of the same sex and age. Increases in both ventricular volume and the degree of sulco-gyral atrophy during the course of the illness can be seen (see Fig. 2.4). These changes parallel the general intellectual decline.

PET scans to map the metabolic activity of the brain show a typical pattern of frontal, parietal, and temporal hypometabolism (Fig. 2.6). These changes are not specific to AD and thus they cannot be used in isolation to make a definitive diagnosis. A similar pattern can be seen with SPECT imaging. These approaches have been used as correlates of specific cognitive deficits (aphasia and apraxia). However, the technology and software necessary to explore these comparisons are still being developed.

It should be noted that if a patient suspected of having AD does not show alterations in their PET and SPECT scans, additional investigations to search for other causes of their dementia are strongly indicated.

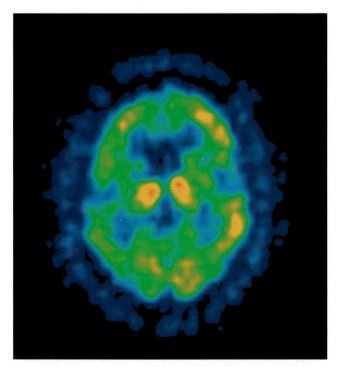

Fig. 2.6 Hypometabolism in the frontal, parietal, and temporal regions in AD, as seen by PET scan.

NEUROPATHOLOGICAL CHANGES

A full neuropathological examination is the only way to obtain a definite diagnosis of AD (Fig. 2.7).

Gross Changes in Brain Structure

The brains of patients with AD show evidence of atrophy with marked widening of the sulci and reductions in the thickness of cortical grey matter (Fig. 2.8). These changes can be especially prominent in temporal, frontal, and parietal regions. In addition, enlargement of the ventricular system is readily visible to the naked eye (see Fig. 2.4). These features are easily appreciated on CT and MRI scans of living patients (see Fig. 2.5). A marked loss in brain weight of some 300–400 grams (from approximately 1350 grams to below 1000 grams) is often found. However, in older patients (over 75 years) gross brain structure may be indistinguishable from that of a healthy person of the same age.

Histopathology

The study of appropriately stained sections of brain reveals the characteristic plaques and tangles described by Alzheimer which are pathognomonic of AD (Fig. 2.9). The pathology of the disease is complex and involves extensive neuronal loss, and the appearance and deposition of abnormal protein deposits within the neurons and in the neuropil (Fig. 2.10).

There are three characteristic sites of abnormal fibrous protein deposits (amyloid) within the brains of AD patients. Amyloid is a generic term applied to a group of proteins which share the distinctive property of displaying a green–red birefringence after staining with Congo red (Fig. 2.11). The birefringence is due to a β-pleated sheet structural confirmation which can be exhibited by any of a number of different proteins. When the β-pleated proteins aggregate they form a very stable structure which is insoluble and extremely resistant to protease digestion. The three sites of amyloid deposition are:

- extracellular senile plaques in the neuropil
- the intraneuronal neurofibrillary tangles
- the deposits of amyloid in the walls of cerebral blood vessels.

There is also extensive neuronal damage and loss which approaches 25 per cent of total neuronal number in given areas of cortex. All of these features are also found, to a much lesser degree, in the 'normal' elderly. Thus the relationship between AD and 'normal' ageing remains enigmatic. There has been much debate about the relative importance of these different pathological features and how they relate to each other.

Diagnosis of AD – Neuropathology

Plaque Frequency

Age	None	Few	Moderate	Frequent
<50	N	P	P	P
50–75	N	S	P	P
<75	N	U	S	P

N = normal, U = uncertain histological evidence, S = suggestive histological evidence, P = pathological indicative histological evidence

Probable

Clinical history of dementia and presence or absence of neuropathology likely to cause dementia and on S (suggestive) age-related plaque category.

Possible

Either: a clinical history of dementia and presence or absence of other neuropathology likely to cause dementia and a U-age-related plaque category,

or an S or P-age-related plaque category with an absence of clinical dementia.

Definite

Clinical history of dementia and presence or absence of other neuropathology likely to cause dementia and a P-age-related plaque category. Neurofibrillary tangles are invariably present in the neocortex. The age related plaque category is determined by the most affected neocortical areas (frontal, temporal, or parietal) and the patient's age.

Normal

Either: no clinical history of dementia, no histological evidence of AD (N category) and absence of neuropathology likely to cause dementia,

or no clinical history of dementia and a U-age-related plaque category.

Fig. 2.7 Diagnosis of AD on neuropathological grounds (adapted from CERAD criteria).

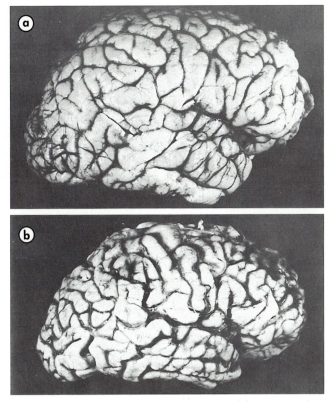

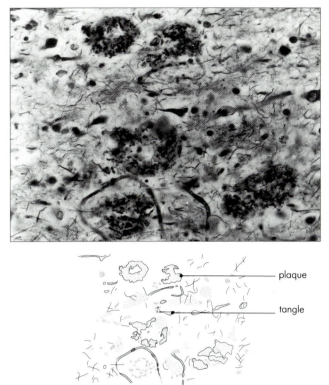

Fig. 2.8 Photographs showing (a) normal brain; and (b) gross atrophy in AD. (Courtesy of Dr CJ Bruton, London.)

Fig. 2.9 Plaques and tangles as seen in sections of the cortex stained with Bielschowsky silver stain.

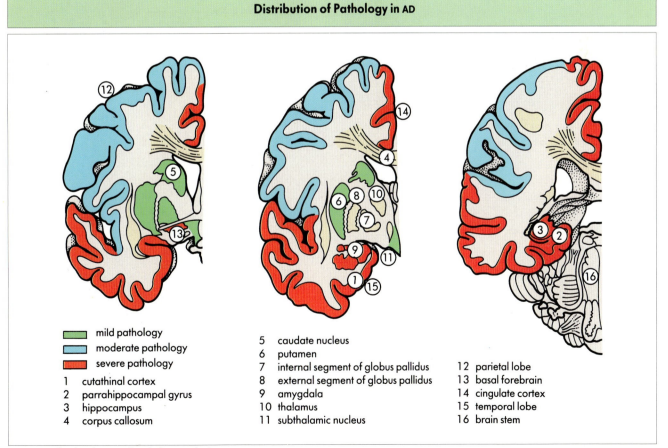

Distribution of Pathology in AD

mild pathology
moderate pathology
severe pathology

1   cutathinal cortex
2   parrahippocampal gyrus
3   hippocampus
4   corpus callosum

5   caudate nucleus
6   putamen
7   internal segment of globus pallidus
8   external segment of globus pallidus
9   amygdala
10   thalamus
11   subthalamic nucleus

12   parietal lobe
13   basal forebrain
14   cingulate cortex
15   temporal lobe
16   brain stem

Fig. 2.10 The distribution of pathology in the brain in AD.

Senile plaques

Senile or neuritic plaques are one of the two pathognomonic diagnostic neuropathological features observed in the AD brain. Plaques are roughly spherical structures found in the neuropil and range in diameter from 5–200μm. They are not easily visible in haematoxylin and eosin preparations but are readily detected by silver impregnation techniques (see Fig. 2.9), by thioflavine S fluorescence, and more reliably by the use of immunocytochemical procedures and specific antibodies raised to known plaque proteins such as the β-protein (Fig. 2.12). The affinity of amyloid for the dye Congo red produces a green birefringence which can be observed using a polarized light source; this is the basis of another commonly used technique for detecting plaques.

Plaques have a varying morphology, which is to some extent dependent on the plane in which the tissue is sectioned, their location, and the stage of development. They can take the form of discrete lesions or in some cases they may coalesce to form larger amorphous deposits. Four main types of plaque have been described (Fig. 2.13).

Primitive plaque The primitive plaque consists of a small number of distended neurites, largely presynaptic or axonal in origin, with just a few amyloid fibrils.

Classical plaque The classical or mature plaque consists of a dense core composed of amyloid fibrils surrounded by a clear halo. Outside this halo is a ring of filamentous and granular

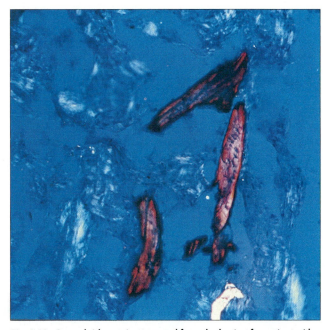

Fig. 2.11 β-amyloid protein extracted from the brain of a patient with AD and stained with Congo red shows green–red birefringence under polarized light.

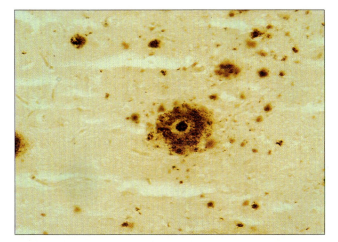

Fig. 2.12 Classic plaque stained with an antibody to the β-amyloid protein.

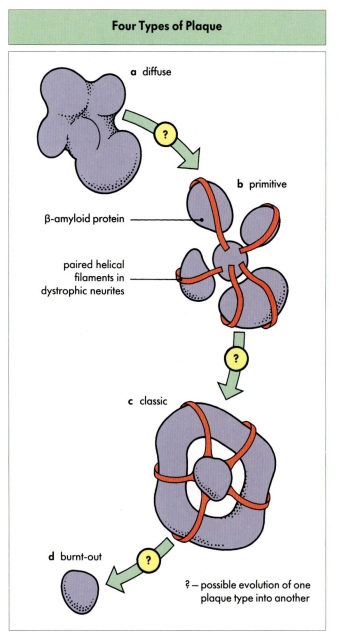

Four Types of Plaque

a diffuse

β-amyloid protein

paired helical filaments in dystrophic neurites

b primitive

c classic

d burnt-out

? – possible evolution of one plaque type into another

Fig. 2.13 Four types of plaque: (a) diffuse; (b) primitive; (c) classic; (d) burnt out.

material made up of distended nerve processes or neurites filled with mitochondria and electron-dense bodies. Ultrastructural studies have revealed that these neurites are intermingled with glial processes, microglia, and surviving normal cortical cell constituents. The plaques are also sometimes associated with an astrocytic response. This can be demonstrated either by using a Holzer stain or immunocytochemically by using antibodies to glial fibrillary acidic protein (GFAP) (Fig. 2.14).

Burnt-out plaque   A third type of plaque is the burnt-out or compact plaque which consists solely of a β-amyloid core.

Diffuse plaque   In recent years, however, the use of antibodies raised against the β-amyloid protein and immunocytochemical techniques have revealed the presence of a fourth type of previously undetected plaque which is now known as a diffuse plaque (Fig. 2.15). This plaque type is characterized as non-Congophilic, and is not generally associated with neuritic or glial elements.

Plaques are found most frequently in the cerebral cortex but are also present in the deeper grey matter of the temporal lobe, striatum, the diencephalon, and the brain stem. Until recently the cerebellum was thought to be unaffected in AD but immuno-staining has revealed that diffuse plaques are a common occurrence in this part of the brain. The hippocampus, parahippo-campal gyrus, and amygdala are preferentially affected by plaque and tangle formation in the early stages of disease.

Plaques and tangles occur to a limited extent in the brains of cognitively normal elderly patients. By the age of 70, plaques are thought to be present in small to moderate numbers in the neocortex of more than 50 per cent of people. Thus, a reliable neuropathological diagnosis of AD is a function of the quantity of plaques present in relation to the age of the patient.

Neurofibrillary tangles and neuritic change

The second major neuropathological change described by Alzheimer in his classic 1907 paper was the presence of numerous neurofibrillary tangles within the neuronal cytoplasm. These tangles are very difficult to see in routine haematoxylin and eosin or Nissl preparations, but can easily be visualized with one of the many silver impregnation techniques available (Fig. 2.9), by utilizing the birefringence properties of Congo red in the presence of polarized light, or by immunocytochemical means using specific antisera (Fig. 2.16). When seen under the light microscope, the tangles appear as thickened, twisted fibrils which, when fully developed, may occupy a large part of the perikaryon of the neuron, displacing rather than destroying the remaining subcellular structures. However, the tangles disrupt protein synthesis and cellular processes, and neurons cannot survive indefinitely with these large intracellular inclusions. In the final stages of tangle formation, the neuron disintegrates, and the nucleus and the cell outline disappear leaving a so-called 'ghost tangle' in the neuropil.

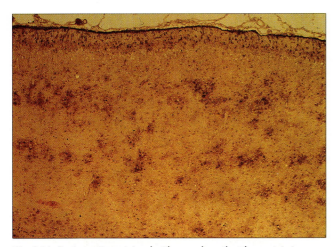

Fig. 2.14 Brain sections stained with GFAP show that the protein is associated with the plaques.

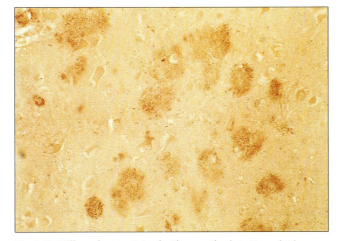

Fig. 2.15 Diffuse plaques stained with an antibody to β-amyloid.

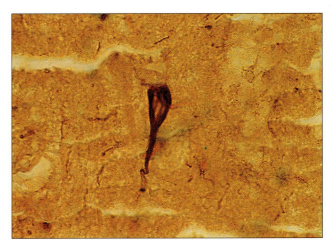

Fig. 2.16 Neurofibrillary tangle stained with an antibody to paired helical filaments.

Tangle structure Tangles show different morphological configurations, determined probably by the type of neuron affected and its anatomical location. Smaller pyramidal cells of the cortex tend to contain triangular or flame-shaped tangles extending from the base of the cell towards the apical dendrite, whereas more complex forms are found in the hippocampal and large cortical pyramidal cells. Tangles in the basal forebrain and in the brain stem often have a more globose configuration.

Tangle components The nature of the tangles has been the source of much debate since Alzheimer's original report. He himself suggested that they originate from the neurofibrils normally present in the neurons; others have proposed a common origin with the amyloid of senile plaque cores.

Tangles are made of a pair of helically twisted tubules each 10nm wide (20nm in total). Recent studies have revealed that the protofilaments of paired helical filaments (PHF) differ from those of normal neurofilaments (Fig. 2.17). PHF protofilaments have larger globular components, and the longitudinal bars between the components are longer than in normal neurofilaments. The precise protein composition of PHF is unknown but immunocytochemical studies have revealed some of the principle components.

One of the most important of the components is an abnormally phosphorylated form of the microtubule-associated tau protein (MW 50–60kDa). Whether the accumulation of modified tau proteins in PHFs and in a diffuse cytoplasmic form in some neurons (pre-tangles) affects the normal cellular functions of tau as a microtubule-binding protein or whether it represents an epiphenomenon of neuronal cytoskeletal reorganization in degenerating neurons is uncertain. PHF can also be found in dendrites and axons of neurons. These neuronal processes often have abnormal morphologies and the general term 'dystrophic neurites' serves to identify them (Fig. 2.17). Dystrophic neurites are an important component of primitive and classic plaques. The temporal lobe contains relatively greater numbers of these neuritic plaques than the frontal lobe. The PHF in both neurite and tangles are often found associated with ubiquitin.

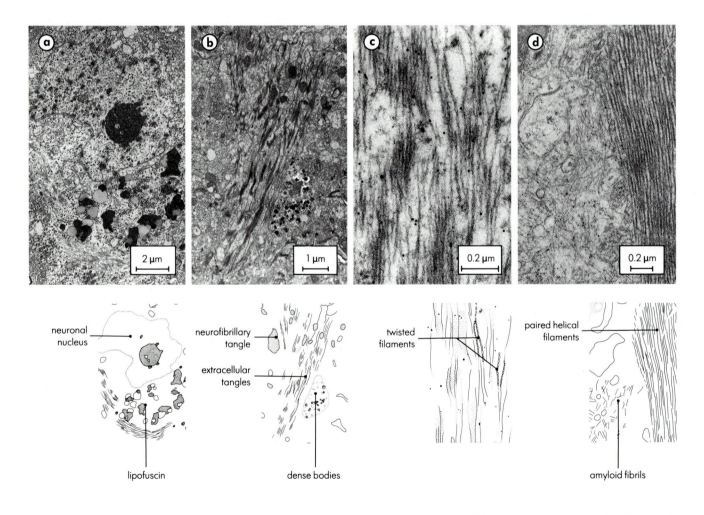

Fig. 2.17 Electron micrographs of neurofibrillary tangle in the cerebral cortex in AD: (a) neurofibrillary tangle within a neuron; (b) extracellular neurofibrillary tangle, with dense bodies and neurofibrillary tangle within a neurite; (c) paired helical filaments immunolabelled with an antiserum to paired helical filaments linked to a gold probe; (d) amyloid fibrils labelled with an antiserum to β-amyloid protein linked to a gold probe; paired helical filaments are not labelled with the antiserum to β-amyloid protein. (Courtesy of Dr C Davis, Manchester.)

Ubiquitin is a cellular protein which is used to maintain the metabolic integrity of cells. Metabolic shock, stress, or disease can result in the formation of abnormal proteins in the cell. These abnormal proteins are conjugated to ubiquitin. This process, akin to an antibody binding to an antigen, tags the protein and marks it for destruction. In a healthy cell, the protein is then destroyed. The association of PHF and ubiquitin indicated that the cell recognizes that the protein component of PHF is abnormal and is actively trying to remove it. However for unknown reasons this process of protein destruction is not effective in AD. Ubiquitin is only found in a proportion of tangles. It is thought that these ubiquitinated tangles are present in neurons which still retain some metabolic potential.

Tangles in other diseases and ageing   Although the presence of large numbers of neurofibrillary tangles is a diagnostic criterion for AD, they are also found in a number of other disorders including the Parkinsonian dementia complex of Guam, dementia pugilistica, and post-traumatic dementia. They are even found, albeit in much smaller numbers, in the normal ageing brain. They are found predominantly in the superficial and middle layers of the anterior frontal and temporal cortex. The areas particularly affected in the anteromedial temporal grey matter include the uncus, amygdala, hippocampus, and the parahippocampal gyrus (Fig. 2.18). Very few if any tangles are seen outside these areas in the normal aged brain. Tangles are found to some extent in most people over the age of 50 and indeed

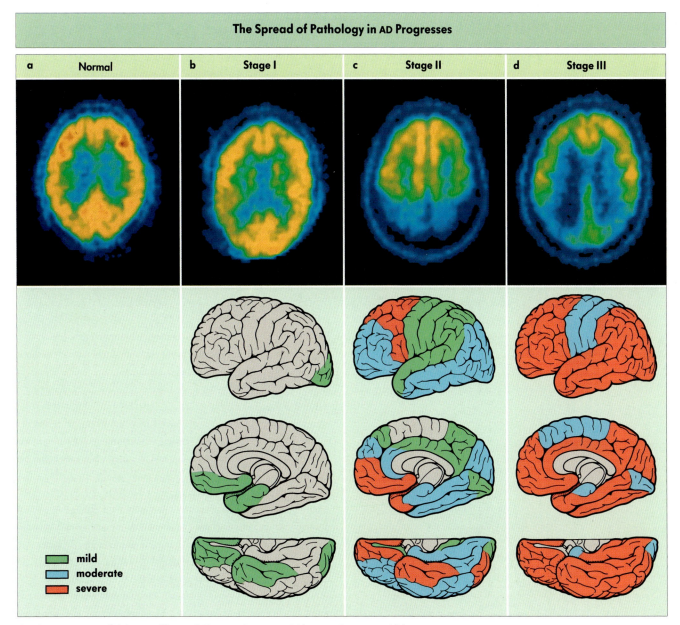

Fig. 2.18   PET scans of: (a) normal brain; (b) brain in Stage I AD; (c) brain in Stage II AD; (d) brain in Stage III AD. The diagrams show the spread of pathology in AD.

there may be extensive involvement of the hippocampus in intellectually normal elderly subjects. In a study based on systematic cell counting in over 200 cases of intellectually normal people, 5 per cent were found to show marked hippocampal tangle formation in their fifth decade while all cases showed this degree of involvement by their 10th decade. In general there is a gradual increase in tangles with age, but there is anything up to a 40-fold difference between the numbers found in normal and demented people.

Relationship between plaques and tangles

In general, plaques are the first and also the most abundant type of pathology seen in the brain in AD. The relationship between plaques and neurite or eventual tangle formation is not clear. It is widely considered that tangles may represent a response to the local toxic effect of plaques. However, it is clear that this is not an invariant response and some brain regions (e.g. the cerebellum) show significant plaque depositions with no appreciable tangle formations.

Cerebral amyloid angiopathy

Cerebral amyloid angiopathy (CAA) is a disorder characterized by the abnormal deposition of amyloid in the walls of cerebral blood vessels. It was first reported in 1938 by Scholz, who described the presence of amyloid in small cerebral vessels in approximately 10 per cent of people dying over the age of 70. It can affect leptomeningeal vessels, pial and cortical arterioles, and occasionally intracortical capillaries. It is generally more prevalent in the parietal and occipital cortex than in fronto-temporal cortical areas. The cerebellar cortex and deep grey matter may also be affected but the brain stem is usually spared.

When viewed under the light microscope, the thickened walls of the vessels appear brightly eosinophilic, and they exhibit a green birefringence under polarized light when stained with Congo red, which led to the term 'congophilic angiopathy'. The amyloid fibrils initially accumulate outside the elastic lamina of the vessels, in the media and the adventitia, but deposits can

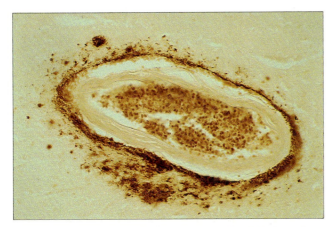

Fig. 2.19 β-amyloid protein deposits around cerebral blood vessels in AD.

also be seen extending in radial spikes into the brain parenchyma. Evidence from ultrastructural studies suggests that the vascular deposits tend to accumulate first in the basal laminae and pericytes. Vascular amyloid in AD is formed from the same protein as the plaque cores – β-amyloid protein (Fig. 2.19). It is not known whether the protein in plaques arises from the same source as that in the vessel walls.

It has been suggested that plaque β-amyloid arises from neurons and vascular β-amyloid from the blood. The fact that the same protein forms two morphologically distinct deposits raises some questions regarding the nomenclature of diagnosis. Mutations in the amyloid precursor protein (APP) gene can cause AD and also Hereditary Cerebral Amyloid Angiopathy (Dutch type). It is not yet resolved whether these conditions should be regarded as phenotypic variations of a single disease process.

There appears to be a close association between CAA and AD with approximately 80 per cent of cases showing some degree of deposition in or around blood vessels, although there are also some reports with large numbers of plaques in the absence of any vascular amyloid. CAA is also seen in the brains of approximately 30 per cent of normal elderly patients and the frequency is thought to increase with age. The disorder is restricted to the cerebral vasculature and is only very rarely seen in conjunction with systemic amyloidosis.

Neuronal loss

There has been debate over the degree of neuronal loss associated with the normal ageing process. This is due to the difficulty in assessing the extent of change in neuronal number unless there is extreme depopulation of cortical neurons with obvious visual evidence of atrophy and gyral shrinkage. Early observations suggested that there was a 15–35 per cent loss of neurons with advancing age, but this is almost certainly incorrect. More recent studies using computer image analysis and stereological methods do not confirm this degree of neuronal loss.

However, a number of quantitative studies have reported a reduction in the extent of the dendritic branching found in neurons. It is this slow progressive loss of neuronal components which probably underlies benign forgetfulness, slower motor performance, and other physiological changes which are common among the elderly. As with the normal ageing brain there has been much debate as to the extent of neuronal loss associated with AD. Some investigators have reported no change in neural number while others have reported 20–30 per cent neuronal loss. However, it now appears that AD is associated with extensive neuronal drop-out which manifests itself as a severe cortical atrophy and thinning of the grey matter ribbon along with a 20 per cent drop in neuropil volume. Cortical cell loss is thought to occur within cortical columns. The loss of cortical neurons, particularly the large pyramidal neurons of layers II and IV, relates directly to the cognitive decline seen in AD. More specific cell loss in discrete subcortical nuclei is also associated with dementia. The loss of a large proportion of the cholinergic cells in the basal nucleus of Meynert and the septum is thought to disrupt memory pathways, and loss from the locus coeruleus may contribute to the sleep disorders and insomnia suffered by older people.

Synaptic loss

A marked loss (approximately 40 per cent) of synapses occurs in affected cortical areas. Traditionally the integrity of synapses would have been assessed by electron microscopy, although this is laborious and time-consuming. A new approach to the assessment of synaptic density has been developed; this utilizes computerized image analysis and immunocytochemical markers to synapse specific proteins (e.g. synaptophysins). Such methods greatly enhance our ability to detect and quantify synaptic loss and demonstrate how plaques and tangles affect synaptic density. Synaptic loss is the best correlate of increasing dementia (r = < 0.7). It is probable that synaptic loss is the primary morphological basis of the cognitive deficits in AD.

The destruction of synapses is associated with the release of β-amyloid precursor proteins into the extracellular spaces.

Other changes

In addition to the neuropathological changes mentioned above there are a number of other more minor changes associated with the ageing brain and AD.

Granulovacuolar degeneration   This phenomenon is essentially restricted to the hippocampus, in the cytoplasm of pyramidal neurons (Fig. 2.20). The vacuoles are 3.5 μm in diameter and each contains a small argyrophilic granule. There may be one or more of these inclusions in a single neuron. They contain similar abnormally phosphorylated proteins to those detected immunocytochemically in neurofibrillary tangles. This form of degeneration is rarely found below the age of 65, but by the ninth decade it is present in 75 per cent of brains. In the normal aged brain, approximately 9 per cent of cells in the Sommer sector of

the hippocampus are affected, whereas in demented patients this proportion rises to over 20 per cent. Granulovascular damage occurs in other disorders apart from AD but its occurrence is generally related to ageing rather than to any specific disease process.

Hirano bodies   Hirano bodies were first identified in cases of the Parkinsonian dementia which is endemic on the Pacific island of Guam. These intensely eosinophilic structures are confined largely to the hippocampus, and measure up to 30 μm in length and 8–10 μm in diameter (Fig. 2.21). EM studies have revealed a structure composed of parallel filaments alternating with thicker, sheet-like material, which does not immunostain with antibodies to neurofilaments. However the presence of cytoskeletal proteins such as actin, vinculin, and tropomyosin suggests that they are caused by a derangement of the neuronal cytoskeleton. The precise cellular localization of these lesions is still disputed because, although they are often found in association with neurons, they have also been observed in the stratum lacunosum of the hippocampus, an area which is neuron-free. They are found to some extent in the brains of intellectually normal elderly people but are generally much more abundant in the brains of demented patients.

Lewy bodies   Lewy bodies are eosinophilic hyaline bodies which can be found within brain stem nuclei such as the substantia nigra and local coeruleus, and throughout the cerebral cortex (Fig. 2.22). Until relatively recently they were generally considered to be a neuropathological feature peculiar to cases of idiopathic Parkinson's disease. However, with more sensitive immunocytochemical detection techniques using ubiquitin and neurofilament antibodies, it now seems that they are much more prevalent than first thought; they appear to be present in 2 per cent of the normal elderly population and they may be present in up to 30 per cent of all dementia cases (see Chapter 5).

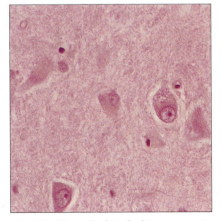

Fig. 2.20 Granulovacuolar degeneration in the pyramidal cells of the hippocampus in AD. (Courtesy of Dr J Lowe, Nottingham.)

Fig. 2.21 Hirano body in the hippocampus in AD. (Courtesy of Dr J Lowe, Nottingham.)

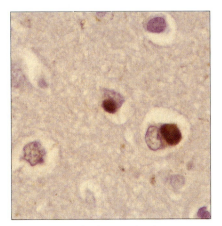

Fig. 2.22 Lewy body stained with an antibody to ubiquitin in AD. (Courtesy of Dr J Lowe, Nottingham.)

NEUROCHEMISTRY

Extensive studies have been undertaken to determine which neurotransmitters might be specifically affected in AD. Almost every transmitter system and every type of transmitter has been implicated (Fig. 2.23), yet it would appear that at the end stage of the disease there is no good evidence for transmitter-specific neuronal loss in AD. Despite the initial reports of marked losses in cortical acetylcholine and the hope that this would lead to a treatment (analogous to replacing dopamine in Parkinson disease), attempts to ameliorate amnesia and cognitive deficits with cholinergic agents have been marginally successful at best.

In addition to cholinergic fibres, non-cholinergic, serotonergic, and possibly dopaminergic fibres which innervate hippocampal and cortical areas are all severely affected by the disease. In addition, glutamatergic and peptide transmitters are also affected (Fig. 2.24). Several studies have shown that deficits associated with plaque and tangle formation, or transmitters found in abnormal neurites tend to reflect the normal distribution of transmitters within that region (Fig. 2.25). These findings indicate that the pathological processes in AD which produce tangles and plaques involve local transmitters in a non-specific fashion, although some classes of neurons or patterns of neuronal connections remain relatively unaffected.

In the light of recent studies, the neurochemical data indicate that, whilst correlations between transmitter deficits and pathology or clinical symptoms undoubtedly exist, they are probably indirect reflections of the extent of local pathology and tell us little about the underlying nature of the disease process.

In terms of possible pharmacological treatments, it is clear that AD does not follow the neurochemical model of Parkinson's disease. Therefore, it seems very unlikely that AD can be meaningfully ameliorated or treated by single or even multiple neurotransmitter replacement therapy.

β-AMYLOID PRECURSOR PROTEIN AND AD

A key diagnostic feature of AD is the presence of plaques. The principle component of the plaque is a peptide of approximately 40–42 amino acids which is referred to as β-amyloid protein (β-APP) (Fig. 2.26). This peptide is now known to be a breakdown product of a much larger protein – β-amyloid precursor protein encoded by a host gene on the long arm of chromosome 21. This gene is expressed in many different species and has been highly conserved through evolution. APP is found in many tissues within the body (liver, lung, kidney, muscle, and brain). The levels of APP mRNA expression differ widely from tissue to tissue, and expression within the brain also varies during the course of development. The regulation of APP gene expression is complex, as the gene has at least 18 exons and these are used to generate at least five transcripts of APP by alternative splicing. This process produces a family of APP proteins of which the APPs of 695, 751 and 770 amino acids in length are the most abundant. APP 695 mRNA is enriched in mammalian brain, whereas APP 751 and 770 are the main type found in non-neuronal tissue.

APP molecules have a large extracellular amino terminal domain with a short carboxyl terminal cytoplasmic tail, tyrosine-sulphated residues and N- and O-linked carbohydrates. APPs are associated with synaptic membranes and are axonally transported.

Causes of AD

Epidemiological studies have consistently shown that family history is a risk factor for developing AD. In addition, there are numerous reports of families in which AD is inherited as an autosomal dominant disorder. Genetic linkage studies have shown that the pathogenic locus for some families is on the proximal long arm of chromosome 21. It is now clear that one locus on chromosome 21 is the APP gene, and that mutations in this gene

Neurochemistry of AD			
Type	**Transmitter**	**System**	**Change in AD**
Monoamine	*Acetylcholine	Basal nucleus of Meynert, and other forebrain cholinergic cell clusters to cortex	Loss of cholinergic cells in forebrain; loss of cholenergic terminals in cortex
	Dopamine	Midbrain to cortex and stratun.	Reduction in dopamine metabolites
	*Noradrenaline	Locus coeruleus to cortex	Loss of noradrenergic cells in brain stem; loss of noradrenaline in cortex
	Serotonin	Raphe nuclei to cortex	Reduced 5HT in cortex
Amino acid	Glutamate	Pyramidal cells in corticocortical and corticofugal pathways	Glutamate binding and uptake sites reduced
Neuropeptide	*Somatostatin and other neuropeptides	Cortical interneurons	Reduced cortical levels
*Found in dystrophic neurites in plaques			

Fig. 2.23 Neurochemistry of AD.

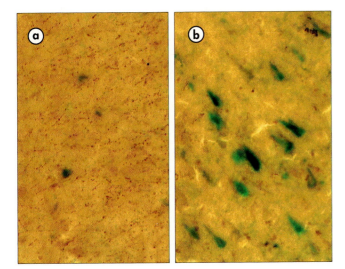

Fig. 2.24 Neurotransmitter deficits due to AD pathology:
(a) somatostatin fibres (brown) in the frontal cortex in a control;
(b) tangle formation (blue) in the frontal cortex in AD with marked loss of somatostatin fibres.

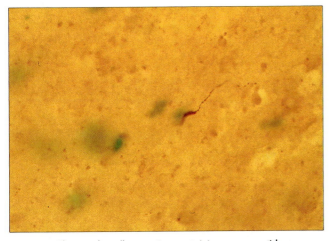

Fig. 2.25 Abnormal swollen neurites containing neuropeptide Y (brown) in an area of temporal cortex containing tangles (blue) in AD.

APP as a Cell-surface Glycoprotein

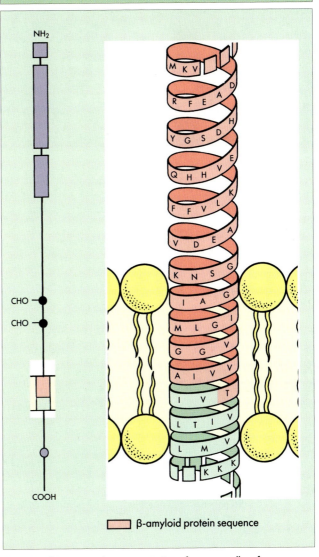

☐ β-amyloid protein sequence

Fig. 2.26 Diagrammatic representation of APP as a cell-surface glycoprotein.

resulting in substitution of valine with other amino acids at codon 717 (residue 642 in APP 695) (Fig. 2.27) give rise to the disease in some families. APP 717 mutations have been detected in English, American, and Japanese families with early onset AD. It is likely that further APP gene mutations remain to be discovered in other kindreds with autosomal dominant familial AD. Linkage with other genetic markers on or outside chromosome 21 (e.g. chromosome 19) could be explained by mutations in regions of DNA having some influence on APP metabolism (e.g. APP-producing enzymes or their inhibitors).

It should be stressed that the proportion of cases in which AD is acquired as a single gene, autosomal dominant disorder is very low, and that there is a substantial body of evidence indicating that the neuropathological changes of AD can also be triggered (most likely in genetically susceptible individuals) by various environmental factors (see Chapter 5). However, the fact that an APP gene mutation can give rise to all of the neuropathological hallmarks of AD without any preceding underlying neuronal pathology or any other defect strongly suggests that amyloid deposition is the primary or at least the seminal event in the pathogenesis of all cases of AD. This proposal is strongly supported by the observation that transgenic mice that over-express a portion of the human APP gene can show deposits of β-amyloid protein similar to those seen in the human brain.

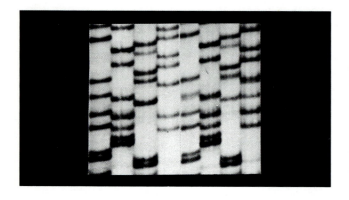

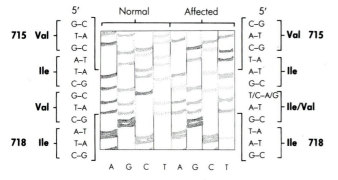

Fig. 2.27 Photograph of a DNA sequence gell demonstrating the change in codon 717 (adenine to guanine) of the APP protein in a patient with autosomal dominant AD. (Courtesy of Dr J Hardy, London.)

Functions of APP

APPs are involved in protease inhibitions (important during development and growth), responses to neuronal stress and damage, and the regulation of cell to cell interactions. Some APPs are released from neurons as carboxyl-terminally truncated molecules. The 751 and 770 secretory forms of APP have the Kunitz-protease inhibitor insert and show the same N-terminal sequence and molecular weight as protease nexin II (a regulatory molecule secreted by fibroblasts). These forms of APP combine with serine proteases (e.g. trypsin, chymotrypsin) to produce stable complexes, which could play a role in blood clotting by inhibiting appropriate coagulation pathway enzymes, including coagulation factor XIa (Fig. 2.28).

Release of APP from neurons is thought to occur via proteolytic cleavage in the middle of the β-amyloid sequence close to the extracellular membrane (see Fig. 2.28). Secreted APP has been detected in CSF, human serum, and the conditioned media of various cultured cells. Cells transfected with cDNA constructs that encode full-length APP 695 and APP 751 release secretory forms of APP that terminate at residue Gln 15 of β-amyloid, leaving behind a C-terminal membrane-bound fragment commencing at leucine. Thus, the 'APP' secretase cleavage enzyme acts at the Gln 15–Lys 16 or Lys 16–Leu 17 bonds, leaving Lys 16 to be excised by an aminopeptidase or carboxypeptidase, respectively.

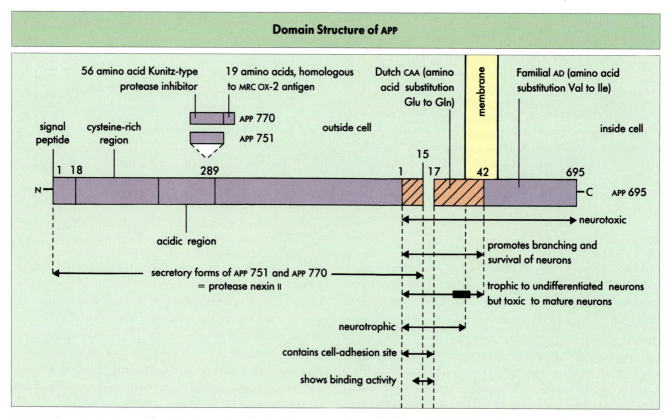

Fig. 2.28 Domain structure and functional map of APP showing the location of β/A4 region. Only the three most abundant isoforms are shown; minor isoforms include APP 714, with 19 amino acid insert, and the APP 563 form, which lacks the β/A4, transmembrane, and cytoplasmic regions. (Courtesy of Dr J Hardy, London.)

Abnormal cleavage of the APP molecule to produce the β-amyloid protein is considered to be a central feature of AD. This may occur *de novo* as a result of disease or be caused by the routing of APP through a little-used alternative processing pathway (involving cleavage at two sites on either side of β-amyloid sequence to liberate the peptide).

APP Regulation and Amyloid Deposition

The APP gene has been shown to be up-regulated by a variety of factors including the cytokine interleukin-1β. Up-regulation occurs within hours of a neuronal stressor such as ischaemia or head injury. The increased amounts of APP produced after such events or during the over-expression of the APP gene in Down's syndrome (due to a 50 per cent increase in gene dosage) is thought to produce the pool of excess APP that is available for conversion into β-amyloid. It is possible that, in Down's syndrome and susceptible individuals, this is a consequence of an excessive amount of APP causing overloading of the normal proteolytic processing pathway. This leads to a rerouting of the APP into an alternative, amyloid generating, pathway.

Abnormal processing of APP could also occur as a result of mutations within the APP gene. Pathogenic mutations are clustered around the normal proteolytic cleavage site within the β-amyloid protein fragment (see Fig. 2.28). The APP 693 mutation in hereditary congophilic angiopathy (Dutch type) lies close to this site, whilst the APP 717 mutation in familial AD is just beyond the carboxyl terminus of the β-amyloid protein region. These mutations may influence APP proteolysis and lead to inappropriate degradation and β-amyloid protein deposition. It is also possible, if several alternative pathways exist for processing APP but most are not utilized under normal conditions, that mutations of the APP protein bias the protein to enter one of these pathways.

The abnormal processing of APP is thought to lead to an accumulation of the β-amyloid protein within cellular lysosomes. Such accumulations would seriously affect the normal processes of protein degradation within neurons. Fusion of the lysosomes at the neuronal membrane would lead to the extrusion of amyloid into the extracellular space. Confocal microscopy demonstrates that this extrusion occurs preferentially at synaptic sites and leads to compromised synaptic function. The reason why large amounts of β-amyloid are deposited in the cortex is unknown. However, large amounts of β-amyloid protein leading to reduced cortical synaptic function probably represent the pathological substrate of emerging dementia.

DIFFERENTIAL DIAGNOSIS

Progressive cognitive impairments, deterioration in social function and personality, and mood changes are common in other kinds of dementia. In addition, hearing difficulties and impaired sight can result in the confusion and apparent lack of comprehension that are frequently found in older patients. These factors can work together to make a clear diagnosis of AD difficult. Several of the main confounding conditions and principal alternative diagnoses are discussed below.

Cerebrovascular disease and multi-infarct dementia

Distinguishing features are abrupt onset, fluctuating course, history of stroke, focal symptoms or signs, and stepwise deterioration (see Chapter 3). If such features are prominent, then a dementia of vascular origin should be investigated (and treated). One of the simplest ways of assessing the likelihood of cerebrovascular disease is to use the checklist devised by Hachinski *et al* (see Chapter 3) to calculate an ischaemia score. This scale is widely used, although some items are difficult to score accurately. Imaging studies are often useful in differentiating AD from cerebrovascular disease. The latter is characterized by the presence of multiple, discrete, high intensity foci on MRI scans. On PET and SPECT scans, multiple discrete areas of hypofunction are readily visible.

However, it should be borne in mind that post-mortem studies have demonstrated that about 20 per cent of patients dying with dementia show pathological changes characteristic of both AD and cerebrovascular disease. Thus, both types of disease process can readily occur in the same patient.

Acute confusional states

A range of conditions and illnesses can lead to confusional states in older people; examples are chronic cardiac disease and respiratory or urinary tract infections. A thorough clinical history should reveal the presence of concurrent infections that are of relatively recent origin. In addition, periods of clouded consciousness, marked variations in the degree of confusion, disorientation, or the presence of lucid intervals with restored cognitive function should signal the presence of a confusional state. Occasionally, an acute confusional state precedes the onset of degenerative dementing process.

Other conditions

There are several relatively common and potentially treatable causes of dementia syndromes. These include drug toxicity, AIDS, hypothyroidism, neurosyphilis, alcoholism, nutritional deficiencies, space-occupying lesions and normal-pressure hydrocephalus. Appropriate investigations will confirm or exclude most of these possibilities.

Major mood disorder – depression

The appearance of depression in the elderly may be extremely difficult to distinguish from the apathy, loss of initiative, reduced social activity, and general decline in performance that can characterize the early course of AD. In most cases, dementia can be differentiated from depression on the basis of the clinical history if attention is paid to the duration, mode of onset, and the nature of the early symptoms. A previous history of depression and the presence of variable or inconstant cognitive impairments suggest depression as a possible diagnosis. Clinical folklore suggests that patients with pseudodementia typically complain of cognitive difficulties; patients with dementia often do not

EARLY DETECTION OF AD

Establishing a firm diagnosis of AD is difficult, even when the behavioural changes are well established; often the chronicity of the condition is used to underpin diagnostic certainty. Making a firm diagnosis is even more difficult in the early stages of the disease, because the range of competence in older people varies dramatically with age, and because memory difficulties, language impairments, and physical disabilities are a common consequence of age. Given these factors, it has proved difficult to establish absolute categories of 'normality'. In the light of this, there are as yet no clear diagnostic criteria for mild AD, and estimates of the prevalence of such conditions in the community vary widely from study to study (e.g. from 2.6 per cent in Britain to 52.7 per cent in Japan). A further complication is encountered by the supposition that AD may be overdiagnosed in patients with low intelligence (e.g. Down's syndrome) or poor education.

Early diagnosis of dementia is important, despite the absence of effective treatment. Early detection is needed to understand the natural history of the disorder, to engage family members in supportive care, and to allow early intervention which can avert crises and sustain viability within the community. Finally, when they become available, early diagnosis will allow pharmacological treatments at a stage when they are most likely to prove effective.

SUMMARY

(i)   AD is the commonest cause of dementia in old age.

(ii) AD can be caused by a variety of different factors, including mutations in the APP gene, head trauma, and trisomy 21.

(iii) Diagnosis is based on progressive cognitive impairment with clear consciousness, although other psychological, psychiatric, and neurological symptoms may also be present.

(iv) Definite diagnosis of AD is only possible after neuropathological examination to demonstrate the occurrence of plaques and tangles in the cortex.

(v)   Synaptic and neuronal loss occurs by disruption of cellular metabolism and cellular degeneration leading to the formation of plaques and tangles.

(vi) Aberrant metabolism of the β-amyloid precursor protein may initiate cellular degeneration.

(vii) Differential diagnosis involves excluding depressive conditions and multi-infarct dementias. Imaging studies can aid the exclusion of other diseases but not provide a definitive diagnosis.

3 Cerebrovascular Dementias

INTRODUCTION

Diseases of or damage to the blood vessels supplying the brain are among the most frequent serious neurological disorders. Cerebrovascular disease ranks third as a cause of death in adults in the USA and probably first as a cause of chronic functional incapacity. Approximately 2 000 000 people living in the USA (0.8 per cent of the population) are impaired by the neurological consequences of cerebrovascular disease. Many of them are between the ages of 25 and 64.

Interruptions in the vascular supply of the brain can give rise to anoxia, ischaemia, and subsequent infarction. The resulting cerebral degeneration is the second commonest cause of dementia in the elderly. About 25–35 per cent of demented patients over the age of 65 have cerebral ischaemic lesions that are a major factor in the dementing process. The term multi-infarct dementia (MID) has become widely accepted as the most appropriate designation for that form of severe emotional, intellectual, and memory disturbance which results from ischaemic and infarct damage to the brain.

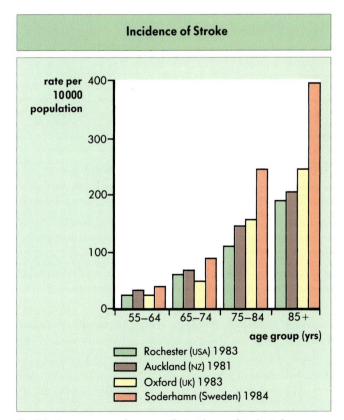

Incidence of Stroke

rate per 10 000 population / age group (yrs)

- Rochester (USA) 1983
- Auckland (NZ) 1981
- Oxford (UK) 1983
- Soderhamn (Sweden) 1984

Fig. 3.1 Average annual age-specific incidence of stroke in four selected studies. (Adapted from Bonita R. *Lancet* 1992;**339**:342.)

These patients frequently have a history of hypertension and one or more strokes, and they also often show neurological signs and symptoms compatible with such a history. The presence of infarcts or focal enlarged sulci is demonstrated by CT and MRI scans, and patchy areas of hypometabolism are often seen on PET or SPECT scans. At autopsy the characteristic picture is of multiple areas of degeneration throughout the cerebral hemispheres.

DEFINITION

Cerebrovascular disease is a condition associated with rapidly developing clinical signs of focal (or global) disturbances of cerebral function, with symptoms lasting 24 hours or longer or leading to death, and with no apparent cause other than a vascular origin (World Health Organization). This definition includes subarachnoid haemorrhage but excludes transient ischaemic attacks (TIA), subdural haematomas, and the complications of infections or tumours.

The reduction or compromise of cerebral blood flow leads to either reversible functional changes (ischaemia) or irreversible neuronal damage (infarct). The terms stroke or cerebrovascular accident refer to the clinical signs and symptoms which result.

EPIDEMIOLOGY

There has been a steady decline in the incidence of major cerebrovascular disease over the last few decades. This may well be because of improved treatment of hypertension and changes in diet, which are major risk factors. However, these advances should not obscure the observation that the risk of a stroke rises with age and that some 1 per cent of the population suffer from the consequences of this disease (Fig. 3.1).

About 30 per cent of patients with dementia have a vascular component. Thus, there are some 1 400 000 patients in the USA whose dementia has a significant vascular component.

Risk Factors

The risk of cerebrovascular disease is increased by:
- hypertension;
- head trauma;
- interruptions in cardiac output;
- amyloid angiopathy.

Other risk factors include smoking, obesity, diabetes, birth

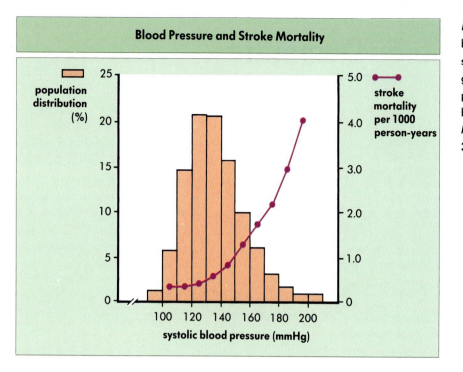

Fig. 3.2 Population distribution of systolic blood pressure (bars) and age-adjusted stroke mortality per 1000 person years (line graph). Numbers over the bars represent the percentage of excess stroke deaths in each blood pressure category. (Adapted from Marmot MG, Poulter NR. *Lancet* 1992; **339**:346.)

control pills, collagen–vascular disease, migraine headaches, high salt diets, high alcohol consumption, and hypothyroid disorders.

Hypertension

Raised blood pressure is the biggest risk factor for cerebrovascular disease. It has been calculated that about 40 per cent of strokes can be attributed to a systolic pressure of more than 140 mmHg (Fig. 3.2). It is unusual for autopsy to reveal a vascular basis for dementia in the absence of a clinical record of marked hypertension (often above 180/110 mmHg). In a large survey of autopsy-proven cases, the blood pressure in cases of MID was considerably greater than in cases of Alzheimer's disease (mean 173/98 and 137/85 respectively), which further underlines this point.

Head trauma

Gross tearing of blood vessels leading to intracranial bleeding and pressure on the surface of the brain are common sequelae of head trauma. It is sometimes overlooked that ischaemic brain damage up to and including infarction is also found in up to 80 per cent of patients with severe head trauma (see Chapter 5).

Head trauma is a common event in westernized nations and is a leading cause of death in those aged under 45. In survivors of severe head trauma it has been estimated that 1–5 per cent remain vegetative, and that 5–18 per cent still have a severe disability more than six months after their accident. Advances in trauma medicine continually improve survival rates, which results in an accumulating problem of disabled and ageing survivors (approximately 750000 in the United Kingdom and 2000000 in the United States of America).

Interruptions in cardiac output

Episodes of cardiovascular disease which disrupt the blood supply to the brain are an obvious cause of ischaemic damage. Such interruptions are not only disease related, but can also occur as a result of various therapeutic procedures (e.g. cardiac by-pass surgery, heart transplantation). Clinically significant episodes of brain ischaemia occur in an estimated 60 per cent of patients undergoing such procedures.

Hereditary cerebral haemorrhage with amyloidosis

Amyloidosis is a generic term to denote the deposition of abnormal fibrillar forms of normal body proteins in extracellular and intracellular spaces. Abnormal deposits of protein (amyloid) around and within the walls of cerebral blood vessels (Fig. 3.3) occur in several autosomal-dominant inherited types of cerebral amyloidosis, e.g. Dutch-type (mutations in β-amyloid precursor protein), Icelandic-type (mutations in Cystatin C protein). The proteins involved vary, although the pathological mechanism is thought to be similar. Amyloid deposits are thought to reduce the efficiency of the vascular system and also to weaken the structure of vessel walls, thus increasing the probability of ischaemia and strokes.

Genetic disorders of this type are rare. However amyloid deposits in the walls of blood vessels are found in many older patients and such sporadic deposits may be associated with 5–10 per cent of intracerebral haemorrhages.

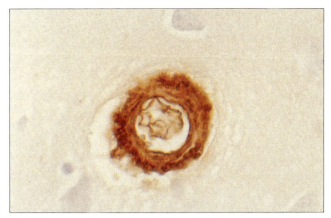

Fig. 3.3 Immunostained cortical blood vessel showing abnormal deposits of amyloid around and within the walls. (Courtesy of Dr MLC Maat-Schieman, Leiden.)

Clinical Characteristics of Cerebrovascular Dementia

Presentation

Acute episodes/abrupt onset
Hypertension
Focal neurological signs or symptoms

Course

Stepwise progression
Confusional states
Emotional lability (depression, aggression, agitation)
Preservation of insight
Preservation of personality
Transient ischaemic attacks
Dizziness
Patchy intellectual deficits

Pathology

Focal hyperintensities (on CT, MRI)
Hypometabolic regions (on PET, SPECT)

Fig. 3.4 Criteria for the diagnosis of multi-infarct dementia.

Ischaemic Score

Clinical feature	Score
Abrupt onset	2
Stepwise progression	1
Fluctuating course	2
Nocturnal confusion	1
Relative preservation of personality	1
Depression	1
Somatic complaints	1
Emotional incontinence	1
History of hypertension	1
History of strokes	2
Evidence of associated arteriosclerosis	1
Focal neurological signs	2
Focal neurological symptoms (score over 10 indicates cerebrovascular disease)	2

Fig. 3.5 The Hatchinski score.

DIAGNOSIS

The clinical diagnosis of multi-infarct (as opposed to a degenerative or Alzheimer-type) dementia is made on the basis of:

- sudden onset;
- the occurence of one or more strokes; and
- a tendency for a fluctuating course with some day-to-day variation, as well as some evidence of spontaneous improvement in the early part of the illness (Fig. 3.4).

A stepwise progression is seen with sudden worsening of the mental state. In addition there is often:

- hypertension;
- evidence of coronary or other major arterial disease;
- a labile emotional state; and
- a tendency for a degree of psychological insight to be retained for much longer than occurs in other neurodegenerative diseases.

The presence of these features is frequently used to construct an 'ischaemic score' as a diagnostic aid to the differentiation of the vascular dementias (Fig. 3.5).

Cerebrovascular disease is a frequent complication of diabetes and hypothyroidism, and a history of these disorders plus dementia indicates that further investigations, particularly using MRI, PET, and SPECT imaging procedures, would also be valuable.

MRI typically reveals (T2 weighted images) multiple focal signal hyperintensities (Fig. 3.6) of variable size and distribution consistent with focal infarction. PET and SPECT show scattered areas of hypofunction, presumably reflecting reduced blood flow or reduced glucose metabolism. The pattern of large regional reductions in metabolism characteristic of Alzheimer's disease is not normally found.

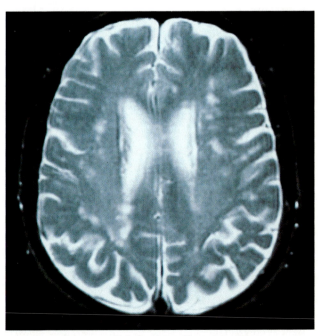

Fig. 3.6 MRI showing multiple focal signal hyperintensities.

Classification of Stroke

Increased understanding on the pathology and physiology of stroke allows for a degree of classification as to the cause, clinical category, and site of the stroke (Fig. 3.7). Such an approach may well prove valuable in:

- predicting progosis;
- helping to treat the effects of the stroke and reducing the risk of subsequent stroke; and
- planning supportive care and rehabilitation.

CLINICAL FEATURES

The main clinical features of cerebrovascular disease are:

- hypertension;
- fluctuating cognitive impairments;
- neurological abnormalities;
- attenuation and atrophy on CT scanning; and
- multiple high intensity focal lesions on MRI scanning.

Cerebrovascular disease is a common feature in patients aged over 60. Men and women appear to be equally affected, although the changes in incidence due to treatment for hypertension and alterations in diet may alter the pattern of disease onset in the future. Although uncommon, it is not unknown for patients to be affected in their late 30s. These cases are invariably familial and are often due to inherited amyloid angiopathies (e.g. Dutch-type and Icelandic-type).

A wide range of cognitive deficits and psychiatric symptoms are seen. In content and severity, these overlap to a great extent with those seen in Alzheimer's disease and dementia with cortical Lewy bodies, and as such they may not be particularly helpful in establishing a correct diagnosis.

The most effective clinical features in distinguishing cerebrovascular disease from other neuropsychiatric conditions are those derived from the pathological effects of hypertension or the compromise in the vascular supply of focal brain regions. As a result of this type of pathology, the presence of circumscribed neurological abnormalities is a more accurate guide to differential diagnosis than cognitive or psychiatric abnormalities.

Particular attention should be paid to the presence of signs and symptoms that indicate focal brain damage:

- unequal tendon reflexes;
- presence of plantar extensor reflexes;
- impaired pupillary reactions;
- amnesic syndrome;
- aphasia, dysphasia;
- motor disturbance (e.g. parkinsonian, pseudobulbar palsy);
- epilepsy.

The presence of these types of clinical features indicates the need for additional investigations using imaging techniques. CT and MRI often reveal a typical picture: a variable degree of cerebral atrophy with a more obvious enlargement of the ventricular system (Fig. 3.8). In many cases, the latter feature is the only

NINDS Classification of Stroke	
Mechanism:	thrombotic; embolic; haemodynamic
Clinical:	atherothrombotic; cardioembolic; lacunar
Arterial site:	internal carotid; middle cerebral; anterior cerebral; vertebral; basilar; posterior cerebral

Fig. 3.7 National Institute of Non-communicative Disorders and Stroke (NINDS) pathophysiological classification of stroke.

obvious abnormality. However, atrophy and ventricular enlargement on CT and MRI can be unreliable ways of differentiating cerebrovascular disease from Alzheimer's disease. Additional features of CT scans that help to differentiate the two are areas of low attenuation (resulting from old and recent infarcts), focal or unequal enlargement of the ventricular system, and focal areas of gyral or sulcal atrophy.

MRI can improve diagnostic discrimination. Old cerebral infarcts appear as focal areas of high signal intensity on T2-weighted images. Multiple areas of such lesions are typical of MID. Acute non-haemorrhagic infarctions are usually invisible with CT until five to ten days after the stroke. On MRI, they may be observed within 24–48 hours. In contrast, CT reveals acute haemorrhagic stroke, which is difficult to differentiate from oedema with MRI.

Imaging of the structure or function of major blood vessels (e.g. carotid angiography) can give valuable information on disease or stenosis.

Investigations using EEG can also be useful. Focal abnormalities (e.g. low amplitude delta focus or asymmetrical patterns) can be found in the vicinity of large infarcts or when the patient experiences episodes of delirium. The presence of focal or lateralized EEG abnormalities is a diagnostic indicator of MID, as patients with Alzheimer's disease and similar cognitive deficits do not demonstrate these types of EEG pattern.

Abnormalities in CSF can be detected in some cases. Most cases show elevations in the enzyme neuron-specific enolase. Generalized elevations in protein levels are seen in 20 per cent of cases. CSF changes are marked in patients that have had recent infarcts and in those with uraemia or congestive cardiac failure.

Course and Outcome

The characteristic course of cerebrovascular disease is:

- sudden onset;
- stepwise progression;
- focal deficits; and
- intact personality.

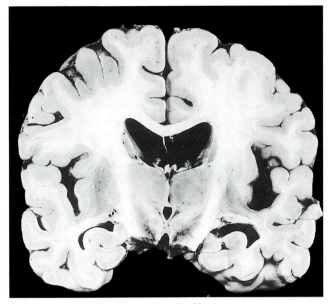

Fig. 3.8 Photograph showing ventricular dilation.

The sudden appearance of neurological and cognitive deficits and the clinical history of a step-like progression – the appearance of clinical symptoms, a period of stability, and then further deterioration or the appearance of other symptoms – is a reliable pattern that distinguishes the dementia of cerebrovascular disease.

Patients often present with the effects of a sudden cerebrovascular accident (e.g. loss of speech, paralysis). In cases with a more gradual onset, changes in personality or emotional state often occur before more obvious evidence of cognitive decline. Complaints of somatic symptoms such as headache, dizziness, tinnitus, and syncope are also common and may precede the appearance of neurological symptoms.

The uneven progress of cerebrovascular disease is in marked contrast to the relatively smooth descent into dementia seen in Alzheimer's disease. The onset of symptoms can be followed by a period of improvement and temporary remission. These periods may last for months in the initial stages of the disease. The dynamics of this clinical pattern are governed by the frequency and size of the subsequent cerebral infarcts.

As the disease progresses, the increasing degree of neuronal destruction is marked by a succession of symptoms such as apraxia, dysphasis, ataxia, visual disturbances, or paralysis. Explosive emotional outbursts are common and easily provoked. These outbursts (weeping or laughter) can occur without the patient appearing to experience appropriate changes in mood.

Over time, the periods of improvement and remission decline and the patient accumulates neurological and cognitive deficits. The types of neurological deficits are variable and depend on the site and extent of the brain lesions. They include ataxia, dysarthria, and motor and sensory disturbances.

The end stage is a combination of parkinsonian features, pseudobulbar palsy (dysarthria, dysplasia, and emotional lability), and a variable degree of cognitive impairment. In some cases, cognitive impairment progresses in the relative absence of focal neurological symptoms.

Personality and the capacity for judgement are often preserved until the final stages of the disease (in contrast to Alzheimer's disease). As such, insight is retained and patients remain aware of the extent and speed of their decline. This leads to states of anxiety and depression of considerable severity.

The time course of the disease is variable, and ranges from the slow accumulation of neurological deficits to the occurrence of a few catastrophic infarcts. The average length of illness is approximately seven years, and progress is usually slower than that seen in Alzheimer's disease. Death is due to ischaemic heart disease (approximately 50 per cent of patients); the remainder die as a direct result of cerebral thrombosis or renal complications.

Types of Stroke

There are three types of stroke (Fig. 3.9):
- occlusive;
- haemorrhagic; and
- embolic.

Occlusive strokes

Occlusive strokes are caused by closure or blockage of blood vessels. Most occlusive strokes are due to atherosclerosis and thrombosis. Very large lesions may result from internal carotid or middle cerebral artery thrombus or from occlusion of the temporo-occipital territory of the posterior cerebral artery (Fig. 3.10). In the latter case extensive damage can occur to the medial temporal cortex and hippocampus.

Haemorrhagic strokes

Haemorrhagic strokes are caused by bleeding from a vessel either at the brain surface – extraparenchymal (e.g. rupture of congenital aneurysms at the circle of Willis, causing subarachnoid haemorrhage) or within the brain – intraparenchymal (e.g. rupture of vessels damaged by long-standing hypertension) (Fig. 3.11). Haemorrhage may result in ischaemia or infarction, leading to further damage. Subarachnoid haemorrhage may cause reactive vasospasm of cerebral surface vessels. The mass effect of an intracerebral haematoma may limit the blood supply of adjacent brain tissue.

Hypertensive intra-axial haemorrhage and rupture of saccular aneurysm are common types of haemorrhage. They occur at specific anatomical locations and cause characteristic clinical symptoms.

Hypertensive intercerebral haemorrhage These commonly occur when the walls of the small penetrating vessels of the corona radiata, internal capsule pons, cerebellum, thalamus, and putamen are damaged. The walls of these blood vessels are weakened and eventually rupture (Charcot–Bouchard microaneurysms). Significant haemorrhages in the midbrain cause paralysis, stupor, and hemiplegia and are associated with a high mortality rate.

Saccular aneurysms Congenital saccular aneurysms are caused by weaknesses in the walls of the blood vessels located at:

- the junction of the anterior communicating artery and anterior cerebral artery;
- the junction of a posterior communicating artery and an internal carotid artery; or
- the first bifurcation of the middle cerebral artery in the Sylvian fissure.

Rupture of the aneurysm in each case causes severe headache and a characteristic syndrome. Rupture of the posterior communicating artery causes a haematoma on the oculomotor nerve that results in ipsilateral pupil dilation and loss of the reflex response to light. The rostral bifurcation of the basilar artery (Fig. 3.12) or the origin of the posterior inferior cerebellar artery are common sites of posterior fossa aneurysms. These are associated with a variety of cranial nerve deficits and signs of brain stem damage. Middle cerebral artery aneurysm can produce the same clinical picture as middle cerebral artery stroke (by formation of a haematoma or secondary infarction) with few or no focal signs, but reduced alertness and behavioural changes. The sudden rupture of an aneurysm anywhere within the skull can produce a marked increase in intracranial pressure and disrupt

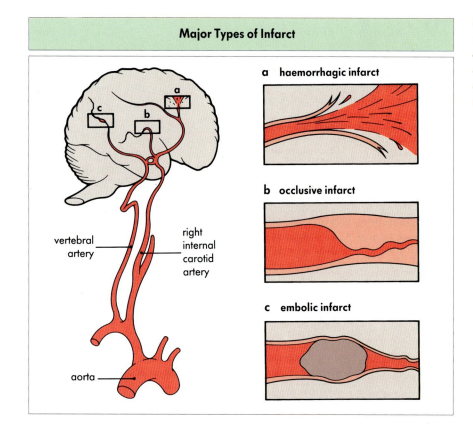

Major Types of Infarct

a **haemorrhagic infarct**

b **occlusive infarct**

c **embolic infarct**

vertebral artery

right internal carotid artery

aorta

Fig. 3.9 Schematic Illustration of the brain, showing a haemorrhagic infarct in the anterior cerebral arterial distribution, an occlusive infarct in the middle cerebral arterial distribution, and an embolic infarct in the posterior cerebral arterial distribution.

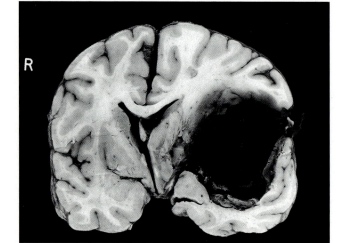

Fig. 3.10 Photograph of an infarct caused by a ruptured cerebral aneurysm. (Courtesy of Dr CJ Bruton, London.)

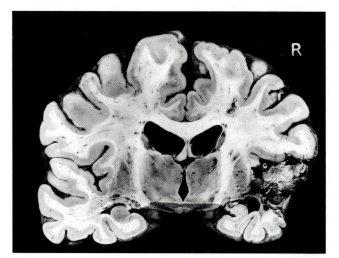

Fig. 3.11 Photograph of an infarct caused by occlusion of the middle cerebral artery. (Courtesy of Dr CJ Bruton, London.)

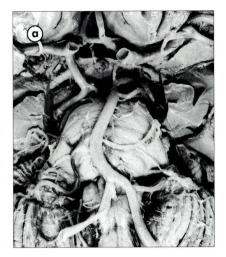
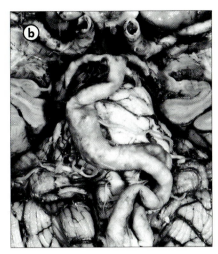

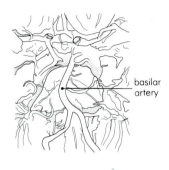

Fig. 3.12 Photograph of (a) normal basilar artery and circle of Willis; (b) aneurysm of the basilar artery in severe cerebrovascular disease.

basilar artery

Sources of Cardiogenic Embolism to the Brain

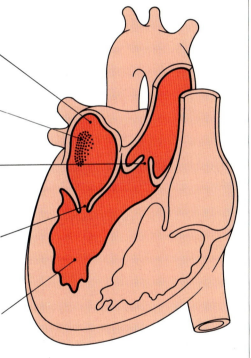

left atrium
atrial fibrillation, myxoma, atrial septal aneurysm

paradoxical emboli
patent foramen ovale, atrial septal defect

aortic valve
calcific stenosis, infective endocarditis, prosthetic valve

mitral valve
infective endocarditis, myxomatous valvulopathy, annulus calcification, prosthetic valve, vegetations due to prothrombotic states

left ventricle
ischaemic dyskinesis, non-ischaemic cardiomyopathy, thrombi due to prothrombotic states

Fig. 3.13 Sources of cardiogenic embolism. (Adapted from Hart RG. *Lancet* 1992; **339**:589.)

the homoeostatic activity of brain stem structures. This results in the sudden onset of coma.

Both occlusive and haemorrhagic strokes can occur at any age from many causes; these include cardiac disease, trauma, infection, neoplasm, blood dyscrasia, vascular malformation, immunological disorder, and exogenous toxins. Diagnostic strategies and treatment should vary accordingly.

Embolic strokes

Occlusion or haemorrhage secondary to embolism, often from the heart, is a third cause of cerebral infarction. This phenomenon was first documented in 1847 by the pathologist Virchow.

Many cardiac disorders can give rise to emboli (Fig. 3.13) and this type of pathology may cause some 20 per cent of ischaemic stroke. Recognizing this pathological process has important practical implications, since cardiac disease is often apparent early on and antithrombic treatments are effective (Fig. 3.14). Thus, early treatment of the underlying condition can significantly reduce the risk of subsequent stroke.

The size of the embolus and thus the size of the stroke lesion can vary with the particular cardiac disorder (Fig. 3.15). Emboli from valvular sources (e.g. mitral valve prolapse, thrombotic endocarditis) tend to be small. Such pathology is associated with transient ischaemic attacks, small subcortical infarcts, or episodes of cortical blindness.

Sources of Cardiogenic Embolism

Valvular diseases

Rheumatic mitral stenosis
Prosthetic valves
Calcific aortic stenosis
Mitral annulus calcification
Non-bacterial thrombotic (marantic) endocarditis (associated with malignancy, diffuse intravascular coagulation, antiphospholipid antibodies, and other prothrombotic states)
Myxomatous mitral valvulopathy with prolapse
Infective endocarditis
Inflammatory valvulitis: Libman–Sacks endocarditis, Behçet's disease, syphilis

Myocardial ischaemia with ventricular thrombi

Acute myocardial infarction
Left ventricular akinesis/aneurysm

Arrhythmias with atrial thrombi

Atrial fibrillation
Sick sinus syndrome

Non-ischaemic dilating cardiomyopathies

Hypertrophic
Amyloid
Rheumatic myocarditis
Neuromuscular disorders
Catecholamine-induced
Doxorubicin hydrochloride
Idiopathic
Viral
Peripartum
Contusion
Hypereosinophilic
Sarcoid
Alcoholic
Chagas' disease
Crack cocaine use
Oxalosis
Echinococcosis

Intracardiac thrombi related to prothrombotic states

Polycystic disease
Myeloproliferative disorders and thrombocythemia
Malignancy
Antiphospholipid antibodies

Cardiac tumours

Primary
Metastatic

Paradoxical emboli

Atrial septal defects
Patent foramen ovale
Ventricular septal defects
Pulmonary arteriovenous fistulas

Miscellaneous sources

Post-cardiac catheterization and valvuloplasty

Fig. 3.14 Causes of cardiogenic embolism. (Adapted from Hart RG. *Lancet* 1992;**339**:589.)

Risk of Embolism from Cardiac Disorders

Major risk sources (substantial risk of stroke)

Atrial fibrillation
Prosthetic valve
Mitral stenosis
Recent myocardial infarct
Left ventricular thrombus
Atrial myxoma
Infective endocarditis
Non-ischaemic dilating cardiomyopathy
Marantic endocarditis

Minor risk sources (low risk of stroke, or incompletely established as a direct source of embolism)

Mitral valve prolapse
Severe mitral annulus calcification
Patent foramen ovale
Atrial septal aneurysm
Calcific aortic stenosis

Fig. 3.15 Degree of risk of embolism from various cardiac disorders. (Adapted from Hart RG. *Lancet* 1992;**339**:589.)

Emboli from the chambers of the heart (left atrium and ventricle) are much larger and are associated with cortical branch artery symptoms (homonymous hemianopia, aphasias, etc) and pan-hemispheric strokes.

ANATOMY

Each cerebral hemisphere is supplied by an internal carotid artery, which arises from a common carotid artery beneath the angle of the jaw, enters the cranium through the carotid foramen, traverses the cavernous sinus (giving off the ophthalmic artery), penetrates the dura, and divides into the anterior and middle cerebral arteries (Fig. 3.16).

Blood also reaches the brain through the vertebral arteries. Each vertebral artery arises from a subclavian artery, enters the cranium through the foramen magnum, and gives off an anterior spinal artery and a posterior inferior cerebellar artery. The vertebral arteries join at the junction of the pons and the medulla to form the basilar artery, which at the level of the pons gives off the anterior inferior cerebellar artery and the internal auditory artery, and at the midbrain gives off the superior cerebellar artery and the posterior cerebral artery.

Anterior cerebral artery

The large surface branches of the anterior cerebral artery supply the cortex and white matter of the inferior frontal lobe, the medial surface of the frontal and parietal lobes, and the anterior corpus callosum. Smaller penetrating branches supply the deeper

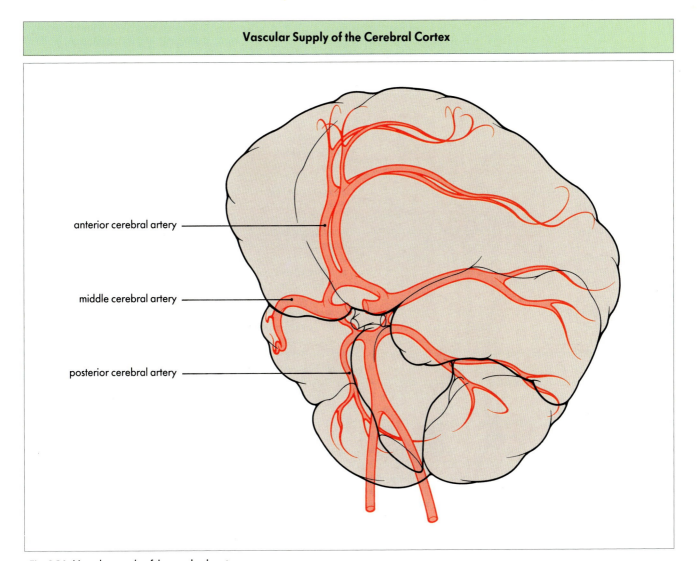

anterior cerebral artery

middle cerebral artery

posterior cerebral artery

Fig. 3.16 Vascular supply of the cerebral cortex.

cerebrum and diencephalon, including limbic structures, the head of the caudate, and the anterior limb of the internal capsule.

Middle cerebral artery

The large surface branches of the middle cerebral artery supply most of the cortex and white matter of the hemisphere's convexity, including the frontal, parietal, and temporal lobes, and the insula. Smaller penetrating branches (the lenticulostriate arteries) supply the deep white matter and diencephalic structures such as the posterior limb of the internal capsule, the putamen, and the outer globus pallidus.

As the carotid artery emerges from the cavernous sinus, it also gives off the anterior choroidal artery, which supplies the anterior hippocampus and, at a caudal level, the posterior limb of the internal capsule.

Posterior cerebral artery

The basilar artery then divides into the two posterior cerebral arteries, which supply the inferior temporal and medial occipital lobes and the posterior corpus callosum. The smaller penetrating

branches of these vessels (the thalamoperforant and thalamogeniculate arteries) supply diencephalic structures, including the thalamus and the subthalamic nuclei, as well as parts of the midbrain.

Anastomoses

Both the carotid and basilar arteries join an arterial ring – the circle of Willis. The circle of Willis gives rise to the anterior, middle, and posterior cerebral arteries which supply each cerebral hemisphere (Fig. 3.17). The anastomosis provided by the circle of Willis provides an overlapping blood supply whereby alterations in supply from the carotid or basilar system can be smoothed out and compensated for. A congenitally incomplete circle, which is relatively common in the general population, is much more frequent in patients who have had strokes. Other important anastomoses include connections between the ophthalmic artery and branches of the external carotid artery through the orbit, and connections at the brain surface between branches of the middle, anterior, and posterior cerebral arteries (sharing border zones or watersheds). The small penetrating vessels arising

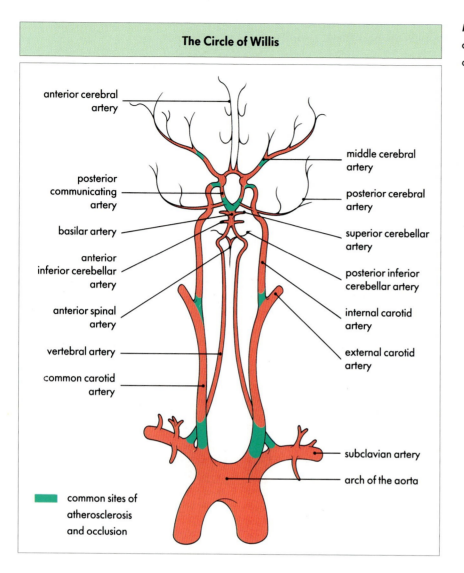

The Circle of Willis

anterior cerebral artery

middle cerebral artery

posterior communicating artery

posterior cerebral artery

basilar artery

superior cerebellar artery

anterior inferior cerebellar artery

posterior inferior cerebellar artery

anterior spinal artery

internal carotid artery

vertebral artery

external carotid artery

common carotid artery

subclavian artery

arch of the aorta

common sites of atherosclerosis and occlusion

Fig. 3.17 The circle of Willis, showing common sites of atherosclerosis and occlusion.

from the circle of Willis and proximal major arteries tend to lack anatomoses. The deep brain regions they supply are therefore called end zones (see Fig. 3.16).

PHYSIOLOGY

The human brain has a high metabolic rate; as a result, the volume of blood flow is extensive and the parameters of this flow are impressive:

- the brain is 2 per cent of body weight but receives 15 per cent of cardiac output;
- brain metabolism accounts for 20 per cent of body oxygen consumption;
- total blood flow to the brain is 750–1000 ml per minute (350 ml through each carotid artery and some 100–200 ml through the vertebrobasilar system); and
- blood flow of grey matter is greater than white matter (approximately 4:1 per unit mass).

Different cognitive tasks result in altered patterns of blood flow. Cerebral blood vessels alter their diameter (autoregulation)

in at least two ways in response to physiological stimuli, thus ensuring that additional metabolic demand is met and that the pattern of blood flow is controlled. Vessels respond to arterial pressure by constricting when it is raised and dilating when it is lowered. These responses ensure an even blood flow that remains almost constant between arterial pressures of 60 and 150 mmHg. Beyond these limits, there are linear rises and falls in blood flow.

Autoregulation also occurs in response to changes in blood gases and pH. Such regulation is very sensitive, and increased arterial concentrations of carbon dioxide cause increased cerebral blood flow because of arteriolar dilatation. The effect is thought to be mediated by alterations in extracellular pH and also by factors such as nitric oxide and the neuropeptide NPY. However, the exact mechanisms are still being investigated.

Reduced concentrations of oxygen have an opposite effect. Changes in arterioles to altered oxygen concentrations are less marked. Breathing 100 per cent oxygen lowers cerebral blood flow by about 13 per cent; breathing 10 per cent oxygen raises it by 35 per cent. The autoregulation of arterioles enables the brain to meet the fluctuating demands for oxygen and glucose metabolism that accompany normal brain activities. For example,

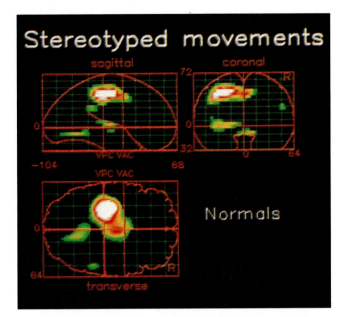

Fig. 3.18 C^{15}O$_2$ PET scans. The coloured areas show changes in regional cerebral blood flow (rCBF) associated with repetitive movements of the right hand and arm in normal subjects. rCBF is portrayed as statistical parametric maps (SPMs) which represent significant increases in rCBF over the resting condition. The major increases in rCBF are in the upper limb area of the contralateral primary motor cortex and in the supplementary motor areas.

repetitive movements of the right arm causes increased oxygen use in the contralateral primary motor cortex (Fig. 3.18). As a result, carbon dioxide concentrations increase and pH drops in the area. This causes an immediate local increase in blood flow. Increased blood flow can also protect the brain by supplying oxygen and removing toxic metabolites after hypoxia, ischaemia, or tissue damage.

Hypoperfusion and border zone infarcts

Global reduction in blood flow (hypoperfusion) can occur as a consequence of shock. This phenomenon can lead to widespread regions of ischaemia or infarction in particular regions. Neurons in the border zones between territories supplied by the main arteries and supplied by the end zones of deep penetrating vessels are particularly vulnerable (see Fig. 3.16). Clinical signs tend to be bilateral after episodes of hypoperfusion. Bilateral infarction of the sensorimotor cortex in the border zones of the anterior and middle cerebral arteries can cause paralysis and sensory loss in both arms. Damage in the border zones of the middle and posterior cerebral arteries (occipital and temporal cortex) can lead to disturbances in memory or vision (cortical blindness). Movement disorders can arise as a result of infarcts in the cerebellar border zone (ataxia) or from damage to the basal ganglia regions supplied by penetrating arteries (chorea or myoclonus). These disorders can also occur together and in association with cognitive or other focal deficits.

The normal processes of autoregulation can show marked disturbances after an infarct, and these disturbances can amplify the damage caused by the initial event. Additional damage can be caused by:

- vasomotor paralysis;
- intracerebral steal; and
- inverse intracerebral steal.

Ischaemic damage to neurons causes a loss of the normal responses to alterations in arterial pressure and increased carbon dioxide or decreased oxygen concentrations. This type of damage can lead to aberrant responses to vasodilators, during which blood flow is increased at distant brain sites but not in the vicinity of the infarct. Thus, blood is diverted from the ischaemic lesion to 'normal' brain tissue (intracerebral steal).

Vasoconstrictors can lead to the reduction of blood flow in the unaffected brain regions but have no effect on vessels in the damaged area (inverse intracerebral steal). This phenomenon explains the common appearance of red venous blood draining from infarcts (reflecting decreased oxygen extraction from damaged tissue, coupled with unchanged blood flow – 'luxury perfusion').

The extent of these phenomena varies considerably from patient to patient. Inverse intracerebral steal is not a constant feature of brain infarcts and, when present, it can coexist with reduced perfusion and increased oxygen extraction in adjacent areas. Although intracerebral steal is common in large infarcts, its extent and duration is difficult to quantify or predict. At present, it is not certain whether, in the acute phase, enhancing the blood flow of affected areas leads to short term improvements (increasing tissue oxygen, removing toxic metabolites) or increases the potential for further tissue damage (increasing oedema, mass effect, anastomotic compromise).

The existence of these complicated and sensitive regulatory mechanisms enables the brain to orchestrate its metabolic activity in a dynamic fashion and to respond to changing demand within seconds. Such sensitivity explains the catastrophic effects of arbitrary disruptions in the brain's blood supply.

PATHOLOGY

Old age

Symptomless infarcts are a common feature of intellectually normal old people. About 60 per cent of elderly controls show some evidence of cerebral damage. Generally, this is restricted to very small lesions (often 5 μm or less across) in the white matter or basal ganglia. Estimates put the loss of neuronal tissue at less than 1 ml. Lesions totalling more than 5 ml of destroyed brain are found in less than 10 per cent of patients. Rarely, large infarcts (up to 50 ml) are seen. Infarctions occur most often in the brain regions supplied by the middle and (to a lesser extent) posterior cerebral arteries. Anterior territories are least often affected.

Cerebrovascular disease

Gross pathology

The external appearance is often unremarkable. A visual inspection of the sliced brain will commonly show enlargement of the ventricular system, which may be focal or unilateral.

Multiple regions of infarcted tissue are invariably present. These vary in size from a few millimetres to centimetres in the cortex; occasionally lesions are so large as to cause the near destruction of a whole hemisphere. Both hemispheres will be affected in most cases, with the most obvious lesions in the territory of the middle or the posterior cerebral artery.

Cerebrovascular pathology

The appearance of the vascular system in cerebrovascular disease is characterized by:

- thickening of the vessel walls within the brain; and
- atheroma of large vessels supplying the brain.

Most patients with cerebrovascular disease have also suffered from extended periods of hypertension. The increased blood pressure causes a pathological thickening of vessel walls, because of medial hypertrophy and lipohyalinosis (Fig. 3.19). This leads to a narrowing of the vessel, particularly marked at the entrance to capillary beds, and consequently to reduced blood flow. This type of pathology is often found in the perforating arteries that supply white matter and in the terminal arterial territories of the putamen. The reduction in blood flow renders these regions vulnerable to the development of ischaemia.

Narrowing of the large arteries at the base of the brain (basilar artery and circle of Willis) caused by atheroma is a common finding (Fig. 3.20). The degree of such pathology and its location is variable and can range from the partial occlusion of a single vessel at one anatomical site through to vessels being affected at multiple sites. Total blockage of a large artery, and thus a complete loss of blood flow to a large brain region, is an unusual finding. Such gross pathology is generally found only in those patients who have experienced a massive recent infarct. The atheromatous deposits in arteries result in focal areas of dilatation, kinking and an irregular course (Fig. 3.21). The narrowing (stenosis) of carotid and vertebral arteries in the neck or in the base of the skull is a useful indicator of the presence of cerebrovascular disease. Invariably the occurrence of such pathology in the major vessels supplying the brain is matched by the presence of pathology in the vessels within the brain.

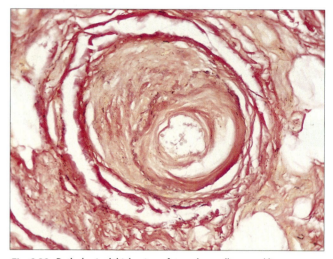

Fig. 3.19 Pathological thickening of vascular wall, caused by hypertension. (Courtesy of Dr J Lowe, Nottingham.)

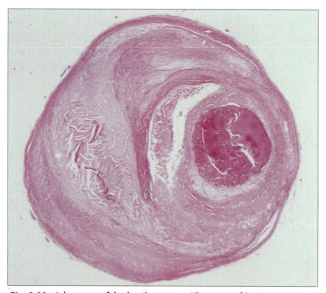

Fig. 3.20 Atheroma of the basilar artery. (Courtesy of Dr J Lowe, Nottingham.)

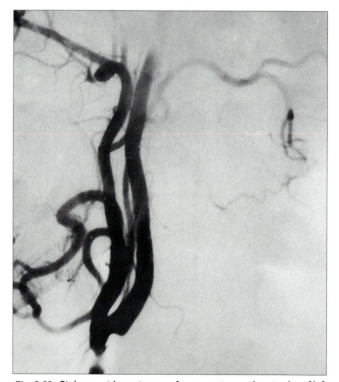

Fig. 3.21 Right carotid arteriogram, from a patient with episodes of left hemiparesis, showing tight stenosis at the carotid syphon and origin of the internal carotid artery.

However, atheroma in the cerebral vessels is a common finding of many normal old people, and the pathological appearance alone is not sufficient to justify a diagnosis.

Systemic vascular pathology

Disease of the vascular system in other organs of the body also occurs in the same patients. The heart and kidneys are most often affected, although the thickening of vascular walls in response to systemic hypertension can be found in organs throughout the body.

Hypertension can lead to myocardial hypertrophy and subsequent cardiac infarction. Such a clinical course would be expected to exacerbate the patients cerebrovascular difficulties. Cardiac disease can also lead directly to cerebrovascular disease, in that emboli from left ventricular or atrial thrombi can lead to the occlusion of major arteries (see Fig. 3.13). The occurrence of atheromatous plaques in the carotid arteries (see Fig. 3.17) favours the formation of multiple thrombi, and this pathological sequence is a frequent cause of cerebrovascular disease.

Pathological studies indicate emboli are not sufficient by themselves to produce typical multi-infarct dementia. The appearance of the full clinical picture of multi-infarct dementia requires the presence of diseased intracerebral vessels in addition to the damage caused by emboli. Exceptionally, bilateral embolic strokes (related to the atrial fibrillation of rheumatic heart disease) that damage large arteries lead to dementia.

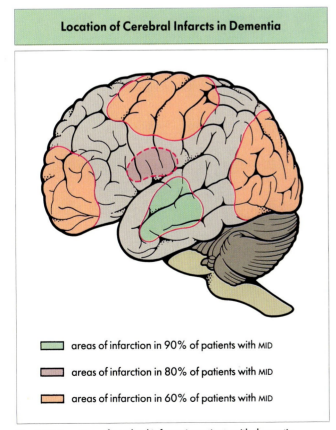

Location of Cerebral Infarcts in Dementia

☐ areas of infarction in 90% of patients with MID

☐ areas of infarction in 80% of patients with MID

☐ areas of infarction in 60% of patients with MID

Fig. 3.22 Location of cerebral infarcts in patients with dementia.

Collagen vascular disease and meningeal infections can also give rise to arterial occlusion or to forms of vasculitis that result in infarction. Meningitis can also cause fibrosis of the basal meninges, which lead to obstructive hydrocephalus and dementia.

Location of infarcts

Small silent infarcts are a frequent finding in old people. This finding, and common sense, suggest that the size, number, and location of the infarcts are important factors in determining whether there will be clinical deficit.

In patients with multi-infarct dementia, almost 100 per cent show bilateral infarcts and 90 per cent have temporal lobe infarcts. In addition, over 80 per cent of patients show infarcts in the basal ganglia white matter (Fig. 3.22). Non-demented patients have fewer and smaller areas of damage and infarcts are often unilateral. White matter involvement occurs in addition to the infarcts in other locations, and this distinguishes MID from the purely lacunar state characteristic of Binswanger's disease.

Parietal, frontal, and occipital infarcts are found in about 60 per cent of patients. Destruction of the corpus callosum or hippocampus is rare in non-demented cases with cerebral softening, but is present in many cases of multi-infarct or mixed multi-infarct Alzheimer's disease. Areas of focal damage are frequently seen in the basal ganglia and thalamus of MID patients. However, they are also a common occurrence in non-demented subjects.

Infarct Volume – Dementia Threshold

Cerebrovascular disease results in dementia if the ischaemic lesions are sufficiently large or if they are in certain locations.

Hatchinski introduced the term 'multi-infarct dementia' and suggested that cerebrovascular disease causes dementia by a series of relatively large infarcts that damage a sufficient volume of brain. Neuropathological studies have suggested that such a threshold exists, and calculations indicate that infarct volumes which total over 50 ml are often associated with dementia, and that a total infarct volume over 100 ml is always associated with dementia. These figures are still regarded as illustrative of the amount of damage required by 'pure' cerebrovascular disease to cause dementia.

Note that many patients with cerebrovascular disease also have Alzheimer's disease or *vice versa* (approximately 20 per cent of Alzheimer's disease cases are 'mixed'). Thus, smaller volumes of infarct could contribute significantly to the dementing symptoms in such patients by causing the destruction of tissues in an already compromised CNS.

Microscopic Pathology

The pathological appearance of lesions under the microscope is variable, and is governed mainly by the site of the lesion the degree of destruction; and the age of the lesion.

Lesions of white matter may be visible by the localized loss of myelin and the presence of activated glial cells and microcystic foci (Fig. 3.23). The appearance of lesions in the cortex is markedly different, with marked loss of neurons from particular cortical laminae or neuronal loss along the track of cortical arteries perpendicular to the pial surface. Ischaemic lesions that are restricted to the cortex can be found in some cases. The cortical ribbon is thinned, and microscopy reveals the presence of many small areas of neuronal loss and scarring which are invariably related to small blood vessels. Occasionally, massive laminar neuronal loss is observed; regions of affected cortex show a massive activation of glial cells and contain lipid-filled macrophages.

Old lesions in areas of extensive destruction form clearly defined cysts filled with clear fluid in both grey and white matter. Close examination often reveals evidence of a zone of damage (penumbra) which extends beyond the readily identifiable region of ischaemia.

PHYSIOLOGICAL CONSEQUENCES OF STROKE

Ischaemia

Following a stroke, the resulting insufficiency of blood supply to brain tissue is called ischaemia. Ischaemia is not synonymous with anoxia, for a reduced blood supply deprives tissue not only of oxygen, but of glucose as well, and prevents the removal of toxic metabolites such as lactic acid. Brief periods of ischaemia can lead to symptoms (e.g. fainting, memory loss) and signs (e.g. paralysis) that are reversible and leave little or no pathological evidence of tissue damage.

When ischaemia is sufficiently severe and prolonged, profound physiological changes take place, and neurons and other cellular elements die; this process is called infarction and the area of damaged tissue is an infarct.

Spectrum of ischaemic damage

The degree of damage caused by ischaemia is related to:
- the magnitude of the reduction in blood flow; and
- period of reduced blood flow.

The interplay between these parameters is obviously complicated and is made more so by the fact that different classes of neurons within the brain have differing vulnerabilities to ischaemic damage.

The delivery of oxygen and glucose is greatly reduced by episodes of ischaemia (strokes) but is rarely cut off completely. This is due primarily to the anatomical organization of blood vessels in the brain, which ensures that vessel anastomoses or collaterals can make up part of the reduction in blood flow, and also to the autoregulatory capacity of vessels, which allows them to dilate in response to reduced flow. These physiological responses act to minimize the effects of ischaemia and to limit the region of the brain that is affected. As a result, the pathology caused by ischaemia shows a typical pattern: a core of severe damage and possibly infarction surrounded by a penumbra of damaged or compromised neurons (Fig. 3.24). The possibility of preserving or restoring function to neurons in the penumbra is of considerable clinical interest.

Mild or transient ischaemia, sufficient to cause a loss of membrane potentials for longer than five minutes, can affect vulnerable populations of neurons within the brain, but leaves glial cells unaffected. Pyramidal neurons within the hippocampus are particularly sensitive, and typical patterns of cell loss in

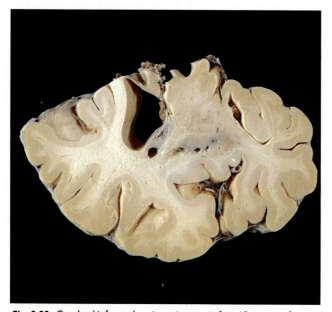

Fig. 3.23 Cerebral infarct, showing microcystic foci. (Courtesy of Dr J Lowe, Nottingham.)

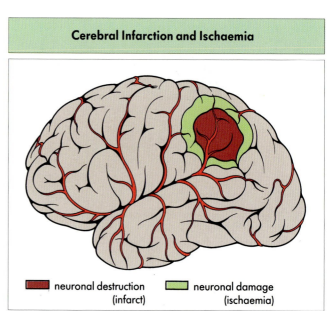

Cerebral Infarction and Ischaemia

■ neuronal destruction (infarct)   ■ neuronal damage (ischaemia)

Fig. 3.24 Cerebral ischaemia results in an area of neuronal destruction, surrounded by a halo of neuronal damage.

this region are seen after transient global ischaemia in patients resuscitated from cardiac arrest or after brief periods of focal ischaemia (e.g. posterior cerebral artery occlusion).

More prolonged periods of ischaemia (up to one hour) result in tissue destruction and the formation of infarcts. Infarcts are characterized by the death of neurons, glia, and other supportive cells within the affected vascular territory. The infarct proper is separated from normal brain tissue by a penumbra of dead, damaged and functionally compromised neurons mixed with surviving glial cells. The size of the penumbra is related to the gradient of ischaemia between the infarct and normal brain tissue.

Prolonged periods of ischaemia (more than one hour) result in the expansion of the area of infarction. The process begins in the centre of the ischaemic region, and the infarct grows in a spherical fashion (see Fig. 3.24), progressively enlarging in a spherical fashion and reaching its maximum size after eight to 24 hours.

Penumbra – clinical relevance

The neuronal tissue within the penumbra of an infarct is of considerable clinical interest. The neurons are damaged and functionally compromised, with membrane abnormalities and aberrant bursts of electrophysiological activity. The abnormal function can cause additional neuronal damage, and this process is thought to cause the progressive neurological deficits that occur in some patients days or weeks after an ischaemic episode. Thus, intrinsic or therapeutic attempts to improve perfusion could exacerbate the instabilities in affected neurons and trigger or enhance the processes which lead to neuronal damage and death. Obviously, if these neurons could be protected in the immediate aftermath of ischaemia, there could be considerable clinical benefits.

Attempts to treat stroke and reduce infarct volume may be clinically beneficial even after the initiating ischaemic event. However, their potential for success is critically dependent on the time between the initiation of infarction and the commencement of treatment.

Molecular pathology of ischaemia

Ischaemia reduces the pool of high energy phosphates (ATP) within neurons. Since these substances rae essential for neuronal metabolism, persistent reductions lead inevitably to neuronal death.

When blood flow falls to about 20 per cent of normal (i.e. approximately 10 ml per 100 g of brain per minute, as opposed to 50 ml per 100 g of brain per minute) following ischaemia, the availability of glucose and oxygen (the mitochondrial electron acceptor) is reduced. As a consequence, the brain's demand for energy (usually supplied by oxidative metabolism) exceeds the available supply. Within minutes, the secondary system for generating (anaerobic ATP generation using stored glucose and glycogen) is exhausted and cellular metabolism is disrupted. Metabolites such as lactate and free hydrogen ions accumulate

in proportion to the degree of anaerobic metabolism which has occurred. This leads to marked changes in neuronal pH and a generalized failure of energy-requiring metabolic processes. Disruption occurs in the mechanisms which maintain membrane integrity and ion gradients (e.g. ion pumps). In turn this leads to the opening of ion channels and equilibrium between intra- and extracellular ions. The disturbances of ionic concentration cause membrane depolarization and result in the release of neurotransmitters including the excitatory amino acids (glutamate and aspartate). These latter transmitters are released in sufficient concentrations to cause neurotoxicity (Fig. 3.25).

Membrane depolarization leads to a rise in intracellular calcium levels and this is thought to accentuate many of the perturbations in cellular metabolism. In particular, calcium activates both nitric oxide synthetase which in turn enhances free radical formation and phospholipases which hydrolyze membrane-bound glycerophospholipids to free fatty acids; these in turn accelerate free radical peroxidation of other membrane lipids (see Fig. 3.25).

Intraneuronal disruptions in metabolism are unlikely to be a complete explanation of cell death nor of the ongoing process of neuronal degeneration which takes place over the next 24 hours or so. Neurons and glia can tolerate marked reductions in oxidative metabolism caused by ischaemia for several minutes (sometimes for over one hour), and make a complete recovery.

It is known that ischaemia triggers a cascade of events which begins with disrupted metabolism within the neuron, leads to membrane depolarization and eventually triggers responses from adjacent neurons and glia. These responses include the up-regulation of genes which code for particular proteins, including membrane proteins (such as the β-amyloid precursor protein), trophic factors (nerve growth factor) and cytokines (interleukins 1 and 6). Together these proteins represent the 'acute phase response' – a cascade of molecular events which occurs within the brain in response to neuronal damage (see Fig. 3.25).

The exact sequence and regulatory mechanisms involved in the acute phase response are under active investigation. However, it is thought that the acute phase response, whilst beneficial and protective in the long run, can cause significant neuronal damage and destruction in the initial, and therapeutically important, stages of ischaemia and infarction.

IMPLICATIONS FOR THERAPY

The realization that the damage triggered by an ischaemic event is progressive and continues for hours after the event has ended has resulted in research designed to slow or stop the degenerative processes unleashed.

Blockade of Calcium Channels

Since the deleterious effects of uncontrolled entry of calcium into cells are well known (Fig. 3.26), considerable effort has been

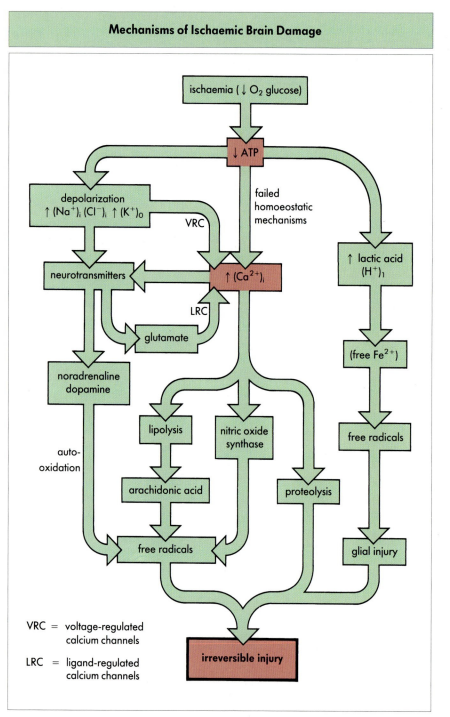

Mechanisms of Ischaemic Brain Damage

ischaemia (↓ O_2 glucose)

↓ ATP

depolarization
↑ $(Na^+)_i$ $(Cl^-)_i$ ↑ $(K^+)_o$

VRC

failed homoeostatic mechanisms

neurotransmitters

↑ $(Ca^{2+})_i$

LRC

glutamate

↑ lactic acid $(H^+)_1$

noradrenaline dopamine

(free Fe^{2+})

lipolysis

nitric oxide synthase

free radicals

auto-oxidation

arachidonic acid

proteolysis

free radicals

glial injury

irreversible injury

VRC = voltage-regulated calcium channels

LRC = ligand-regulated calcium channels

Fig. 3.25 Possible mechanisms of ischaemic brain damage.

expended on ways of blocking the influx of calcium into the cell or its intracellular release. It has been demonstrated that calcium inflow through post-synaptic (L-type) voltage-regulated and glutamate-regulated membrane channels are involved in the production of cell damage. Blockade of N-methyl-D-aspartate (NMDA) and quisqalate (Q) glutamate receptor-channel complexes leads to marked reductions in the size of infarct volumes in experimental animals. However, these drugs disrupt glutamate-mediated synaptic transmission and can lead to considerable side-effects.

Blockade of Acute Phase Response

Substances which inhibit the effects of cytokines have also been shown to reduce markedly the size of infarcts in experimental animals. One such substance is the naturally occurring brain protein (interleukin 1 receptor antagonist – IL-1 RA). This protein is normally manufactured and released by cells after trauma in large quantities. It is believed that it forms part of the regulatory system which acts via negative feedback to reduce and control the acute phase response. Increasing the levels of IL-1 RA thera-

Regulation of Calcium Influx

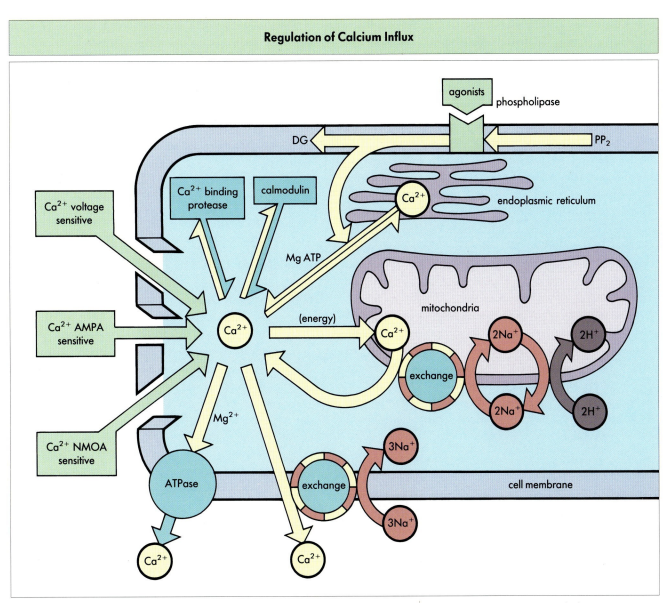

Fig. 3.26 Calcium influx is regulated by voltate-sensitive and ligand-sensitive channels. Energy-dependent regulation of intracellular calcium is by an ATP-dependent pump. Calmodulin and other intracellular proteins control the homeostasis of calcium ions, which is energy-independent. (Adapted from Pulsinelli W. *Lancet* 1992;**339**:533.)

peutically may augment the physiological systems within the brain and help reduce the degree of neuronal degeneration triggered by ischaemia in a way which avoids disruption of normal synaptic activity.

OTHER ISCHAEMIC DEMENTIAS

Binswanger's Disease

Subcortical arteriosclerotic encephalopathy was the name given by Olszewski (1962) to a dementing condition characterized by:

- cerebral white matter infarcts;
- cerebral demyelination; and
- relative sparing of cortical grey matter.

The disease is named after Binswanger, who originally reported on eight similar cases in 1894 and first attributed the pathology in the white matter to reductions in blood flow.

The clinical course of patients with this disorder is similar to that of other types of cerebrovascular disease. Typically, they are hypertensive and present with symptoms in their 50s. Disease progression is marked by a series of cerebrovascular episodes after which neurological deficits (e.g. pseudobulbar palsy) and motor signs are common. Remissions, with partial recovery of function, can occur. Later in the course of the disease, a progressive dementia emerges. Differential diagnosis to exclude Alzheimer's disease is extremely difficult on clinical grounds although the presence of subacute neurological deficits suggests a diagnosis of Binswanger's disease. Diagnostic confirmation requires CT or MRI (Fig. 3.27) to demonstrate widespread attenuation of white matter, and obvious infarcts may be present. Ventricular dilatation is almost always marked and there may be sulcal atrophy. The degree of ventricular enlargement relative to cortical atrophy is significantly greater than that usually seen in Alzheimer's disease.

Leucoaryosis

The clinical significance of white matter damage due to infarcts (leucoaryosis) has not been widely studied, and cases in which this type of pathology contribute significantly to the patient's dementia (excluding Binswanger's disease) used to be considered rare by pathologists. Leukoaryosis is a variant of multi-infarct dementia in which the majority of the clinically significant lesions are found in the white matter, although other regions, including the cortex, are also affected. When examined, the brain is slightly atrophic and areas of cortical infarction may be found. Ventricular enlargement is generally marked owing to the destruction and retraction of adjacent white matter.

The white matter of the frontal and parietal lobes is generally more affected than the temporal and occipital regions. Within white matter tracts, a range of ischemic lesions, both partial and cystic, is found; their appearance and extent relate to the severity and length of clinical course. Substantial areas of infarction in the cortex and basal ganglia occur in less than half of patients diagnosed in life. However, small regions of ischaemic damage in these areas can be seen with a microscope.

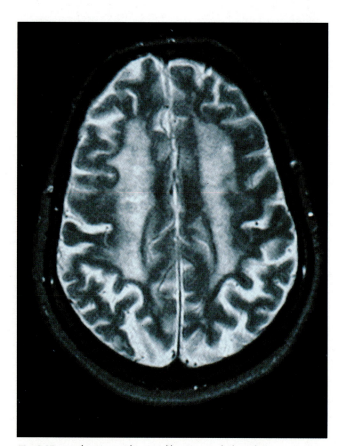

Fig. 3.27 MRI showing widespread leucoencephalopathy in Binswanger's disease.

The relationship between the degree and location of white matter damage and the nature and severity of clinical symptoms is uncertain. The nature of the deficits might owe more to the consequences of cortical disconnection (loss of linking fibre tracts) than to cortical destruction (loss of cortical neurons). It is possible that this pathological mechanism generates a particular profile of neuropsychological deficits which, if discernible, could be of considerable diagnostic utility.

It is expected that growing use of CT and MRI imaging as a means of diagnostic investigation will lead to a significant increase in the number of patients diagnosed as having this disorder.

DIFFERENTIAL DIAGNOSIS

Cerebrovascular Dementia and Alzheimer's Disease

Cerebrovascular disease is second only to Alzheimer's disease as a cause of progressive intellectual impairment in older patients. Differentiating between the two on clinical grounds is difficult. It is probable, however, that there is a considerable tendency to overdiagnose cerebrovascular disease during life. Doubtless this is due in part to the potential for therapeutic intervention that such a diagnosis implies. In the middle-aged adult, the clinical diagnosis is encountered much more often than is justified by the eventual pathological findings. In the older patient with Alzheimer's disease the diagnosis may also be made erroneously, since minor infarctions will readily produce clinical evidence of focal disorder when the reserves of the brain are reduced.

The presence of arteriosclerosis in the peripheral or retinal vessels cannot be taken as a firm guide towards the diagnosis. Peripheral changes are common with advancing age and will frequently be found when the dementia has some other basis; conversely, after middle age, cerebral arterial pathology cannot be excluded even when there is no evidence of arteriosclerosis elsewhere.

Hypertension is perhaps a more reliable guide but can similarly be misleading. It is most unusual for autopsy to reveal a vascular basis for dementia in the absence of marked hypertension (over 210/110 mmHg). In a large survey of autopsy-proven cases, the blood pressure had been significantly higher in those with multi-infarct dementia (mean 173/98) than in those with Alzheimer's disease (mean 137/85). The stepwise clinical progression and fluctuations in cognitive status together with focal lesions on MRI and PET or SPECT scans offer the best approach to firm diagnosis.

Transient Ischaemic Attack

Transient ischaemic attacks (TIA) are acute episodes of reduced or inadequate cerebral blood flow that result in a focal loss of cerebral or visual function lasting less than 24 hours.

TIAs cause a local degree of ischaemia that is sufficient to cause membrane abnormalities in neurons, with a consequent loss of normal electrophysiological function, but not enough to lead to neuronal death and the formation of an infarct. They can be caused by micro-emboli leading to temporary occlusion of vessels, or by systemic conditions, such as postural hypotension, that cause reduced blood flow.

The symptoms associated with TIAs are extremely variable. There is a general consensus that TIAs can be divided into those that affect:

- territories supplied by the internal carotid artery, which cause complete or partial loss of vision in one eye, aphasia, numbness of the face or arm, or partial paralysis of a limb; and
- territories supplied by the vertebrobasilar system, which cause bilateral blindness or homonymous hemianopia, bilateral paralysis and loss of sensation, dizziness or vertigo, or diplopia.

Determination of the territory affected is of clinical importance, as vertebral angiography is hazardous yet carotid endoarterectomy to remove atheromatous deposits or to correct stenosis is beneficial in up to 20 per cent of patients.

TIA and stoke

Episodes of TIA are short, usually lasting no more than an hour. They may occur once or as repetitive phenomena. Recovery, by definition, is essentially complete. However, the more numerous the attacks, the more likely that a permanent deficit will develop.

Differential Diagnosis of TIAs
Migraine
Epilepsy
Structural brain lesions
Tumours
Chronic subdural haematoma
Vascular malformation
Other non-vascular causes
Hypoglycaemia
Menière's disease
Multiple sclerosis
Hysteria
In patients with transient monocular symptoms
Giant cell arteritis
Malignant hypertension
Glaucoma
Papilloedema
Other orbital and retinal non-vascular disorders

Fig. 3.28 Differential diagnosis of TIAs. (Adapted from Bamford J. *Lancet* 1992;**339**:400.)

Correct diagnosis of TIA is of considerable clinical importance, since patients who experience several TIAs have a higher risk of a subsequent stroke than the general population. In one large series:

- 50 per cent of TIAs had strokes within three years; and
- 60 per cent had strokes within six years.

The occurrence of TIAs can be taken as a warning signal and indicates that prophylactic measures (reducing alcohol intake, change in diet, anti-hypertensive therapy, or surgery) could significant reduce the risk of stroke.

Given the short-lived nature of a TIA, diagnosis can be difficult in the presence of other transient conditions that are also characterized by a sudden onset (Fig. 3.28). Of these migraine and epilepsy are the most frequently encountered.

TIA and migraine

TIA and migraine can both be accompanied by headache and both can occur in the absence of headache. Migraine is the likely diagnosis when:

- a serial progression of symptoms gradually build up over 30 minutes or so; and
- positive symptoms (e.g. scintillating scotomas) occur.

TIAs generally result in a fast onset of symptoms which affect many parts of the body simultaneously and involve negative symptoms (losses of function).

TIAs and epilepsy

TIAs related to carotid territories can cause involuntary irregular shaking of a limb. This type of presentation can be confused with focal epileptic attacks. Focal motor seizures with pronounced postictal weakness can be confused with TIA. However, most focal epileptic seizures result in positive phenomena, in contrast to the negative phenomena evoked by TIAs.

A diagnosis of TIA may well be superfluous when reduced or inadequate cerebral blood flow occurs as a direct result of a known disease process (e.g. arteritis, coagulation disorder), because therapy will be dictated by the presence of the other condition.

SUMMARY

(i)   Almost 1 per cent of the population of the USA are impaired by the neurological consequences of cerebrovascular disease.

(ii)   Cerebrovascular disease is caused by hypertension, other vascular diseases, head trauma, interruption in cardiac output, and inherited disorders.

(iii)   Clinically, it is characterized by a sudden onset, stepwise progression, neurological abormalities, and a relatively intact personality.

(iv)   The loss or compromise of the brain's blood supply leads to altered physiological conditions, ischaemia, and infarction. This leads to neuronal destruction. Altered physiological processes persist after the interruption or compromise in blood supply is removed.

(v)   The site and amount of ischaemia or infarction determine the clinical symptoms of the patient. Infarctions totalling more than 100 ml in volume are associated with dementia.

(vi)   Cerebrovascular disease and Alzheimer's disease share many similarities and can often occur together in the same patient.

(vii) The effects of cerebrovascular disease can be ameliorated by long-term treatment with anti-hypertensives and also by the acute administration of glutamate antagonists and cytokine inhibitors.

(viii) Leukoaryosis (white matter infarcts) is a particular form of cerebrovascular disease.

(xiv) Transient ischaemic attacks cause deficits lasting less than 24 hours and are an indicator of increased risk for stroke.

4 Cortical Lewy Body Disease

INTRODUCTION

Extensive examination of the neuropathology of Alzheimer's disease has shown that as many as 20 per cent of cases have rounded eosinophilic inclusion bodies (Lewy bodies). These Lewy bodies are found within brain stem nuclei (in a manner identical to that which characterizes idiopathic Parkinson's disease) and throughout the cerebral cortex. In addition, many cases of dementia have now been reported in which, despite the presence of numerous cortical plaques and Lewy bodies, few or no cortical tangles are found. This spectrum of pathology is judged to be characteristic of a separate category of dementia known, for lack of a better term, as dementia with cortical Lewy bodies (DCLB). This condition has also been called diffuse Lewy body disease and cortical Lewy body disease.

The clinical symptoms are essentially the same as those seen in Alzheimer's disease, although motor symptoms are more in evidence. Important distinguishing factors are the presence of psychiatric symptoms other than dementia, and the fluctuations in cognitive state throughout the course of the disease.

The status of DCLB as a separate nosological entity is still under consideration since it has been regarded, with good reasons on molecular grounds, as a variant of Alzheimer's disease.

EPIDEMIOLOGY

The epidemiology of DCLB is still under investigation. In general the important factors will probably be similar to those seen in Alzheimer's disease. Approximately 20 per cent of cases clinically diagnosed as Alzheimer's disease are thought to have DCLB.

At present, the only factor to be clearly linked to the occurrence of DCLB is genetic. A mutation in the β-amyloid precursor protein gene on chromosome 21 at codon 717 has been shown to be tightly linked to the disease (see page 4.7). This mutation is also linked to Alzheimer's disease. This finding emphasizes the links between the two conditions.

CLINICAL FEATURES

Diagnosis

The mean age at onset of symptoms is 68 years (range 55–83 years) and the mean duration of illness is five years (range two to 19 years).

Clinical diagnosis is difficult because of the overlaps with Alzheimer's disease and Parkinson's disease. At present, a clear diagnosis can be made only after post-mortem examination. However the presence of parkinsonian symptoms and a fluctuating cognitive state might prove to be useful indicators for the presence of DCLB (Fig. 4.1).

Parkinsonian Features

About 40 per cent of DCLB cases present with symptoms and signs which are typical of and indistinguishable from those of idiopathic Parkinson's disease. They have extrapyramidal rigidity, bradykinesia, resting tremor, and classical gait disturbance. A markedly flexed posture might also be present. Generally, such patients respond well to treatment with levodopa, and deteriorate abruptly when it is withdrawn. Cognitive impairment develops on average about four years after the onset of motor symptoms. However, the length of this interval is very variable, and delays of between one and 19 years have been reported.

A further 20 per cent of patients show similar parkinsonian features together with mild cognitive impairment, either at or shortly after presentation.

The remaining 40 per cent present with neuropsychiatric symptoms and show motor features later in their illness, on average four years after onset.

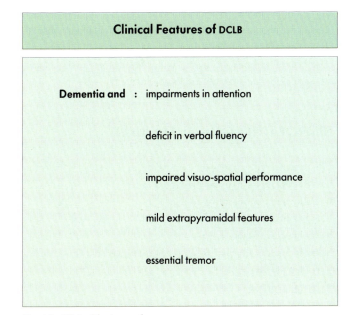

Clinical Features of DCLB

Dementia and : impairments in attention

deficit in verbal fluency

impaired visuo-spatial performance

mild extrapyramidal features

essential tremor

Fig. 4.1 Clinical features of DCLB.

Neuropsychiatric Features

Almost half of the patients present with neuropsychiatric disturbances such as:

- memory impairment alone, or memory impairment with overvalued ideas;
- dementia alone;
- dementia with paranoid ideas;
- dementia with auditory and visual hallucinations;
- dementia with both paranoid delusions and hallucinations.

All cases eventually show some neuropsychiatric disturbance with varying degrees of memory impairment from mild to severe. Detailed neuropsychological assessment demonstrates cortical deficits including dysphasia; dyscalculia; and visuo-spatial, constructional, and ideomotor dyspraxia (Fig. 4.2). Disturbances in language and praxis have also been reported.

Patients presenting with parkinsonian symptoms often have depression, and many patients presenting with dementia have auditory or visual hallucinations or delusions with a paranoid content.

Fluctuation in cognitive state

A marked contrast between DCLB and Alzheimer's disease lies in the striking fluctuations in cognitive impairment seen in the majority of patients. Patients with DCLB can be cognitively impaired one day and cognitively intact the next. These fluctuations are commonly ascribed to acute confusional states, but investigations generally reveal no underlying cause. Cognitive fluctuations are seen in drug-naïve patients and are not attributable to pharmaceutical treatment. In addition, fluctuations in cognitive state are not associated with fluctuation in motor performance. This observation makes it unlikely that they are related to variations in laevodopa levels (which, in any case, tend to occur over hours rather than days).

In fact, fluctuation in the severity of cognitive impairment appears to be the only early clinical feature which distinguishes the dementia associated with DCLB from other forms of cortical dementia.

Late features of DCLB

Regardless of the mode of presentation, the late features of DCLB are dementia and parkinsonism. This, together with the fluctuations in cognitive impairment, has frequently led to an erroneous clinical diagnosis of multi-infarct dementia. However, multi-infarct dementia is an unusual complication of idiopathic Parkinson's disease, and vascular disease in general is less common in parkinsonian patients than the general population as judged by case-control studies. Parkinsonian features are also commonly found in other forms of cortical dementia including that judged clinically to be senile dementia of the Alzheimer type. Recent evidence suggests that in these cases the parkinsonian features may in fact be attributable to coexistent Lewy body pathology in the brain stem.

Clearly, further research on this issue is indicated. The need for such clarification is emphasized by recent observations that sub-groups of dementia patients with parkinsonian features have a poorer prognosis than patients with dementia alone.

INVESTIGATIONS

There are no specific diagnostic tests for DCLB. The procedures used are the same as those to determine Alzheimer's disease. MRI and PET scan procedures are useful in establishing the presence of atrophy and metabolic disturbances, but cannot distinguish between DCLB and Alzheimer's disease.

NEUROPATHOLOGICAL FEATURES

The macroscopic appearance of the brain is very similar to that seen in Alzheimer's disease (Fig. 4.3) with:

- a shrunken appearance;
- gyral atrophy; and
- ventricular enlargement.

Microscopically the pathology is characterized by:

- cortical Lewy bodies;
- brain stem Lewy bodies;
- spongiform change;
- cortical plaques (and tangles).

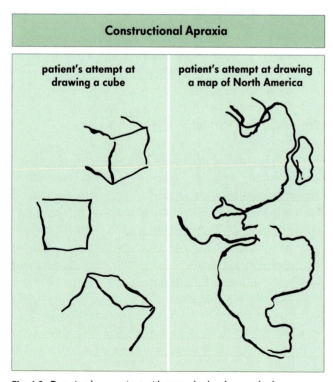

Constructional Apraxia

patient's attempt at drawing a cube

patient's attempt at drawing a map of North America

Fig. 4.2 Drawing by a patient with DCLB who has been asked to copy a diagram of a cube and to draw a map of North America. Note the left-sided neglect.

The central neuropathological feature of DCLB is the presence of Lewy bodies in the cortex (Fig. 4.4). However, substantial numbers of plaques and variable numbers of tangles are also present. All cases show cell loss in the substantia nigra, with classical Lewy bodies in remaining neurons (Fig. 4.5). These changes are indistinguishable from those which characterize uncomplicated idiopathic Parkinson's disease.

The Lewy bodies are found most frequently in small neurons within the deeper layers of the temporal, anterior cingulate, insular, entorhinal, and frontal cortices (Fig. 4.6).

Most cases also show sufficient numbers of neurofibrillary tangles in the hippocampus and temporal cortex to suggest a second diagnosis of Alzheimer's disease.

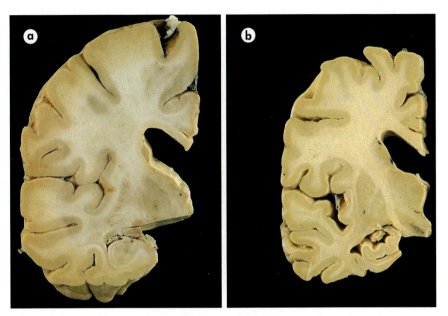

Fig. 4.3 Photographs showing (a) normal brain; (b) generalized atrophy.

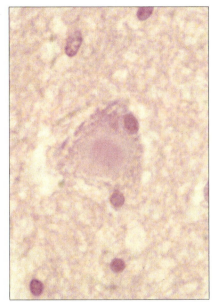

Fig. 4.4 Lewy body in the cortex (haematoxylin and eosin stain). (Courtesy of Dr J Lowe, Nottingham.)

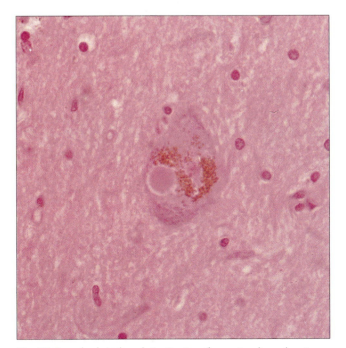

Fig. 4.5 Lewy body in the substantia nigra (haematoxylin and eosin stain). (Courtesy of Dr J Lowe, Nottingham.)

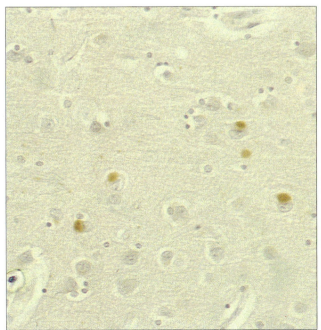

Fig. 4.6 Diffuse Lewy bodies in the cortex, stained with ubiquitin. (Courtesy of Dr J Lowe, Nottingham.)

Lewy Bodies

Lewy body distribution Lewy bodies in cortical cells tend to be most numerous in the temporal, parietal, and frontal lobes and less frequent or absent in the occipital lobe, particularly the striate area (see Fig. 4.6). There are few Lewy bodies in the subiculum and hippocampus. However, they are numerous in the parasubiculum and parahippocampal gyrus. Lewy bodies have been identified in small- and medium-sized pyramidal neurons of the fifth and sixth cortical laminae, and less frequently in the third and fourth laminae (compare with tangle distribution in Alzheimer's disease) (Fig. 4.7).

Lewy body morphology Cortical Lewy bodies are difficult to see using conventional histological stains. The Lewy bodies in the brain stem are much more easily stained. Localization of cortical Lewy bodies is best using immunocytochemical techniques and antibodies to ubiquitin (Fig. 4.8). The use of immunocyto-chemistry has made the cortical Lewy bodies easier to see and quantify and has greatly improved the efficiency of diagnosis.

Cortical Lewy bodies are smaller than those in the brain stem (typically 5–10 μm) and much more variable in shape, which ranges from round to triangular; some have an irregular shape. The less intense staining often gives poor demarcation between the body and halo. Some appear as though they are compressed beside the nucleus. Lewy bodies are almost always found within neurons; it is rare to find them lying free in the neuropil. This is in contrast to tangles.

Ultrastructural studies show that filaments of cortical Lewy bodies are randomly arranged but aggregated towards the centre (Fig. 4.9). The haphazard pattern of filaments contrasts with the structure of classical Lewy bodies in the brain stem which have central cores (often of a granular consistency) and peripheral, radially orientated filaments. The filaments are composed of phosphorylated and non-phosphorylated neurofilaments. The accretion of neurofilaments to form a Lewy body is thought to be a consequence of abnormal protein processing.

Spongiform Change

Spongiform change in the temporal lobe is a common finding in DCLB; it is present in approximately 85 per cent of cases. This change consists of vacuoles of varying sizes which occasionally

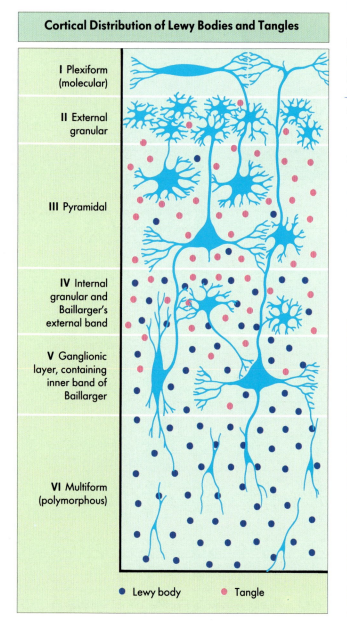

Cortical Distribution of Lewy Bodies and Tangles

I Plexiform (molecular)	
II External granular	
III Pyramidal	
IV Internal granular and Baillarger's external band	
V Ganglionic layer, containing inner band of Baillarger	
VI Multiform (polymorphous)	

● Lewy body   ● Tangle

Fig. 4.7 Distribution of tangles and Lewy bodies in the cortex.

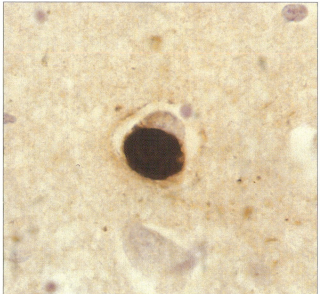

Fig. 4.8 Cortical Lewy body, stained with ubiquitin. (Courtesy of Dr J Lowe, Nottingham.)

coalesce and are indistinguishable from those seen in the cortex in Prion disease (Fig. 4.10).

The major difference between spongiform change in Prion disease and spongiform change in DCLB is that in DCLB it is restricted to the temporal lobe. The vacuoles differ from those seen with oedema and from the microcystic rarefaction seen in the upper cortical layers in Alzheimer's disease. The presence of spongiform change has prompted efforts to determine if DCLB is transmissible. There is as yet no evidence that it is.

Plaques and Tangles

Plaques containing β-amyloid identical to the plaques seen in Alzheimer's disease are found in all cases of DCLB (Fig. 4.11), and the amounts and distribution of amyloid deposited are similar in these two conditions (Fig. 4.12). Approximately 30–40 per cent of DCLB cases will also show significant numbers of tangles in the cortex (Fig. 4.13). The numbers of tangles in such cases is generally lower than found in Alzheimer's disease.

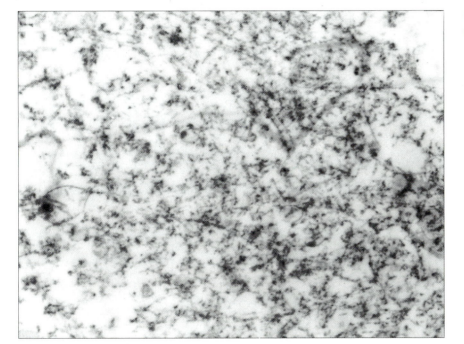

Fig. 4.9 Organization of filaments in a Lewy body.

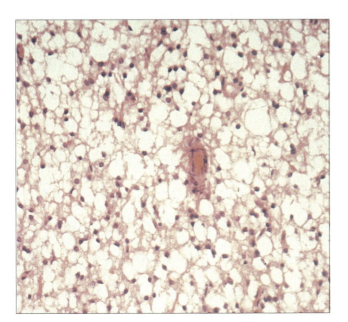

Fig. 4.10 Cortical vacuoles and spongiform change (haematoxylin and eosin stain).

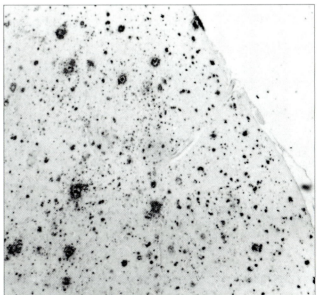

Fig. 4.11 β-amyloid plaque in DCLB.

β-Amyloid Deposition in DCLB

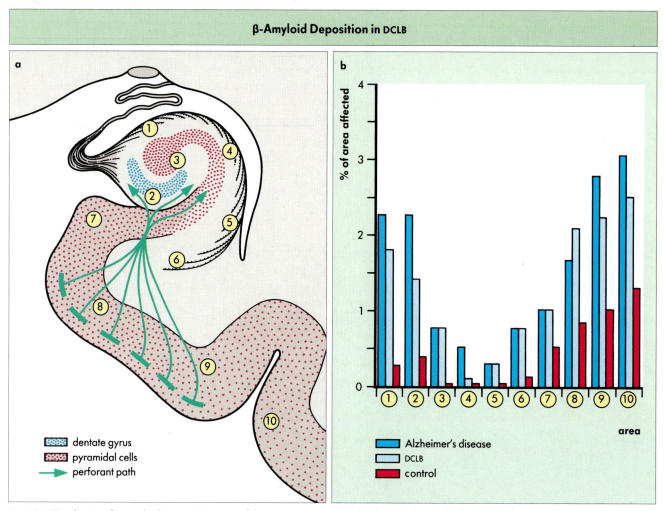

Fig. 4.12 Distribution of β-amyloid in DCLB. (a). Areas of deposition in the medial temporal lobe along the perforant path. (b). Comparison of the distribution of β-amyloid in DCLB, Alzheimer's disease, and controls. The encircled numbers refer to the areas indicated in (a).

Fig. 4.13 Tangles in cortex, stained with Congo red.

NEUROCHEMISTRY

The neurochemistry of DCLB is difficult to define. Provisional studies indicate that the presence of cortical Lewy bodies is associated with losses of acetylcholine and peptide transmitters. The overall picture is reminiscent of that seen in Alzheimer's disease, and it is more than likely that the neurochemistry of DCLB follows the pattern seen in Alzheimer's disease; i.e. that the neurochemical deficit is determined by the transmitter content of the neurons affected.

DCLB, ALZHEIMER'S DISEASE, AND PARKINSON'S DISEASE

The interrelationship between these diseases and the pathologies thought to be characteristic of them is complex, and a number of issues remain unresolved. There is accumulating evidence that, in the elderly at least, brains with Lewy body disorders show an increased tendency towards the development of Alzheimer-type pathology in some regions; this is exemplified by the high concentrations of neocortical plaques accompanied by occasional neurofibrillary tangles in many cases of senile dementia of Lewy body type, and to a lesser extent in Parkinson's disease.

However, it remains to be established whether the reverse tendency applies, and whether Alzheimer's disease itself, particularly in its presenile form, predisposes to the formation of Lewy bodies in susceptible brain areas. Small numbers of early-onset Alzheimer's disease cases do show Lewy bodies in brain stem nuclei, but whether these have developed as a direct or indirect consequence of the Alzheimer disease process, or whether their development represents Lewy body formation occurring in a brain which is (in an as yet unknown way) more susceptible to several neurodegenerative disease processes is not yet known.

Mutations in the β-Amyloid Precursor Protein Gene (β-APP) and DCLB

In this context, it is worth noting the finding that, in a large pedigree with familial Alzheimer's disease and a known mutation at codon 717 of the β-APP gene on chromosome 21, several of the affected patients had numerous cortical Lewy bodies. This finding would suggest that, on molecular genetic grounds, DCLB is best viewed as a morphological variant of Alzheimer's disease (akin to the variants of Prion disease) rather than a disease entity in its own right.

It is of interest that in other rare neurodegenerative disorders, some genetically determined, Lewy body formation has been described in a minority of cases, e.g. Hallervorden–Spatz disease and Pick's disease. The presence of Lewy bodies in these rare neurodegenerative diseases is unlikely to be a chance or coincidental occurrence. Their formation is either part of the primary pathological process or a secondary phenomenon related to a specific type of neuronal or glial degeneration common to the various diseases.

DIFFERENTIAL DIAGNOSIS

Accurate diagnosis is difficult while the nosological status of DCLB is in doubt. However, parkinsonian features followed by dementia, dementia with marked psychiatric symptoms, or a fluctuating cognitive state may prove useful indicators. One proposal for an explanation of the presence of psychiatric symptoms arises as a direct consequence of the pathology. Unlike tangles, Lewy bodies do not rupture the neurons which contain them. It is possible, therefore, that neurons containing Lewy bodies have a functional capability, albeit compromised. This reduced function, rather than outright neuronal destruction, may underlie some of these differences in clinical symptoms.

The presence of Lewy bodies, plaques, and tangles in varying amounts gives rise to a range of disorders (Fig. 4.14). The absolute

The Spectrum of Lewy Body Disorders in the Elderly

Category	Distinctive clinical features	Lewy body prevalence	Alzheimer-type pathology
Parkinson's disease	Classical movement disorder (tremor, rigidity, akinesia) in a broad age range; dementia developing in some (mainly elderly)	Primarily subcortical brain stem; age or dementia-related increase in limbic cortex; very occasional or low densities in some neocortical lobes	Moderate or occasionally high plaque densities in neocortex in some but not all cases; occasional NFT in neocortex mainly in cases developing dementia
DCLB > 65	Fluctuating confusion/dementia in the elderly (over 65), often with visual hallucinations and/or mild extrapyramidal features	Present in brain stem and subcortical areas; moderate numbers in limbic cortex, low densities with variable distribution in neocortical lobes	Most with moderate or high plaque density and sparse NFT in archicortex in the majority
Diffuse Lewy body disease < 65	Dementia, mainly in younger cases, usually associated with extrapyramidal features of Parkinson's disease. Psychiatric, neuropsychiatric presentation	Anatomically widespread; high densities throughout cortex, including limbic and neocortex; also present in brain stem and subcortical regions	High plaque densities and sparse NFT in neocortex, moderate/high plaque and NFT densities in archicortex
Intermediate or combined syndromes	Symptomatology not yet fully defined	Variable: PD or DCLB combined with Alzheimer's or vascular disease	Moderate or high plaque and NFT densities in neocortex and archicortex with or without ischaemic lesions
Preclinical phase	Not known at present. Prospective testing may reveal subtle impairments of movement, or psychiatric disturbances	Some in subcortical nuclei; sparse in neocortex. Preferential neuron loss in locus coeruleus; mild substantia nigra neuron loss may or may not be present	Absent to moderate plaque densities in neocortex and archicortex; sparse or rare NFT in neocortex and/or archicortex

Fig. 4.14 The spectrum of Lewy body disorders in the elderly.

categorization of an individual case within this spectrum is a fine judgement and may not be warranted by our current understanding of the complex pathology.

SUMMARY

(i)   DCLB is a dementing condition characterized by the presence of motor and psychiatric symptoms.

(ii) Clinical diagnosis is at best tentative and needs neuropathological confirmation.

(iii) The condition is characterized by the presence of Lewy bodies in cortical neurons.

(iv) DCLB also shares the pathological spectrum of Alzheimer's disease and Parkinson's disease.

(v)   It is possible that DCLB is a morphological variant of Alzheimer's disease.

5 Head Trauma

INTRODUCTION

Accidents leading to head trauma are common events in our society, and a degree of brain damage occurs in up to 30 per cent of such accidents. The damage arises from the purely physical effects of trauma (such as swelling, herniation, haemorrhage, and axonal shearing), and also from the neurochemical consequences of the ischaemia which invariably accompanies physical brain damage. Brain damage following trauma can be viewed as having two phases of pathology:

- an acute phase resulting from the physical stresses which are involved; and
- an acute–chronic phase driven by physiological response to ischaemia.

A distressing feature of the neurological consequences of head trauma derives from its epidemiology. Many people who suffer trauma-related brain damage are teenagers or young men in their 20s who, if physically or psychiatrically disabled, are likely to require extensive rehabilitation and care for many years. Even when the degree of physical disability is not extensive, intellectual and/or psychiatric problems resulting in neuropsychological deficits or altered personality can lead to considerable difficulties in social functioning.

EPIDEMIOLOGY

The precise incidence of head injury is difficult to determine, as the criteria used to record the various events which can cause head injury differ from country to country (e.g. head injuries can be caused by criminal assaults or suicide attempts, in addition to accidents). However, it is accepted that accidental head injury is the developed world's leading cause of death in people under the age of 45. In addition, head injury is the direct cause of death in 30 per cent of patients who die as a result of trauma. In the UK there are nine deaths from head injury per 100 000 population each year. This accounts for:

- 1 per cent of all deaths;
- 30 per cent of all deaths caused by trauma; and
- approximately 50 per cent of deaths due to road traffic accidents.

The rates of deaths due to head injury are even larger in the USA.

Outcome surveys in the UK, USA, and the Netherlands indicate that for every 100 head injury survivors:

- up to five remain in a vegetative state;
- up to 15 are still severely disabled six months after injury;
- 20 have minor psychiatric or psychological problems; and
- 60 make a good recovery.

Improving the treatment of trauma has resulted in an increased number of disabled survivors, and will continue to do so. There is an estimated prevalence in the USA of 150 per 100 000 of the population with a persisting handicap resulting from trauma-related brain damage (i.e. about 450 000 people). Approximately one family in 300 has a member with such a disability.

CLINICAL FEATURES AND COURSE

Most patients (60 per cent) who sustain a head injury make a good eventual recovery and have no residual deficits. The rest suffer from chronic problems which range from brief periods of amnesia and personality changes through to severe disabilities or a chronic degenerative disease process. A small proportion of patients remain in the vegetative state.

Acute Effects of Trauma

The most common clinical history of the acute effects of trauma consist of the triad of symptoms:

- loss of consciousness;
- a period of mental confusion; and
- amnesic defects.

Loss of consciousness

Consciousness is impaired after all but the slightest impacts in non-penetrating head trauma. Often, loss of consciousness is complete and the patient falls to the ground and has no response to stimuli; there is momentary respiratory arrest, reduced blood pressure, pallor, a loss of corneal reflexes, and contraction of limbs followed by flaccid paralysis and loss of tendon reflexes.

Consciousness returns after a variable interval (related to the magnitude of the trauma), often accompanied by headache, drowsiness, dizziness, and vomiting. The patient's own assessment of the duration of unconsciousness is often inaccurate owing to confusion and post-traumatic amnesia (see page 5.2).

Loss of consciousness is usually more marked when trauma causes the skull to rotate on impact; therefore it is less common in penetrating head injuries and in injuries caused by crushing.

The time spent unconscious is a good predictor of prognosis. However, patients with a loss of consciousness lasting several hours can make uneventful recoveries. In general, the longer the period of unconsciousness and the deeper the level of coma (Fig. 5.1), the greater the likelihood that the patient has suffered brain damage and will suffer neuropsychological and psychiatric sequelae. When unconsciousness persists for weeks or months, some permanent neurological handicap is probable.

Glasgow Coma Scale	
	Score
Eye opening	
Spontaneous	4
To speech	3
To noxious stimulation	2
None	1
Best motor response	
Obeys command	6
Localizes stimuli	5
Withdraws	4
Abnormal flexion	3
Extensor response	2
None	1
Verbal response	
Oriented	5
Confused conversation	4
Inappropriate words	3
Incomprehensible sounds	2
None	1

The score is the sum of individual scores for eye opening, motor and verbal responses – from 3 (poor) to 15 (excellent).

Fig. 5.1 The Glasgow coma scale (from Teasdale G, Jennett B. *Lancet* 1974;**2**:81).

Post-traumatic coma may be deep from the beginning or may deepen in the immediate aftermath of the trauma because of oedema, intracranial haemorrhage, or both. Surgical intervention to evacuate blood from inside the skull is indicated when comatose patients show signs of brain stem compression:

- failing respiration;
- falling blood pressure;
- fixed dilated pupils; and
- muscular flaccidity.

CT and MRI greatly facilitate the assessment of possible brain damage and the presence of intracranial blood.

Confusion (post-traumatic psychosis)

After recovering consciousness, the patient experiences a phase of disorientation and impaired cognitive function before the optimal level of post-trauma performance is achieved. This phase is enormously variable and dependant on the period of unconsciousness and the degree and type of cerebral injury. After periods of unconsciousness lasting several hours, confusion and disorientation may last for several days or weeks. When the patient has experienced a deep and extended period of coma and permanent brain damage is likely, the disturbance may last for

months. These post-traumatic effects are, inevitably, more prolonged and severe in the previously brain damaged, the aged, and the demented.

The nature of the confusional state is variable and spans the spectrum from florid delirium to hyperactivity and irritability to apathetic withdrawal. The factors which dictate the expression of the confusional state include not only the site and extent of brain damage but also the personality of the patient.

These psychiatric phenomena can pose considerable management problems when the failures in cognition result in patients with paranoid ideation who can also be aggressive and uncooperative. Occasionally serious criminal acts are perpetrated as a result of such disturbances. The period of confusion can have important medicolegal consequences when the circumstances relating to the traumatic event become embroiled into the disordered thinking of the patient. The confusional state, or aspects of it, either resolve or become permanent.

Amnesia

Irrespective of the magnitude of trauma which caused the loss of consciousness, on recovery the events immediately pre- and post-trauma are often not remembered. The extent of such trauma-related periods of amnesia is a useful prognostic indicator.

Post-traumatic amnesia (PTA) This has been defined as 'the time from the moment of injury to the time of resumption of normal continuous memory' (Lishman, 1987). This period includes all periods of unconsciousness and overt confusion and additional periods of mnemonic confusion.

Characteristically, the return to normal memory is abrupt; thus many patients can, retrospectively, give an accurate determination of the period of PTA. PTA is absent or much shorter in about 50 per cent of penetrating or crush brain injuries.

Retrograde amnesia (RA) The duration of RA is 'the time from the moment of injury and the last clear memory from before the trauma the patient can recall' (Lishman, 1987).

The time of RA may prove to be very misleading if it is determined soon after injury. Typically, the period may be extensive but shrinks dramatically as the effects of post-traumatic confusion diminish. As a rule, assessment of the RA should not be finalized until the patient's PTA has been firmly established.

The period of RA is typically short, lasting from seconds to a minute in most cases; it is considerably shorter than the period of PTA. Longer periods of RA are usually confined to severe cases of brain damage. Long periods of RA which follow mild trauma are often generated by the patient's psychological state.

Severity of trauma and amnesia The length of PTA is the most useful indicator (more useful than the period of unconsciousness or confusion) for judging the severity of brain damage and the likely prognosis. The period of PTA is a permanent index and is thus available for clinicians to determine long after the acute effects of the injury have resolved.

The length of PTA correlates well with objective measure of brain damage (presence of cognitive impairments, motor disorders, aphasia, etc) and with the time that will elapse before the patient returns to work (Fig. 5.2). Although the period of PTA is usually much shorter in penetrating or crush brain injuries, the relationship between increasing periods of PTA and amount of disability is still present.

Chronic Effects of Head Trauma

As has been noted, 60 per cent of head trauma patients make a complete recovery. However, the remainder suffer from a wide variety of psychiatric and neurological complications.

Psychiatric sequelae
The range of psychiatric symptoms which occur as a consequence of head trauma is wide and includes:
- phobias;
- anxiety states;
- depression;
- schizophreniform psychosis;
- neurotic disorders; and
- cognitive deficits.

These problems are clinically important, as difficulty in obtaining employment and problems of interpersonal or social interaction are more likely to be caused by psychiatric symptoms than by physical handicap. A range of factors affect the extent and form of post-traumatic psychiatric complications (Fig. 5.3).

Post-traumatic syndrome The exact nature and even the existence of this syndrome has been the subject of debate. This syndrome is characterized by the presence of persistent headache, dizziness, and, to a greater or lesser extent, fatigue, insomnia, poor memory, irritability, and emotional lability. The symptoms often persist for months after the traumatic event and are often observed to be aggravated by stress, tension, or depression. In many cases, the symptoms lack clear precipitants and are very resistant to treatment. Several studies have shown that, although physical causes might underlie some symptoms in the immediate aftermath of the trauma, as time goes on a physical cause is less

and less likely to be discovered. It is thought that such long lasting post-traumatic symptoms are likely to be psychogenic in origin. The post-traumatic syndrome is rare in the presence of trauma which causes intellectual impairment or neurological disability. An important observation is the significantly higher symptom rate in patients who blame their employer or large organizations for their accident rather than themselves. This fact is of considerable importance when such issues become the subject of litigation.

Neurological sequelae
Lesions of the cranial nerves are commonly seen (e.g. anosmia, visual field defects, ophthalmopareses), as are motor disorders resulting from cortical and brain stem lesions. Complications arising from intracranial bleeding and penetrating head injuries are likely to give rise to focal neurological damage related to the area of brain damaged (Fig. 5.4).

Post-traumatic epilepsy Epilepsy is one of the commonest chronic sequelae. A clear distinction can be made between:
- early epilepsy (during the first weeks after injury); and
- late epilepsy (developing after a delay of months).

Early epilepsy rarely occurs in the absence of prolonged PTA, depressed fracture of the skull, or intracranial bleeding. It occurs more commonly in children under the age of six, and it may be a major complication. Early epilepsy in children can progress to status epilepticus which, if not rapidly and adequately controlled, results in variable amounts of irreversible hypoxic brain damage.

The occurrence of early epilepsy considerably enhances the risk of late epilepsy. In late epilepsy, the first fit occurs 12 months or more after the trauma in 50 per cent of patients. It is the most frequent delayed complication of a non-penetrating head injury. The risk is greater in patients who suffered:
- an intracranial haematoma;
- a compound depressed fracture;
- early epilepsy;
- focal brain damage; or
- focal brain damage with prolonged unconsciousness.

Late epilepsy is commoner in penetrating head injuries (about 40 per cent) than non-penetrating head injuries (5 per cent).

PTA Length Related to Severity of Injury		
Degree of concussion	**Length of PTA**	**Estimated time before resuming work**
Slight	Less than 1 hour	4–6 weeks
Moderate	1–24 hours	6–8 weeks
Severe	1–7 days	2–4 months
Very severe	More than 7 days	4–8 months

Fig. 5.2 Correlation of the length of post-traumatic amnesia with objective measures of brain damage.

Aetiological Factors in Psychiatric Disturbance after Head Injury	
Premorbid personality	Environmental factors
Amount of brain damage	Compensation and litigation
Location of brain damage	Response to intellectual impairments
Emotional impact of injury	Development of epilepsy
Emotional repercussions of injury	

Fig. 5.3 Factors involved with psychiatric disturbance after head injury.

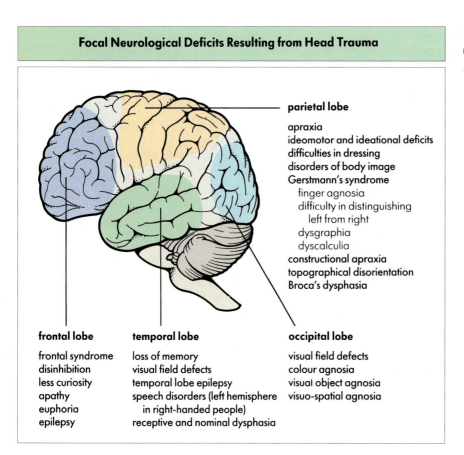

Focal Neurological Deficits Resulting from Head Trauma

parietal lobe

apraxia
ideomotor and ideational deficits
difficulties in dressing
disorders of body image
Gerstmann's syndrome
   finger agnosia
   difficulty in distinguishing
     left from right
   dysgraphia
   dyscalculia
constructional apraxia
topographical disorientation
Broca's dysphasia

frontal lobe

frontal syndrome
disinhibition
less curiosity
apathy
euphoria
epilepsy

temporal lobe

loss of memory
visual field defects
temporal lobe epilepsy
speech disorders (left hemisphere
   in right-handed people)
receptive and nominal dysphasia

occipital lobe

visual field defects
colour agnosia
visual object agnosia
visuo-spatial agnosia

Fig. 5.4 Types of focal neurological deficits, related to the area of the brain which is damaged.

The close relationship between the degree of focal brain damage and the risk of post-traumatic epilepsy implies that direct destruction of brain tissue is the most important cause of post-traumatic epilepsy in any type of head injury.

The incidence of post-traumatic epilepsy has remained surprisingly constant over decades despite improved medical procedures to deal with trauma victims and the prophylactic use of anticonvulsants.

Progressive neurodegeneration   Progressive decline over an extended period of time (10–15 years) has been noted in approximately 15 per cent of patients who have suffered a severe head trauma. The pathophysiological mechanisms that contribute to this process are unknown. Case studies have documented the presence of Alzheimer-type pathological change in the brains of some patients and, as a result, it has been suggested that some forms of primary neurodegenerative disease may be triggered by head trauma. These include:

● Alzheimer's disease;
● Parkinson's disease; and
● motor neuron disease.

Punch-drunk syndrome (dementia pugilistica)   Repeated concussive or subconcussive blows to the head, such as occur to professional boxers, result in minor brain damage. Areas of hypoperfusion in the brain have been demonstrated in amateur boxers using SPECT imaging. CT and MRI studies have demon-

strated focal abnormalities, ventricular enlargement, and cortical atrophy consistent with a more chronic process in professional fighters. The accretion of minor brain damage can lead to the accumulation of neurological signs and induce a progressive neurodegenerative syndrome. This condition, known as dementia pugilistica or the punch-drunk syndrome, becomes clinically obvious years after the last fight. It can be described in three stages:

● stage 1 – affective disorder, mild inco-ordination;
● stage 2 – dysphasia, apraxia, agnosia, apathy, blunting of affect, and neurological signs;
● stage 3 – global cognitive decline and parkinsonism.

The syndrome is present in about 20 per cent of older professional boxers (those over 50). It is more likely to develop in boxers with long careers who have been dazed, if not knocked out, on many occasions. The brains of these patients have a characteristic pattern of brain damage, the principal features of which are:

● fenestrated septum (Fig. 5.5a);
● degeneration of the substantia nigra (Fig. 5.5b);
● neuronal loss in cortex and cerebellum;
● cortical neurofibrillary tangle formation (Fig. 5.5c); and
● cortical diffuse β-amyloid plaques (Fig. 5.5d).

The molecular pathology of the punch-drunk syndrome appears to be very similar to that seen in Alzheimer's disease. This observation has been used to argue that severe or repeated head trauma can trigger Alzheimer's disease (see Chapter 2).

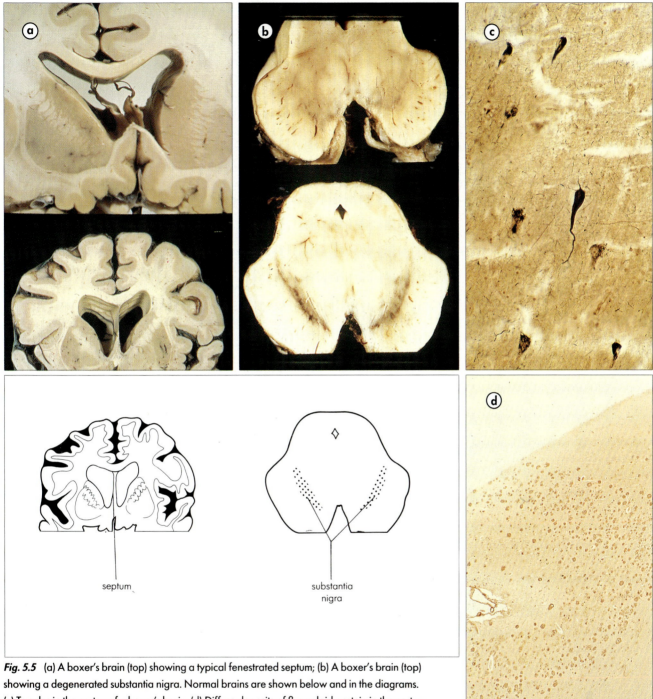

Fig. 5.5 (a) A boxer's brain (top) showing a typical fenestrated septum; (b) A boxer's brain (top) showing a degenerated substantia nigra. Normal brains are shown below and in the diagrams. (c) Tangles in the cortex of a boxer's brain. (d) Diffuse deposits of ß-amyloid protein in the cortex of a boxer's brain.

Normal-pressure hydrocephalus Subarachnoid haemorrhage is a common consequence of many types of head injury. These haemorrhages can lead to the filling of the subarachnoid space with blood, which can result in the development of normal-pressure hydrocephalus and the onset of a dementia syndrome. Prompt surgical intervention to evacuate the blood will relieve this condition.

Severe disability and coma

Even patients with severe focal brain damage can make a very good recovery, provided that appropriate treatment is instituted early. However, many patients have lasting neurological deficits and may experience an extensive period of coma. Clinicopathological studies and experimental investigations indicate that severe disability after head injury (in patients that survive their

injury for more than one month) and the occurrence of a prolonged episode of coma (more than one week) or deep coma
(vegetative state) is caused by the presence of diffuse brain
damage (diffuse axonal injury and hypoxic brain damage; see
page 5.12).

Clinical effects of head injury in children

The human brain continues to develop for some 20 years after
birth. This development is characterized by processes of neuronal
death or dropout (apotosis), formation and plasticity of synaptic
connections, and myelination of nerve tracts. The activity of
these processes in the brains of children accounts for the differences in the responses of children and adults to head trauma.

The structure of the skull and its contents is thought to be less
rigid and more elastic in children. As a result, the physical
effects of an injury are absorbed better, and rises in intracranial
pressure are less disruptive.

Children show a reduced incidence of chronic cognitive deficit
following head trauma, and when cognitive defects occur, they
resolve much faster than the equivalent deficit in an adult. It is
thought that this recovery is related to the enhanced synaptic
plasticity of the developing brain.

The post-traumatic syndrome and neurotic reactions to head
injury are very rare in young children. Aspects of these reactions
are seen in older children, and these approximate to the adult
responses as age increases.

Behavioural disturbances are chronic sequelae of head injury
in children. Difficulties in learning, anti-social behaviour, and
hyperactivity have been described. Behaviour disturbances can
occur even in the absence of obvious cognitive or neurological
deficits, and often lead to low educational attainment and subsequent difficulty in social adjustment.

Types of Head Injury

There are two main types of head injury:
- blunt, non-missile, or non-penetrating head injury; and
- missile or penetrating head injury.

The essential difference rests on whether the agent of trauma
(e.g. a bullet) actually penetrates the skull.

The two types of head injury are distinguished because of the
clinical problems that relate to the breaching of the skull and the
focal nature of the brain damage in penetrating head injury.
Patients with penetrating head injury have:
- higher immediate mortality rates; and
- greatly increased rates of post-traumatic epilepsy.

Features of head injury

The commonest form of head injury is the non-penetrating kind.
The main feature of this type of head injury have been exhaust-
ively documented (Hume Adams, 1992) and are described briefly
here. Additional features specific for penetrating head injury are
dealt with briefly at the end of this section.

Lesions of the scalp

Laceration and/or bruising of the scalp is common, and is a
good indicator of the site of the trauma. Lacerations bleed
copiously and are often the site of, or the route of entry for,
subsequent infections.

Lesions of the skull

The skull is a rigid structure of great mechanical strength. A
skull fracture indicates that the head has suffered a localized
traumatic event of considerable force. The type of fracture found
is dictated in part by the shape of the object that has made
traumatic contact with the skull:
- flat shapes produce fissure fractures, which can extend into
  the base of the skull;
- angled or pointed objects produce a localized fracture.

Fractures of the base of the skull can give rise to later episodes
of infection. Such fractures often pass through the middle ear or
the anterior cranial fossa, and cause leakages of CSF through the
nose, mouth, or ear. Infection can spread along the routes followed
by leakage of CSF. Up to 30 per cent of patients that have
leakages of CSF develop tumour-like complications when the
resulting cavity becomes distended owing to trapped air (aerocoele). In addition, the presence of a skull fracture is associated
with a significantly increased risk of intracranial haematoma.

Many patients with a skull fracture recover fully with no
residual neurological symptoms.

Traumatic injuries due to sharp or angled objects can produce
localized fractures in which regions of the skull are pushed in
or depressed by at least the thickness of the skull (depressed
fracture). The depressed fragments of bone may actually tear
the dura and rupture blood vessels in the immediate vicinity.

Contrecoup fractures (i.e. fractures that are located at a distance
from the point of injury and that are not direct extensions of a
fracture originating at the point of injury) occur principally in
the roofs of the orbits and the ethmoid plates after falls that
cause trauma to the back of the skull.

Skull fractures in infants and young children can give rise to
subsequent clinical difficulties owing to the phenomenon of
'growing fractures'. In children, the dura is closely attached to
the inner surface of the skull and is easily ruptured after a
depressed fracture. This can cause meninges or neuronal tissue
to 'ooze' between the fractured bone, which can delay or stop
healing, leaving a swollen mass of brain tissue under the surface
of the scalp.

NEUROPATHOLOGY

Gross Changes

The physical effects of the trauma result in the tearing of blood
vessels. This leads to haemorrhages and the bruising of brain
tissue. These effects are visible on CT and MRI scans and on

visual inspection of the brain post-mortem. The main types of gross pathology are:

- intracranial haemorrhages; and
- contusions.

Intracranial haemorrhages

These are the commonest cause of clinical deterioration and death in patients that have experienced a lucid interval after their injury. The risk of such haemorrhages can turn even an apparently trivial head injury into a life-threatening condition.

After a head injury, haemorrhages can occur into:

- the extradural, subdural or subarachnoid spaces;
- the brain; and
- the ventricles.

Extradural, subdural, and intracerebral haematomas cause expanding intracranial lesions, which increase intracranial pressure and compress the surface of the brain. Subarachnoid haemorrhage is often associated with the formation of contusions, and intraventricular haemorrhage is often seen in patients with diffuse axonal injury.

Extradural haematoma   This type of lesion is found in:

- 2 per cent of all head-injured patients; and
- up to 15 per cent of patients with fatal head injury.

Most patients with an extradural haematoma also have a 'skull fracture (although this is not necessarily the case with children). Ruptured vessels in the meninges (often the middle meningeal artery following temporal bone fracture) are the source of the haemorrhage, and as the haematoma swells it causes pressure on the adjacent brain and eventually distorts it (Fig. 5.6). In fatal cases, death is a result of cerebral compression and transtentorial herniation.

Extradural haematomas can be difficult to manage, for the initial injury may appear slight, and the patient be fully conscious with little neurological damage. The lucid period can last for 12–24 hours or even longer before the swelling of the haematoma produces symptoms. Extradural haematoma is sometimes bilateral, and may occur in conjunction with other brain damage. In this latter case, patients may be unconscious from the time of the original injury.

Serial CT scanning studies have demonstrated that extradural haematomas continue to increase in size (up to 50 per cent) until some 10 days after the injury. This is followed by a period of one to two months, during which time the haematoma resolves.

Intradural haematoma   Three forms can be distinguished:

- subdural haematoma;
- intracerebral haematoma; and
- combination.

Subdural haematoma   These usually occur when the veins crossing the subdural space (linking cerebral hemispheres to the sagittal sinus) rupture; rarely, cortical arteries are also involved. Rupture of these vessels can follow slight accidents, or even whiplash injuries, in which no direct trauma to the head has occurred. Blood from the ruptured vessels spreads freely through the subdural space, and can envelop the entire hemisphere (subdural haematomas are much more extensive than extradural haematomas). The widespread nature of the haemorrhage leads to an even increase in pressure over the surface of the affected hemisphere (in contrast to the focal pressure and flattening seen with extradural haemorrhages). However, the presence of an acute subdural haematoma is associated with swelling of the ipsilateral cerebral hemisphere. Thus, CT and MRI reveal an

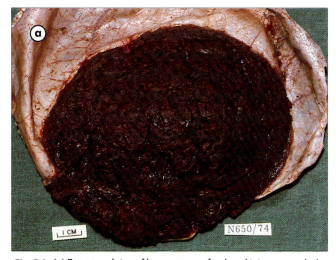

Fig. 5.6 (a) Extent and size of haematoma after head injury, revealed by exploratory surgery. (Courtesy of Professor DI Graham, Glasgow.)

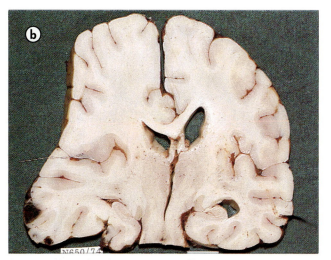

(b) Coronal brain slice showing pressure effects of extradural haematoma. (Courtesy of Professor DI Graham, Glasgow.)

almost normal pattern of sulci and gyri in the affected hemisphere, although some gyral flattening can be seen in the contralateral hemisphere.

Subdural haematomas have been defined as being acute, subacute, and chronic:

- acute haematoma is composed of clotted blood (at least 48 hours);
- subacute haematoma is a mixture of clotted and fluid blood (over 48 hours);
- chronic haematoma is fluid (over three weeks).

Although most small subdural haematomas resolve spontaneously, this is not always the case. Occasionally, subdural haematomas become surrounded by a membrane and continue to expand slowly until their size produces a degree of brain distortion and raised intracranial pressure that precipitates clinical symptoms. The reason why some subdural haematomas become chronic is not known, but this phenomenon is commoner in older patients, in whom there can be considerable distortion of the brain structure before the onset of symptoms. If the condition is untreated, the increasing intracranial pressure eventually leads to death.

Intracerebral haematoma   Intracerebral haematomas are generally considered to be those that occur within the brain and that are not directly related to the surface of the brain. They are caused by the rupture of the internal blood vessels of the brain, often deep within the cerebral hemispheres (particularly frontal and temporal regions) at the time of injury. Sequential CT scan studies have shown that haemorrhages are often multiple, and their appearance on CT and MRI scans is often delayed, becoming apparent only several hours after admission.

The use of CT and MRI in the routine examination of head-injured patients has shown that many patients have multiple small haematomas scattered throughout the deep grey matter, especially in the basal ganglia. Patients with this pattern of haematoma formation tend to have been unconscious or barely conscious from the time of injury. Such patients are often found to have experienced a significant degree of contusional damage and diffuse axonal injury.

Multiple lesions   Several types of pathology – e.g. subdural haematoma and intracerebral haemorrhage, or extradural haematoma and contusions (see page 5.7) on the surface of the brain – are often seen in severe cases. This constellation of damage is commonly referred to as a 'burst' lobe, and is usually located in the frontal and temporal lobes.

Contusions

Contusions are a form of bruising of the brain, and are a characteristic pathology seen in non-penetrating head injury. Contusions are easily and reliably identified, so allowing both recent and past episodes of head injury to be documented.

Contusions have a characteristic distribution, whatever the site of the original injury. They are located in the gyral crests (Fig. 5.7) of:

- the frontal poles;
- orbital surfaces of the frontal lobes;
- temporal poles;
- lateral and inferior surfaces of the temporal lobes; and
- cortex adjacent to the sylvian fissures.

Contusions are not usually found in the parietal and occipital lobes nor in the cerebellum, unless there is a skull fracture in these areas.

The appearance of contusions evolves with time through three stages. Initially the contusion is visible as microscopic regions of perivascular haemorrhage following the track of small vessels in the cortex, usually running perpendicular to the cortical surface (Fig. 5.8). It is thought that this type of pathology can occur within seconds or minutes of the injury.

With time, blood continues to seep into the adjacent cortex, and neurons in the immediate vicinity begin to degenerate (Fig.

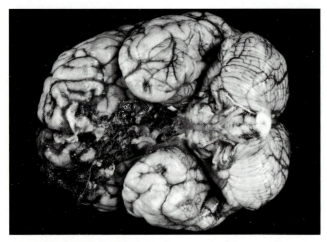

Fig. 5.7 Undersurface of the brain showing typical patterns of contusion in temporal and frontal poles after head injury. (Courtesy of Professor DI Graham, Glasgow.)

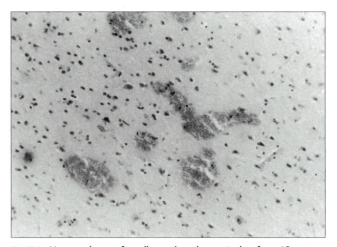

Fig. 5.8 Haemorrhage of small vessels at the cortical surface. (Courtesy of Professor DI Graham, Glasgow.)

5.9). The destruction of neurons causes glial activation and the formation of a glial scar. In some cases, haemorrhage will extend into the white matter, causing the demyelination of axons and the loss of fibres in tracts.

Finally, necrotic tissue is removed and the contusion metamorphoses into a shrunken and gliosed scar (Fig. 5.10). The scar is often brownish, owing to residual haemosiderin-filled macrophages. Old contusions often have a triangular shape, with the point in the depths of the cortex and a wider base extending up to the crest of a gyrus (Fig. 5.11).

It is worth noting that contusions can be distinguished from the foci of old ischaemic damage, as the latter are almost invariably more severe within the depths of sulci (Fig. 5.12).

Gliding contusions Although most contusions are related to the surface of the cortex, a class of contusions can be found deeper at the margins of the grey and white matter. These contusions are known as gliding contusions, and are defined as 'focal haemorrhages in the cerebral cortex and subjacent white matter at the superior margins of the cerebral hemispheres' (Hume Adams, 1992).

Gliding contusions are usually seen bilaterally, although their overall distribution is invariably asymmetrical. Gliding contusions are thought to be caused by the action of shear forces on the structural interface between grey and white matter. Gliding contusions are always found in association with other diffuse brain damage.

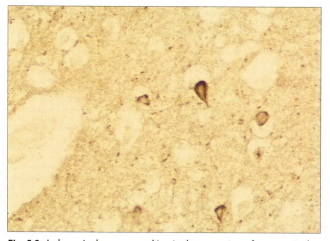

Fig. 5.9 Ischaemic damage, resulting in degeneration of neurons in the cortex. (Courtesy of Professor DI Graham, Glasgow.)

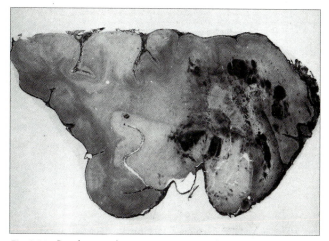

Fig. 5.10 Post-haemorrhagic scar. (Courtesy of Professor DI Graham, Glasgow.)

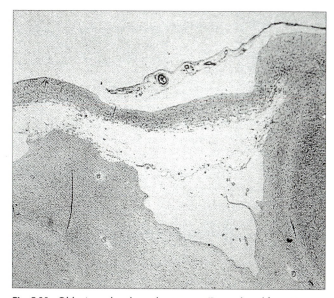

Fig. 5.11 Old, triangular-shaped contusion. (Reproduced from Hume Adams J. *Greenfield's Neuropathology*, 5th edition, 1992.)

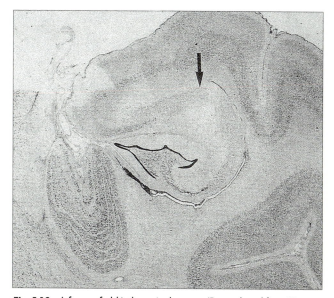

Fig. 5.12 A focus of old ischaemic damage. (Reproduced from Hume Adams J. *Greenfield's Neuropathology*, 5th edition, 1992.)

Mechanisms of Brain Damage

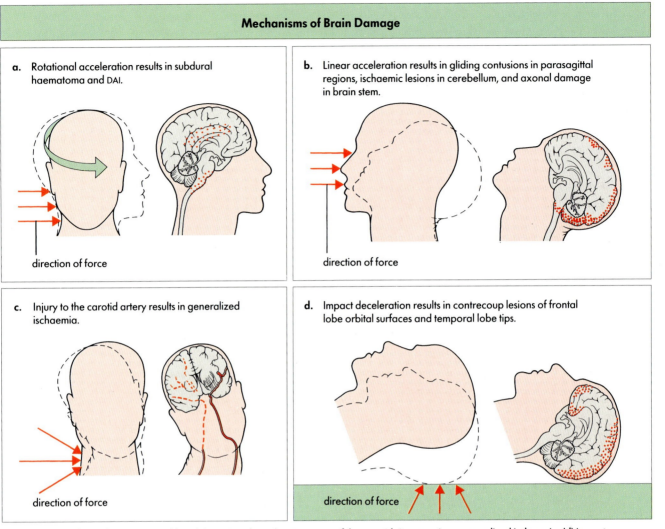

a. Rotational acceleration results in subdural haematoma and DAI.

direction of force

b. Linear acceleration results in gliding contusions in parasagittal regions, ischaemic lesions in cerebellum, and axonal damage in brain stem.

direction of force

c. Injury to the carotid artery results in generalized ischaemia.

direction of force

d. Impact deceleration results in contrecoup lesions of frontal lobe orbital surfaces and temporal lobe tips.

direction of force

Fig. 5.13 Acute brain damage caused by: (a) rotational acceleration; (b) linear acceleration; (c) injury to the carotid artery and compression of the carotid sinus causing generalized ischaemia; (d) impact deceleration caused by falls against an unyielding surface.

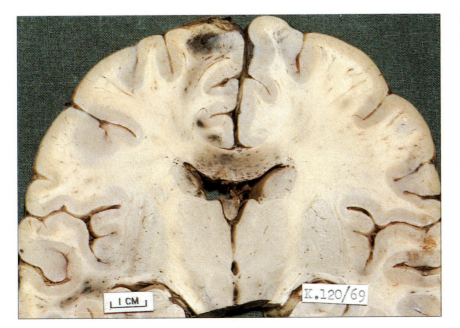

Fig. 5.14 Coronal section showing cystic damage in the corpus callosum.

I CM

K.120/69

Pathogenesis of contusions Contusions are thought to be due to the external (injury-causing) force applied to the head, and to the inertia of the brain inside the skull. Applying force to the head causes the skull to accelerate in either a linear or rotational fashion. However, owing to the brain's inertia, it lags behind the acceleration of the skull and often comes into contact with the internal surface of the skull (Fig. 5.13). When the head is involved in an impact, the skull's acceleration and rotation are abruptly halted, but within the skull the brain continues in the same direction of motion. As a result, there may be impact between the brain and the inner surfaces of the skull, and shearing stress, due to the obstruction by the skull of the rotational movements of the brain, occurs. This explains why contusions are common adjacent to the frontal and temporal poles, since the brain comes into contact with the anterior and middle fossae of the skull. The shear forces within the brain can then lead to gliding contusions and diffuse axonal damage.

Infection

Infection is a complication of skull fractures. Fractures of the calvaria or skull base can provide a route for bacteria to pass from the major air sinuses into the subarachnoid spaces, and thus lead to meningitis. Such fractures are often associated with leakages of CSF or the formation of an aerocoele.

Focal sites of infection, such as intracerebral abscesses, are relatively common in penetrating head injury, since infected material can readily gain access to the cranial cavity.

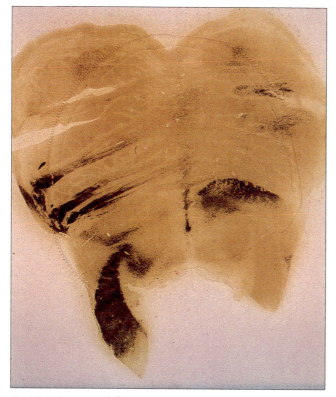

Fig. 5.15 A pontomedullary rent.

Focal Brain Damage

The shape and structure of the head and neck leads to some common patterns of damage after a head injury. Structures affected include:
- carotid and vertebral arteries;
- corpus callosum;
- hypothalamus;
- medulla; and
- cranial nerves.

Carotid and vertebral arteries

Hyperextension of the neck as a result of trauma can stretch the carotid artery and cause a traumatic thrombosis. The thrombosis can lead to a major infarct and hemiplegia hours after the injury. Rupture of the vertebral artery after trauma can also occur. This is invariably accompanied by bruising or injury behind and below the ear, and occasionally by fracture of the transverse process of the first cervical vertebra. The rupture produces a massive subarachnoid haemorrhage, which is often fatal.

Corpus callosum

This large white matter tract can be the site of extensive diffuse axonal injury (see page 5.12) and ischaemia caused by a loss of blood supply from the pericallosal arteries. The first stage of pathology is a series of small (2–3 mm diameter) perivascular haemorrhages, which can be found scattered along the corpus callosum on either side of the midline. The haemorrhage expands over six to 48 hours and infiltrates surrounding tissue. Eventually, the lesion loses definition and shrinks to a glial scar with scattered haemosiderin-filled macrophages (Fig. 5.14).

Hypothalamus

During the traumatic movement of the brain within the skull, the infundibulum (pituitary stalk), which links the pituitary to the hypothalamus, can stretch. Excessive strain can snap the infundibulum, leading to the disconnection of the hypothalamus and pituitary and the loss of some of the pituitary's blood supply. As a result, infarction of the anterior pituitary can occur.

Damage to the hypothalamus and pituitary can also occur a considerable time after head injury as a result of intracranial bleeding (e.g. in chronic subdural haematoma). These types of expanding lesions raise intracranial pressure and lead to compression and distortion of the normal brain structure.

Brain stem

Traumatic injuries that cause twisting or extension of the neck can lead to damage within the brain stem and associated fractures of the base of the skull and upper cervical vertebrae. The shear forces involved stretch and sever long nerve tracts travelling through this region, and can also cause localized haemorrhages, such as a tear at the junction of the pons and medulla (Fig. 5.15).

Cranial nerves

The cranial nerves pass from the brain and exit through various holes in the skull. Their fine structure and finite length make them susceptible to tearing by the rotation of the brain within the skull after trauma. The nerves most often damaged are:

- olfactory (I) nerve;
- optic (II) nerve;
- facial (VII) nerve; and
- auditory (VIII) nerve.

This damage is often related to the presence of fractures in the bones which the nerves pass through or travel over.

Diffuse Brain Damage

Loss of consciousness or loss of neurological function can occur seconds after a head injury. It is thought that this sudden loss of function, and a great deal of the chronic neurological damage, is due to the diffuse brain damage that occurs at multiple sites throughout the brain. Neuropathology has defined four main types of diffuse brain damage that arise at the moment of injury or that develop as a slow response to the trauma:

- diffuse axonal injury;
- diffuse vascular injury;
- ischaemia; and
- raised intracranial pressure and brain swelling.

Diffuse axonal injury

Diffuse axonal injury (DAI) is a distinct diagnostic entity. There are three distinctive features in the pathology of diffuse axonal injury in its severest form:

- a focal lesion in the corpus callosum;
- focal lesions in the dorsolateral quadrant of the rostral brain stem adjacent to the superior cerebellar peduncles; and
- diffuse damage to axons.

The first two types of pathology can be identified macroscopically and have been well described. Diffuse damage to axons can only be seen microscopically (Fig. 5.16) and an appreciation of the severity of axonal injury will require microscopic examination, particularly in cases that do not have obvious macroscopic axonal damage.

The histological appearance of axonal damage depends on the length of survival after injury. DAI is difficult to demonstrate in patients that survive less than 15 hours. This is a point of considerable forensic interest. Patients who survive for several days show the presence of many localized axonal swellings (retraction balls of Cajal seen by silver stains). These are seen in white matter tracts, particularly in:

- the white matter of the cerebral hemispheres;
- the corpus callosum;
- the subcortical fibre tracts (fornix, internal, and external capsules);
- the cerebellum (cerebellar peduncles); and
- the brain stem (corticospinal tract, medial lemnisci, medial longitudinal bundles, and central tegmental tracts).

Fibre tracts which travel in a parasaggital plane are usually the worst affected because of the rotational forces involved (see Fig. 5.13a). Lesions are often asymmetrical.

Pathogenesis   The physical forces generated by the trauma stretch the axons in the white matter, and so damage the axolemma or related axoplasm at the injured node of Ranvier. As a result, the membrane properties of the axon are compromised and control over ion exchange is lost. Disruption of this type triggers a cascade of changes (see Chapter 3), which disrupts metabolic activity, causes localized disorganization of axonal cytoarchitecture, and interferes with axonal transport. The focal interruption of axonal transport leads to a build-up of axonally transported proteins and organelles at the site of the lesion. As a result, the axon swells and forms a retraction ball. Finally, axotomy occurs and the axon distal to the lesion degenerates.

Experimental studies have suggested that this process of axotomy takes a considerable period of time to develop fully (analogous to the consequences of ischaemia; see Chapter 3); as a result, treatment may be developed to slow or even halt the process of axotomy.

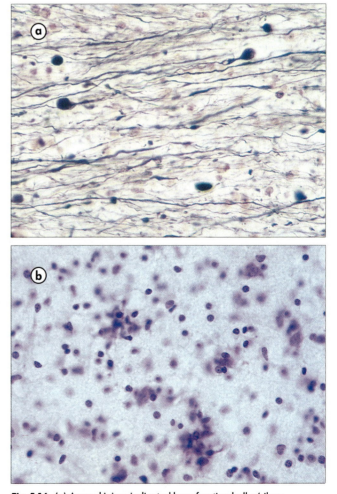

Fig. 5.16   (a) Axonal injury indicated by refraction bulbs (silver impregnation); (b) Foci of reactive glial cells (haematoxylin and eosin stain). (Courtesy of Professor DI Graham, Glasgow.)

With longer survival times (months) axonal swellings eventually disappear and the lesion site becomes marked by an extensive glial reaction. Finally, cystic lesions can occur in the way already described above for the corpus callosum.

Patients that sustain severe diffuse axonal injury are unconscious from the moment of impact, do not experience a lucid interval, and remain unconscious, vegetative, or at least severely disabled, until death. The clinical picture has been described as primary brain stem injury.

Diffuse vascular damage

The occurrence of many small haemorrhages scattered throughout the brain is another common consequence of head injury. They are particularly prominent in the white matter of the frontal and temporal lobes, thalamus, and brain stem. All parts of the vascular system are affected, and haemorrhages can be seen in arteries, veins, and capillaries.

Ischaemic damage

Infarction and widespread hypoxic ischaemic brain damage is commonly seen after head trauma, usually in the hippocampus and basal ganglia. The cortex and cerebellum are less often affected. The damage is thought to occur by:
- temporary occlusion of the posterior cerebral arteries; and
- reduced blood flow due to raised intracranial pressure.

Ischaemic damage is likely in patients that have had clinically evident hypoxia (as a systolic blood pressure of less than 80 mmHg for at least 15 minutes) or episodes of raised intracranial pressure (over 30 mmHg) at some time after the injury.

Ischaemic damage is focal in the hippocampus and basal ganglia, and widespread in the cortex. Cortical damage is often seen in the border zones between the major cerebral arterial territories (Fig. 5.17; see Chapter 3), usually between the anterior and middle cerebral arteries. Damage is bilateral in most cases. A diffuse pattern of cortical damage in both hemispheres can also occur. However, focal damage restricted to the territory supplied by a single artery is comparatively rare.

The common occurrence of cortical damage and its pattern suggest that it is caused by periods of reduced blood flow. This proposal is supported by the fact that cardiac arrest and status epilepticus are also known to give rise to similar patterns of cortical damage.

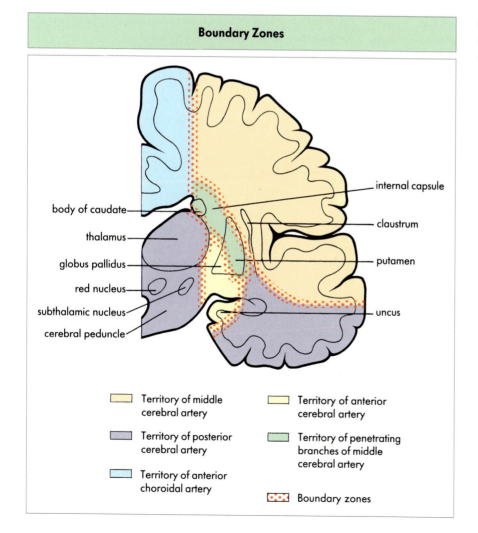

Boundary Zones

body of caudate
thalamus
globus pallidus
red nucleus
subthalamic nucleus
cerebral peduncle

internal capsule
claustrum
putamen
uncus

Territory of middle cerebral artery

Territory of posterior cerebral artery

Territory of anterior choroidal artery

Territory of anterior cerebral artery

Territory of penetrating branches of middle cerebral artery

Boundary zones

Fig. 5.17 Diagram showing the boundary zones between the territories of the major cerebral arteries.

Pathogenesis The occurrence of ischaemia produces membrane disruption, which leads to depolarization, the release of excitatory amino acid transmitters, and the acute-phase protein response. Both types of physiological cascade can enhance the degree of neuronal damage (see Chapter 3).

This type of brain damage is (after DAI) the commonest pathology found in the brains of severely disabled patients.

Raised Intracranial Pressure and Brain Swelling

The pressure of CSF is constantly changing, rising and falling in response to two different rhythms:
- the change in arterial pressure over the cycle of a heartbeat;
- the change in central venous pressure related to the pattern of respiration.

As a result of these fluctuations, the intracranial pressure is usually expressed as a mean; the normal range is 0–15 mmHg in patients undergoing continuous monitoring. The upper limit of normal is lower in children (e.g. newborn babies: 3 mmHg; five year olds: 5 mmHg).

The volume of the skull is finite. When expanding mass lesions occur (e.g. haematoma), either surplus volume within the cranial vault is filled, or regions of the brain are compressed to accommodate the lesion. However, this ability for 'spatial compensation' is limited, and once it is exceeded, intracranial pressure begins to rise. The most important mechanism for spatial compensation appears to be a reduction in the volume of CSF within the cortex.

Pressure Waves

These increases in pressure are usually seen in the form of pressure waves, of which there are two main types. The most important type clinically are A waves and B waves.

A waves
These are increases in pressure, which can be abrupt and which last from five to 20 minutes before subsiding to normal. They are common in expanding lesions and obstructive hydrocephalus, and their occurrence is related to sudden deteriorations in the patient's condition (from worsening headache to decerebrate rigidity). They are thought to be caused by changes in cerebrovascular vasodilatation.

B waves
These are seen more frequently, but because they rise as a sharp peak and decline within tens of seconds, they are not a cause of brain damage. They are thought to be caused by changes in cerebral blood volume and cerebrovascular tone.

When pressure begins to exceed the upper range of normal for minutes at a time, brain damage may occur. In general:
- mild rises to 15–22 mmHg are reasonably well tolerated;
- moderate rises to 30 mmHg require intervention;
- severe rises above 37.5 mmHg are associated with ischaemic brain damage;

- pressures above 60 mmHg often indicate a terminal state;
- when intracranial pressure reaches arterial pressure, cerebral blood flow ceases and all neurological functions fail.

Herniation

Reduced volume of intracranial CSF is an important mechanism in spatial compensation. However, when CSF volumes are reduced in particular regions, the localized reductions in pressure cause brain substance to flow into the space (away from the increased pressure produced by the lesion). This can result in the movement of brain tissue from one cranial compartment into another – herniation. There are three sites at which this often occurs, to give supracallosal, tentorial, or tonsillar herniation.

IMAGING

CT and MRI can give reliable indications of raised intracranial pressure, and also indicate the site of the problem by showing:
- displacement of brain structures across the midline;
- unilateral ventricular enlargement;
- bilateral reductions in ventricular size;
- reduction or loss of the third ventricle;
- herniation of brain tissue.

Brain swelling

Brain swelling occurs in about 75 per cent of cases, and is a major factor contributing to an increase in intracranial pressure (along with haemorrhages). Three principal types of brain swelling are encountered in patients with a head injury:
- swelling adjacent to contusions on the surface of the brain;
- diffuse swelling of one cerebral hemisphere; and
- diffuse swelling of both cerebral hemispheres.

Brain swelling is thought to be caused in two ways: by cerebral vasodilatation and a consequent increase in cerebral blood volume (i.e. congestive brain swelling), or by an increase in the water content of neuronal tissue (i.e. cerebral oedema).

Congestion
Diffuse swelling of one cerebral hemisphere is often seen after surgical evacuation of an ipsilateral acute subdural haematoma. The brain simply expands to fill the space. It is thought that this is due to vasodilatation, with the overfilling of a non-reactive vascular bed in which the mechanisms of autoregulation have been damaged by the trauma-induced ischaemia. The initial vasodilatation is sometimes followed by cerebral oedema as a result of the breakdown of the blood–brain barrier.

Diffuse swelling of the entire brain is usually seen only in children and adolescents. It is thought to be caused by a global increase in blood volume, and it is associated with epileptic activity and the occurrence of status epilepticus.

Cerebral oedema

There is often swelling of white matter near contusions and of tissue near intracerebral haematomas (Fig. 5.18). Next to the contusion, there is a zone containing vessels that have been physically disrupted and that show increased capillary permeability together with a loss of normal physiological regulation at the arteriolar level. This disruption allows water to enter and causes local oedema.

The delayed clinical deterioration (two to three days after injury) in patients with a subdural haematoma is more likely to be caused by brain swelling and a subsequent increase in intracranial pressure than by enlargement of the haematoma itself.

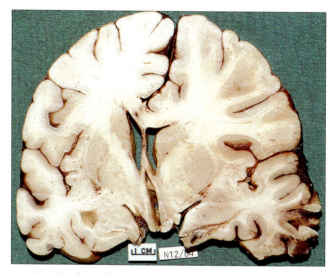

Fig. 5.18 Swelling of the brain after haematoma, showing distortion of the midline. (Courtesy of Professor DI Graham, Glasgow.)

PENETRATING AND NON-PENETRATING HEAD INJURY

The mechanics of the two types of head injury differ, and they give rise to different types of damage and thus a characteristic set of clinical problems.

Penetrating injuries are caused by objects falling or being propelled through the air. Penetrating injuries generally cause focal damage. Diffuse damage is not usual because the element of rotational injury is missing. The extent and depth of a penetrating injury is a function of the shape and speed of the missile and the location of impact. The injury may be classified as:

- depressed;
- penetrating; and
- perforating.

In depressed injuries, the object itself does not penetrate the skull but it can cause a depressed fracture and focal contusions. Consciousness is rarely lost.

In penetrating injuries (Fig. 5.19), the object does enter the skull. Small sharp objects (e.g. a spike) can cause minimal injury, and damage may be overlooked if the missile is no longer embedded in the skull. Brain damage is focal and its severity is often related to the depth of penetration. There is often no history of loss of consciousness. Penetrating head injuries carry a high risk of infection (abscess, meningitis). Such injuries are also associated with a high degree of risk for the development of post-traumatic epilepsy, which occurs in about 40 per cent of cases.

Perforating injuries are characterized by the missile (often a bullet) entering, traversing, and leaving the skull. High-velocity bullets can pass through the skull without knocking the victim down or causing impairment of consciousness. Exit wounds are generally larger than entry wounds. Brain damage is often severe. Low-velocity missiles are more likely to fragment within the skull, and can cause fragments of cloth, bone, and scalp to be pushed into the brain.

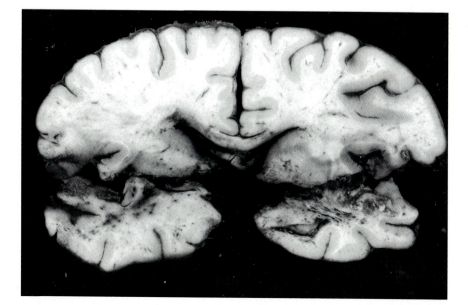

Fig. 5.19 A coronal section of brain, showing a bullet track after a perforating head injury.

The velocity of the missile passing through the brain can cause remote contusions, affecting the frontal and temporal poles, the undersurface of the cerebellum, or (occasionally) contrecoup fractures in the orbital plates. Typically, only 10 per cent of patients shot in the head survive for more than 24 hours, and 5 per cent for more than seven days.

SUMMARY

(i)   Head trauma is the commonest cause of death in people aged under 45.

(ii) Of patients suffering head trauma, 60 per cent recover, 20 per cent have psychiatric or psychological problems, 15 per cent have severe brain damage, and 5 per cent remain in a vegetative state.

(iii) Acute effects of head trauma are: loss of consciousness, confusion, and amnesia.

(iv) Chronic effects of head trauma are amnesia, psychiatric symptoms, motor disorders, focal brain damage, and epilepsy.

(v)   Head trauma can trigger a progressive neurodegenerative Alzheimer-type disease.

(vi) Head trauma can be divided into penetrating and non-penetrating injuries.

(vii) Pathological features are lesions of scalp and skull, contusions, intracranial haemorrhages, diffuse axonal injury, and ischaemic damage.

(viii) Diffuse axonal injury and ischiaemic damage are associated with chronic neurological deficits.

(ix) Raised intracranial pressure is caused by expanding lesion and brain swelling.

6 Aids Dementia

INTRODUCTION

AIDS – the acquired immunodeficiency syndrome – was recognized as a clinical syndrome in the early 1980s, and the putative causal agent, the human immunodeficiency virus (HIV), was isolated in 1984. Despite its brief history as a disease, AIDS has already caused a profound change in clinical practice because of its infectivity (15 000 000 infected worldwide), and it has led to substantial changes in the sociology of sexual behaviour because of its association with sexual activity.

Almost all patients infected with HIV undergo seroconversion between one and five years after infection and then suffer from severely compromised immune system function. The clinical course is one of increasingly frequent and serious bacterial and viral infections which, ultimately, cause wasting and death. Patients can show a range of neurological and psychiatric symptoms including a dementing syndrome – AIDS dementia complex. Approximately 10 per cent of AIDS patients show this syndrome.

Differential diagnosis from Alzheimer's disease and other dementias on the basis of symptomatology is difficult. The presence of HIV or HIV-immunoreactivity in serum or brain tissue is diagnostic of AIDS and this, in conjunction with cognitive decline, indicates the diagnosis of AIDS dementia complex.

The projected increase in the numbers of AIDS patients and the common involvement of the CNS in infection indicate that the dementia associated with AIDS is likely to grow as a clinical problem in the next few decades.

Worldwide, some 15 000 000 people are already infected with the HIV and the World Health Organization (WHO) estimations predict a figure of 40 000 000 infected patients by the year 2000 (Fig. 6.1). At least 1 000 000 patients in the USA are already infected with HIV, some 200 000 have developed AIDS and of these 130 000 have died (figures to the end of 1991). In 1991 in New York City, AIDS was the commonest cause of death in young women.

Changes in sexual practices and the use of condoms have been advised in an effort to halt the spread of infection. However, HIV already infects more than one in three adults in some central African cities. Preliminary reports suggest that, in the Western world, AIDS infectivity will escape the confines of the 'high-risk groups' and the pattern will become closer to that seen in central Africa – a heterosexually transmitted disease associated with multiple sexual partners (e.g. via prostitution). It has also been proposed that the presence of compromised or deficient immune system function (i.e. such as that seen in drug abusers, or patients on immunosuppressive therapy) is also a significant risk factor. The exact extent of HIV infectivity and thus of AIDS will be determined finally by the epidemiologists of the next millennium.

Careful clinical investigations and follow-up studies of AIDS patients have demonstrated that the CNS is affected by the virus in many cases. The CNS involvement gives rise to a wide range of psychiatric symptoms which includes an AIDS dementia complex. Estimating the incidence and prevalence of HIV-associated dementia complex is difficult, since such estimates are influenced

EPIDEMIOLOGY

The epidemiology of AIDS is complicated by the associated social factors and the inevitable politicization of research data which might be held to reinforce or create social or cultural stereotypes.

The demographic characteristics vary from continent to continent. In central Africa, AIDS affects males and females equally and is transmitted through heterosexual activity. In the USA and Europe, AIDS is still largely confined to well-defined 'high risk' groups (essentially male homosexuals and intravenous drug abusers).

HIV is transmitted in at least four ways:

- through sexual contact;
- from mother to infant before or during birth;
- through blood transfusion, organ donation, or the use of contaminated instruments which pierce the skin (e.g. iatrogenically, or needle sharing in illicit drug abuse); and
- direct contact with bodily fluids.

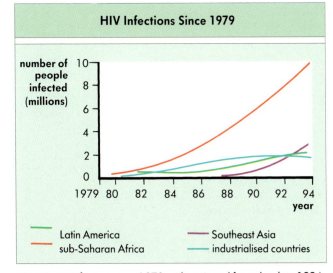

Fig. 6.1 HIV infections since 1979, with projected future levels to 1994. Areas not shown have, so far, fewer infections.

by the demographics and location of the patient sample, the stage of infection, and the criteria used for the diagnosis. However approximately 10 per cent of AIDS patients show an HIV-associated dementia complex. Of this group, approximately one third had symptoms of dementia as the only early manifestation of AIDS. The incidence rates of AIDS dementia complex increase significantly with age, even in patients less than 50 years old.

Diseases of the Central Nervous System Associated with HIV Infection

Opportunistic and other infections

Caused by viruses

Progressive multifocal leucoencephalopathy
Cytomegalovirus encephalitis, myelitis, retinitis
Herpes simplex (type 2) meningitis, myelitis
Herpes simplex (type 1) encephalitis
Immunosuppressive measles myelitis, encephalitis
Varicella-zoster encephalitis, myelitis

Caused by fungi

Cryptococcosis
Candida albicans
Aspergillus fumigatus
Mucormycosis
Coccidioidomycosis
Histoplasmosis

Caused by bacteria

Mycobacterium avium intracellulare
Whipple's disease
Nocardia (abscesses)

Caused by protozoa

Toxoplasma gondii (toxoplasmosis)

Caused by spirochaetes

Syphilis

Neoplasms

Lymphoma – primary or systemic

Metastatic Kaposi's sarcoma

Caused by HIV

Encephalopathy

Vacuolar myelopathy

Aseptic meningitis

Vascular causes

Cerebral haemorrhage

Cerebral infarction

Fig. 6.2 CNS diseases associated with HIV infection.

CAUSE OF AIDS DEMENTIA

The dementia is a complication of a CNS infection with the HIV virus. Brain pathology in AIDS patients can also be caused by a large number of opportunistic infections (Fig. 6.2). However, the pathological stigmata associated with these other infections can be separated from that characterizing the AIDS dementia complex (see page 6.8).

CLINICAL COURSE

The initial event is infection with the HIV. The patient is generally asymptomatic until seroconversion occurs some one to four years after infection (Fig. 6.3). Following seroconversion, the disease progresses into full-blown AIDS through a series of stages (Fig. 6.4) in some 90 per cent of patients. During the course of the disease, patients often manifest psychiatric or neurological symptoms and can develop AIDS dementia.

Psychiatric Symptoms

The most common psychiatric presentation in HIV-infected people are those due to the sociological stresses arising from the discovery that they are infected. These can be categorized as:
- adjustment reactions (acute stress reactions);
- adjustment disorders;
- affective disorders (mood disorders);
- schizophreniform (acute psychotic) disorders; and
- paranoid disorders.

It is important to distinguish psychological reactions to HIV infection from the symptoms caused by infection of the central nervous system (i.e. chronic impairment in intellectual functioning and eventual dementia), because of possible treatment implications. Unfortunately, this is a difficult distinction, for mood disturbance and/or psychotic features often occur as the presenting symptoms of an organic brain syndrome.

Adjustment reactions Adjustment reactions (acute stress reactions) occur as a response to the trauma of diagnosis of HIV infection. Such reactions involve expressions of despair, grief, guilt, anxiety, protest, anti-social behaviour, depression, suicidal activity, and hypochondriasis. These reactions are similar in severity and content to those generated by other traumatic life events or disease diagnoses. Generally, these reactions do not result in chronic functional impairment and their course and severity can be greatly ameliorated by appropriate counselling and psychosocial support.

Adjustment disorders When the features described as adjustment reactions are intense and long lasting (over six months), they can be described as adjustment disorders. Psychotherapeutic and/or psychopharmacological interventions are successful in dealing with most presentations. In severe cases, hospitalization

Natural History of HIV Infection

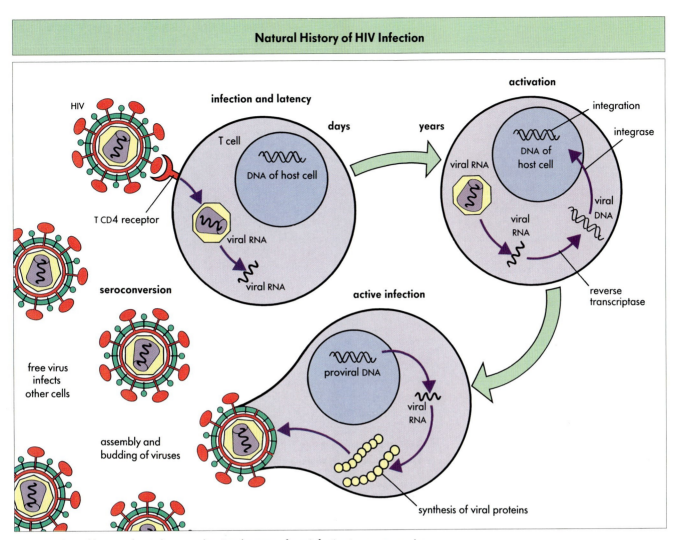

Fig. 6.3 Natural history of HIV in humans, showing the stages from infection to seroconversion.

may be required. A prior psychiatric history is strongly associated with the onset of adjustment disorders.

Affective disorders   Depression is commonly reported in stages 2 and 3 (see Fig. 6.4), but is rarely quantified. It has been suggested that the appearance of depression often reflects the dynamic tension between uncertainty and adjustment to life with HIV, and should therefore be expected in a majority of patients at some time in the history of their infection. The onset of clinical depression is usually gradual and is mediated by psychosocial factors such as lack of social support, lack of social and health-care infrastructures, guilt or lack of acceptance about sexuality or lifestyle, lack of adequate accommodation, and problems with finance and employment. Suicide is a significant risk. Manic episodes are very rare in the absence of organic brain syndromes in HIV infected people.

Psychiatric disorder and stage of illness   Staging of the clinical illness is significantly related to the risks of psychopathology. People with AIDS-related complex (ARC) appear to experience greater psychological morbidity than those who remain asymptomatic or who have AIDS in the first few months after diagnosis. Those with mid-stage manifestations of HIV disease have a greater level of uncertainty about whether they will progress to AIDS and then on to death.

Schizophreniform and paranoid disorders   Anecdotal reports have described HIV-infected patients (with and without AIDS) who have acute psychotic illnesses and hallucinations, paranoid or grandiose delusions, and thought disorders. It is not known whether these are prodromal appearances or neuropsychiatric disturbances or coincidental occurrences. Their appearance is relatively infrequent.

Suicide   Suicide attempts following the news of a positive HIV test are a relatively frequent occurrence. Care is required when informing patients of a positive HIV test, since the risk is increased in the period of stress following a positive test and in situations where social support and counselling are inadequate or unavailable. Several factors have been identified as indicating an increased

Staging Scheme for the AIDS Dementia Complex	
Stage	**Characteristics**
Stage 0 (normal)	Normal mental and motor function.
Stage 0.5 (equivocal/ subclinical)	Minimal or equivocal symptoms (cognitive or motor dysfunction) or signs (snout response, slowed extremity movements) characteristic of ADC, but without impairment of work or capacity to perform activities of daily living (ADL).
Stage 1 (mild)	Unequivocal evidence of function intellectual or motor impairment, but able to perform all the more demanding aspects of work or ADL. Can walk without assistance.
Stage 2 (moderate)	Cannot work or maintain the more demanding aspects of daily life, but able to perform basic self care. Ambulatory, but may require a single prop.
Stage 3 (severe)	Major intellectual incapacity (cannot follow news or personal events, cannot sustain complex conversation, considerable slowing of all output), or motor disability (cannot walk unassisted, requiring walker or personal support, usually with slowing and clumsiness of arms).
Stage 4 (end-stage)	Nearly vegetative. Intellectual and social comprehension and responses are at a rudimentary level. Nearly or absolutely mute. Parapatetic or paraplegic with double incontinence.

Fig. 6.4 Scheme for staging the AIDS dementia complex (ADC).

risk of suicide attempts (Miller and Riccio, 1990):

- multiple psychosocial stresses;
- perceived social isolation;
- perceiving oneself as a victim;
- denial;
- substance abuse; and
- perceived lack of social support.

In addition it has been reported that depressed alcoholic homosexual men may attempt to infect themselves with HIV as a form of attempted suicide.

Delirium

Acute organic brain syndromes or confusional states (delirium) occur in almost half of all AIDS patients. Such states are particularly common in patients with histories of brain damage or substance abuse. Delirium is characterized by:

- clouding of consciousness;
- reduced attention capacity; and
- increased psychomotor activity.

Delirium usually occurs as the result of a concurrent infection (e.g. meningitis), space occupying lesions (e.g. lymphoma) or disturbances in electrolyte balance. When the underlying condition is controlled, patients invariably recover.

AIDS DEMENTIA COMPLEX

Recently the brain has been recognized as a target for HIV infection. The virus appears to enter the central nervous system shortly after infection, as shown by the occurrence of CSF abnormalities:

- pleocytosis;
- protein elevation; and
- intrathecal synthesis of specific antibodies.

These changes are seen in about 60 per cent of asymptomatic, immunologically intact HIV infected people. HIV (HIV-1 type) can be isolated from the CSF of 30 per cent of asymptomatic seropositive people, and the presence of psychiatric symptoms and a dementing syndrome has been extensively documented in patients with AIDS. Neuropathological studies have reported a varying degree of pathology in over 65 per cent of patients who have died of AIDS.

A disorder characterized by cognitive dysfunction, neurological, and behavioural deficits has often been described in patients with AIDS. This syndrome has been given several names, including subacute encephalitis, AIDS dementia complex, HIV-1 encephalopathy, HIV-1 associated dementia, and HIV-1 associated dementia complex. The term AIDS dementia complex appears to be the most appropriate designation for this syndrome.

Symptoms

The onset of AIDS dementia complex is usually insidious and can occur before, during, or after the onset of other peripheral or CNS manifestations of the disease.

Psychiatric symptoms

Early cognitive and behavioural symptoms include:

- forgetfulness;
- loss of concentration and mental slowing;
- difficulties with sequential mental tasks (e.g. following a recipe);
- apathy;
- reduced emotional responsiveness and social withdrawal; and
- malaise and loss of sexual drive.

Depressive mood disorders and psychosis are relatively rare.

Neurological symptoms

Early motor symptoms include problems with:

- balance;
- clumsiness; and
- leg weakness.

Typically these symptoms manifest themselves by dropping things, by tripping and falling, and as problems in manual dexterity and deterioration in writing ability.

Appropriate examination usually reveals the presence of motor signs such as ataxias, tremor (e.g. when holding the arms and fingers outstretched) and hyperreflexia. Frontal release signs (snout reflex, palmar grasp), and dysarthria may also occur. Deficits in eye movements may also be present, with interruption of smooth pursuit movements and slowing or inaccuracy of saccades.

In the early stages, mental status tests may be normal, except for slowing of verbal or motor responses and difficulties in delayed recall. Neuropsychological examination of patients demonstrates prominent deficits in fine motor control and sequential processing (e.g. trail making). Deficits in visuo-spatial problem solving (block design), verbal fluency, and visual memory can be present but are less prominent. In general, slowness in completing tasks is the most obvious defect, although errors can also occur. However, naming and vocabulary skills are largely preserved even in the most advanced cases, in contrast to Alzheimer's disease.

As the syndrome progresses, global deterioration of cognitive functions occurs and there is severe psychomotor retardation. Speech is affected, with slowing and word finding difficulties. Difficulties in talking can progress to mutism. Gradually, patients become bedridden and doubly incontinent. Loss of insight occurs, and apathy and indifference become prominent. Peripheral neurological signs and symptoms can appear as a result of sensory neuropathy. Seizures can develop in the later stages of the disease.

Operational diagnostic criteria (WHO, American Academy of Neurology) have been developed to try and maintain diagnostic consistency and allow a distinction to be made between the AIDS dementia complex and other types of dementia. These criteria (based on criteria for dementia in International Classification of Diseases, 10th ed) emphasize:

- the presence of motor signs and symptoms; and
- the lack of aphasia, apraxia, and agnosia.

Course

Onset is insidious and the course is very variable. The factors that control the rate of progression of neurological deficits are not understood. Predicting progression and short term outcome is complicated by the inevitable occurrence of multiple episodes of opportunistic infections. Depending on the extent and severity of such infections, the deficits may fluctuate, stabilize, or progress rapidly to severe deterioration and death. Death is usually due to pneumonia or massive systemic infection.

Investigations

Blood and CSF

Blood tests will usually demonstrate the presence of antibodies to HIV. In CSF, mononuclear pleocytosis can occur and the ratio between the T-lymphocyte subsets (CD4:CD8) may be reversed (Fig. 6.5). HIV can be detected using the polymerase chain reaction. HIV-1-specific antibodies and the HIV-1 antigen p24 may also be present. CSF B_2-microglobulin levels have been reported to relate to the degree of dementia. Opportunistic infections can also be detected (e.g. cytomegalovirus or herpes simplex virus).

EEG Investigations are usually negative in the early stages. Diffuse slowing has been reported in the later stages.

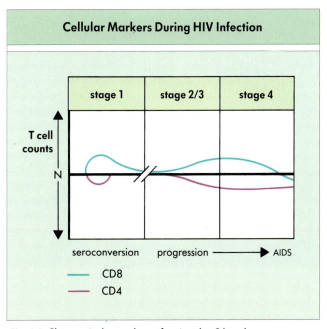

Fig. 6.5 Changes in the numbers of CD4 and CD8 lymphocytes, compared to normal levels, during the course of HIV infection.

CT and MRI   CT and MRI scans show signs of cortical atrophy with widened cortical sulci and a variable degree of ventricular enlargement. MRI frequently shows diffuse or focal regions of high signal intensity in the white matter. The appearance of these features can alter over time and it has been suggested that some features of the pathology may be partially reversible. These reversible changes have been linked to improvements in cognitive function after treatment with zidovudine (AZT).

PET and SPECT   These scans show reduced metabolism in subcortical (thalamus and basal ganglia) structure in the early stages of AIDS dementia complex (Fig. 6.6). A complimentary picture is revealed in SPECT scans with evidence of reduced cerebral blood flow in the same regions. In the later stages of the disease, hypometabolism and reduced blood flow are more prominent in the cortex and are often focal in nature. Imaging can provide useful information to help distinguish AIDS dementia from primary neurodegenerative dementias such as Alzheimer's disease (see Chapter 2).

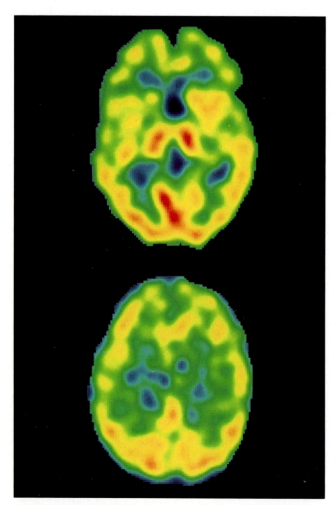

Fig. 6.6 Scans of blood flow measured with 99mTC NMPAO and SPECT of a patient with AIDS dementia complex. The scans reveal patchy areas of hypofunction in the cortex and basal ganglia. Two slices are shown here, one through the basal ganglia (top), and one through the cortex (bottom). (Courtesy of Len Holman, MD, Boston, Massachusetts.)

AIDS INFECTIONS

HIV (HIV-1 and 2) is an RNA-containing virus and is categorized as a lentivirus. HIV is thought to gain entry into the body via latently infected cells and is not thought to infect the host in the form of a free virus (unlike other types of virus that infect the CNS, such as herpes simplex).

Latently infected cells probably have no viral proteins on their surface and, as a result, the HIV can evade the normal mechanisms of immunological control. It is probable that, in circumstances such as blood transfusions and intravenous substance abuse, free virus can be transmitted from person to person.

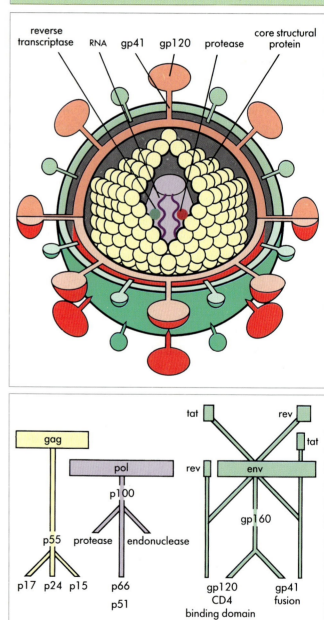

HIV Genes and their Functional Roles

Fig. 6.7 Diagrammatic representation of the structure of HIV-1, and the principal genes of the virus, and their functional roles.

The structure of HIV-1 is now known in some detail (Fig. 6.7). The genetic material of HIV-1 is present in the form of RNA (instead of DNA). In order to translate the viral RNA into DNA, a particular enzyme – reverse transcriptase – is required (the presence of this enzyme categorizes HIV as a retrovirus). HIV can only reproduce within a host cell. The way HIV-1 gains entry into cells is an important part of the biology of HIV-1 infection. Entry into the cell is accomplished by the virus binding to a receptor (CD4) on the surface of cells (see Fig. 6.3). These receptors are found on T-helper lymphocytes, macrophages, microglia, and dendritic cells. Once inside the cell, HIV-1 can either remain dormant or, by inserting its genetic material into the host DNA, can replicate itself and produce new virus particles, which bud off from the cell membrane and infect other cells (Fig. 6.8; see also Fig. 6.3).

One of the keys to the clinical and pathological features of HIV-1 infection (AIDS) lies in the infection of CD4-receptor carrying cells. For instance, HIV-1 infects dendritic cells. Dendritic cells are amongst the first to detect the presence of foreign proteins or infective agents entering the body. They then act to stimulate T-lymphocytes to respond to specific antigens or foreign proteins. By attacking and destroying the cells responsible for the co-ordination of the immune response, HIV-1 evades the body's defence mechanisms and allows other opportunistic infections free access (see Fig. 6.2).

Expression of HIV non-structural genes (e.g. mef, tat, rev) varies with the type of cell and its state of activation or differentiation (see Fig. 6.7). In activated T cells, HIV-1 infection produces large numbers of infectious virions and results in cytolytic cell death. The key viral factor in proliferating cells is tat, which accelerates viral replication. In activated monocytes and macrophages, less tat is expressed and infection results in abundant viral production but delayed cytolysis.

HIV-1 infection of cells that remain unstimulated can result in a 'latent' infection, which can persist for considerable periods of time. This feature is thought to account for the extended periods of time that can occur between infection, seroconversion and the resulting active disease process.

A further feature of HIV has additional clinical import. The virus has a considerable capacity for 'genetic drift'. The mutations within the viral genome permit the generation of novel viral-envelope proteins, which can continue to evade the compromised immune response of the host. This ability to change the signature of the envelope protein ensures that development of vaccines against the virus will be a difficult procedure.

Immunosuppression in AIDS

Infection with HIV leads to immunosuppression, a phenomenon that also occurs in many other viral infections. However, the immunosuppression in AIDS is more severe because HIV selectively binds to and infects key cells in the immune system – dendritic cells, helper T cells, and monocytes.

Infection of dendritic cells leads to compromise of the immune response and reduced T-lymphocyte responses. Activation of infected T cells results in the inversion of the CD4 to CD8 cell ratio and an absolute decrease in CD4-expressing cells. This loss of helper cells cripples the entire immune response, not only to HIV but to other opportunistic infections.

Monocytes are also damaged during HIV infection. Monocytes are important to the co-ordination and function of the immune response and the compromise and loss of monocytes is as critical as damage to helper T cells. In the CNS (and probably all other tissues), infection of monocytes and compromise of monocyte function is thought to lead directly to HIV specific damage.

During the course of the disease, activation of both the humoral and cellular limbs of the immune response occurs. However, this activation is not sufficient to control the spread of infection. Neutralizing antibodies to the variable region of HIV (see Fig. 6.7) develop only late in the course of the disease, and their expression remains at low levels. It has been suggested that even when an early response occurs, this may have the paradoxical effect of enhancing infection because of their interaction with the Fc receptor.

Impairment of T-helper cell activity by viral or immunopathogenic mechanisms would be expected to lead to diminished T cell and B cell proliferative responses, aggravating immune depression. Delayed type hypersensitivity (DTH) reactions may be active in systemic infection with HIV, but are not thought to be very effective in clearing the virus. Although active in initial phases of infection with HIV, cell-mediated immune responses diminish along with the health of the patient.

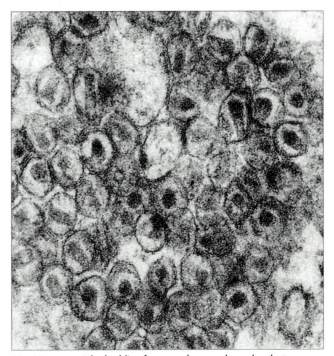

Fig. 6.8 HIV particles budding from membranes, shown by electron microscopy. (Reproduced from *Brain Pathology* 1991;1: No 3.)

HIV Entry into the CNS

HIV probably gains entry into the CNS by way of infected mono-cytes or macrophages. It is quite possible that the activation of the body's normal defence mechanisms caused by opportunistic infections of the CNS provide the stimulus for the infiltration of infected monocytes into the brain. Macrophages and multi-nucleated giant cells can be identified as sites of HIV replication within the brain.

HIV infection can be associated with an acute meningitis. In many patients, infection of the meninges will be the only apparent site of CNS involvement (Fig. 6.9). HIV can be consistently identi-fied in CSF, and this indicates that a chronic low-grade infection of the meninges might be present throughout the course of the disease. The factors that trigger the spread of HIV into the brain are unknown, but responses to concurrent infections are probably involved (as discussed above). Spread of infection from meninges to brain is comparatively rare in other viral infections (e.g. polio) and this represents an important difference between HIV and other viral infections of the CNS.

HIV and Cell Damage

Considerable cellular damage can occur as a consequence of HIV infection. However, the pathological processes that lead to cell-ular damage are the subject of debate. Two main types of process have been suggested:

- direct damage can be caused by interaction between the HIV envelope protein gp120 and the CD4 receptor. This leads to membrane changes and cell fusion. Complexes of gp120 and CD4 accumulate in nuclear pores and disrupt mRNA transport and protein metabolism; or
- indirect damage can be caused by disrupting the function of infected cells. In the CNS, macrophages produce many sub-stances (cytokines, prostaglandins, leukotrienes, kynurenines, oxidative radicals, and protease), and these can be neurotoxic in particular situations (see Chapter 3).

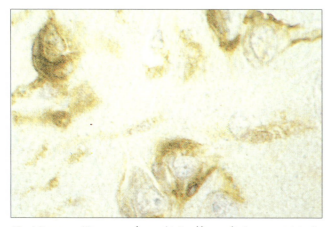

Fig. 6.9 HIV-positive macrophages (stained brown by immunostaining) in the central nervous system. (Reproduced from *Brain Pathology* 1991;1: No 3.)

NEUROPATHOLOGY

Gross Pathology

Ventricular dilatation and gyral atrophy are commonly seen in the brains of patients with the AIDS dementia complex. These findings are consistent with the pattern of atrophy seen in CT and MRI scans. Occasionally, meningeal fibrosis can also be seen. Sectioning of the brain often reveals the presence of patho-logy caused by adventitious infections such as mycoplasma or herpes simplex. Careful examination can also reveal rarefaction of the central white matter. In some cases diffuse or focal micro-vacuolation of the white matter also occurs (Fig. 6.10).

Neuropathology

Opportunistic infections of the CNS are common in patients with the AIDS dementia complex. In view of this the pattern of pathological change that is found in the brain is dictated by a combination of:

- specific AIDS dementia complex pathology; and
- pathology resulting from the opportunistic infection (Fig. 6.11).

Early reports of the brain pathology found in AIDS patients were dominated by descriptions of the effect of cytomegalovirus infections and toxoplasmosis. (The pathological features of such infections have been described many times and will not be reiterated here.) After these early reports, more detailed studies indicated that a constellation of pathological change could be

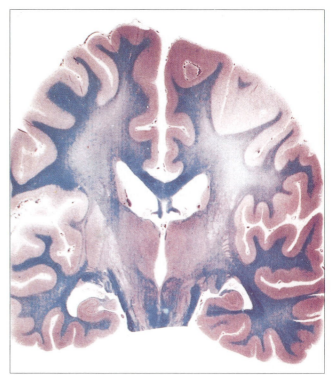

Fig. 6.10 Rarefaction of central white matter (myelin stain). (Reproduced from *Brain Pathology* 1991;1: No 3.)

specifically related to the presence of HIV within the brain. Giant multinucleated cells clustered around blood vessels are present in most cases and are thought to arise as a result of HIV-induced cell fusion, perivascular infiltrates (macrophages, lymphocytes, and microglia, along with multinucleated cells), and they occur in the presence of diffuse astrocytosis (Fig. 6.12). This is accompanied by widespread neuronal loss and dendritic pathology.

A consensus on the main types of CNS pathology specifically related to the AIDS dementia complex has been reached (*Brain Pathology*, 1991) and includes:

- HIV encephalitis;
- HIV leukoencephalopathy;
- vacuolar myelopathy and vacuolar leukoencephalopathy;
- lymphocytic meningitis;
- diffuse poliodystrophy; and
- cerebral vasculitis (including granulomatous angiitis).

HIV encephalitis (HIVE)

Multiple HIVE foci are a characteristic feature within the brain and are found in the white matter, basal ganglia, and cortex (Fig. 6.13). The foci contain large amounts of non-integrated HIV DNA and HIV proteins. Electron microscopy has demonstrated aggregations of HIV within the cytoplasm or associated with the membrane. Necrosis can occur in the centre of large foci. HIVE foci may be associated with sponginess and myelin loss. However, the neurons and neuronal processes in the immediate vicinity of HIVE foci often appear to be unaffected, and obvious associations between foci and neuronal degeneration is rare.

Blood vessels in close proximity to HIVE foci can show fibrinoid extravasation indicating a breakdown in the blood–brain barrier. HIVE is present in about 10 per cent of patients with AIDS brains and a combination of HIVE and HIV leukoencephalopathy is found in a further 10 per cent.

HIV leukoencephalopathy (HIVL)

Progressive diffuse damage to white matter is a second major feature of the neuropathology of HIV-associated cognitive/motor complex. Myelin loss is easily visualized as pallor in myelin stains, usually in a symmetrical distribution. Myelin breakdown products are also commonly found in macrophages in the same regions. Numerous HIV-producing cells are scattered between the damaged myelin (Fig. 6.14). Vacuolar swelling within the myelin (vacuolar myelinopathy) may also be present. HIVL is only diagnosed in the presence of HIV-producing cells; this distinguishes the leukoencephalopathy of AIDS from that seen in conditions such as Binswanger's disease (see Chapter 3).

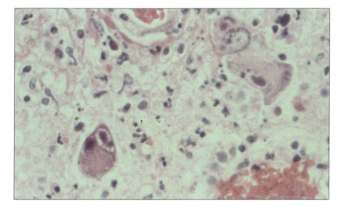

Fig. 6.11 Cytomegalovirus infection of the central nervous system in an HIV patient. (Courtesy of Professor P Lantos, London.)

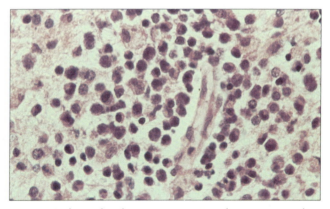

Fig. 6.12 Malignant lymphoma in an HIV patient, showing perivascular clustering of cells. (Haematoxylin and eosin stain.) (Courtesy of Professor P Lantos, London.)

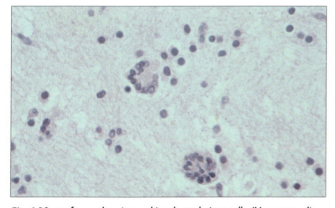

Fig. 6.13 HIV focus, showing multinucleated giant cells. (Haematoxylin and eosin stain.) (Courtesy of Professor P Lantos, London.)

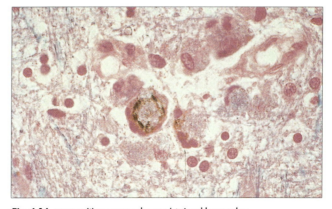

Fig. 6.14 HIV-positive macrophages (stained brown by immunostaining) in the central nervous system. (Reproduced from *Brain Pathology* 1991;1: No 3.)

Vacuolar myelopathy

This pathology is not specific to AIDS, and should only be diagnosed in the presence of HIV-producing cells.

Vacuolar leukoencephalopathy

This is relatively uncommon, and mainly affects the white matter of the cortex, basal ganglia, and brain stem.

Lymphocytic meningitis

As previously discussed, the spread of HIV infection from meninges to brain is not understood.

Diffuse poliodystrophy

Diffuse glial reaction is common in the brains of patients with AIDS. Often there is a separation between sites of HIV-producing cells and regions of gliosis. It is possible that the diffuse glial reaction marks the site of neuronal loss and dendritic atrophy (see below).

Cerebral vasculitis

The relationship between this pathological phenomenon and other types of pathology or HIV infection is not known.

Neuronal degeneration

Two other types of pathology have also been described and may have considerable clinical significance:
- neuronal loss; and
- dendritic atrophy.

Neuronal loss

Neuronal loss can be marked (e.g. up to 30 per cent in frontal cortex) yet the paucity or absence of productive infection within (or lysis of) neurons and glial cells indicates that a simple direct pathological effect of HIV infection on these cells is not a prominent feature.

Indirect pathological mechanisms of cellular degeneration are probably the main cause of neuronal loss in HIV dementia complex. This is an important pathological characteristic of the condition. A variety of molecular events underlie the mechanism of the indirect pathology:
- the release of toxic substances by infected cells (e.g. cell-coded products like cytokines) or toxic products of viral genes;
- interference of gp120 (HIV envelope glycoprotein) with the trophic properties of neuroleukin; and
- interference of gp120 with neurotransmitter function (e.g. vasoactive intestinal peptide – VIP).

Dendritic atrophy

Recent studies on the prefrontal cortex in patients with HIV-associated cognitive and motor complex has demonstrated a loss of synapses and dendritic pathology. Apical dendrites were dilated and showed evidence of vacuolation. The length and branching of these dendrites was reduced. Basal and oblique dendrites were not affected to the same degree. Spine density was reduced by over 40 per cent along the entire length of the dendrites. These studies indicate that dendritic damage may be a primary change underlying the clinical symptoms of HIV-associated cognitive and motor complex. If correct, this post-synaptic focus of pathology is in marked contrast to the pre-synaptic pathology found in other neurodegenerative dementias.

PATHOGENESIS

HIV-associated cognitive and motor complex is believed to be directly caused by the infection of the brain with HIV-1 for the following reasons:
- Southern blot analysis shows a high frequency and copy number of proviral HIV DNA in the brains of patients with this condition;
- *in situ* hybridization has revealed the presence of viral RNA in these brains;
- immunohistochemistry has detected HIV-1 antigens;
- electron microscopy has identified viral particles; and
- HIV-1 has been directly cultured from the brain and CSF of demented patients.

Immunohistochemical and hybridization techniques have sometimes failed to demonstrate the presence of the virus even in advanced stages of the syndrome, but the more sensitive polymerase chain reaction (PCR) is now able to detect HIV-1 sequences in virtually all patients, and the extent of the proviral sequence distribution in the brain, as detected by this technique, has been found to correlate with the severity of dementia.

The main determinants of the degree of neuronal loss and thus dementia are:
- the virus load; and
- viral neurotoxicity.

Virus Load

HIV replication rates rise during the course of the illness. Extensive replication within the CNS generally occurs late in the disease. It is possible that HIV can enter the CNS only after the compromise of the peripheral immune system or that the amount of HIV entering the CNS rises as a consequence of opportunistic infections of the CNS. The extent of HIV replication within the CNS correlates with the extent of neuropathology and the severity of clinical symptoms.

One important question yet to be answered fully concerns the postulated existence of neurotropic variants of HIV-1. HIV-1 has a high rate of mutation, and the gene coding for the envelope glycoprotein gp120 appears to be particularly variable. It has been reported that viral CSF or brain isolates behave differently from blood isolates in lymphocyte cell cultures. This indicates that there might arise neurotropic strains that preferentially replicate within the CNS. It is possible that neurotropism is required for replication in the CNS and that the lack of neurotropism explains the observation that not all the patients whose brains are infected with HIV-1 and who are significantly immuno-suppressed develop the dementia syndrome. Other possible explanations of the occurrence of severe cognitive decline in some patients but not in others include the synergistic effect of other pathogens, and the genetic susceptibility of the host.

HIV and Neuropathology

The type and extent of pathology seen in AIDS dementia complex poses interesting questions as to its genesis. Neuronal and synaptic loss is regionally selective, and there appears to be no direct correlation between the presence of sites of HIV replication and sites of neuronal loss. For example, neuronal loss in AIDS brains is present in the frontal but not in the parietal cortex, and it is not co-localized with the presence of HIVE-type neuropathology.

Proteins secreted from cell types affected by HIV (e.g. cyto-kines from microglia) can cause damage to neurons and axons if secretion is uncontrolled, and this may be a cause of pathology. However, neurons surrounding HIVE foci are usually unaffected, although damage may only be apparent after prolonged periods of close contact.

Therefore, although increased amounts of HIV in the CNS and the amount of neuronal damage can be related in a global fashion for the whole brain, neuronal loss and HIV replication are not co-localized. This presents a considerable problem for our understanding of the pathophysiology of the disease.

HIV and neurodegeneration

The neurodegenerative effects resulting from HIV infection of monocytes might result from HIV proteins:

- having direct neurotoxic effects;
- blocking essential trophic factor or transmitter receptors; or
- stimulating the release of neurotoxic factors from microglial cells or macrophages.

Factors produced by HIV-infected macrophages can produce degeneration of glia and neurons in cell culture. The HIV tat peptide (basic region 49–57) can modify membrane permeability, and this could lead to degeneration. It is also possible that the process of neurodegeneration occurs over a considerable period of time and progresses through an initial stage of functional impairment before degeneration of neuronal structure. Initial functional impairment with eventual neuronal destruction might explain the observations that patients treated with AZT show improvements in cognitive function.

HIV gp120 proteins, glutamate, and neurotoxicity

At least one of the proteins of HIV has been demonstrated to have neurotoxic effects (Lipton, 1991). The HIV-1 envelop glyco-protein gp120 is shed by the virus. Fragments of gp120 are released from HIV-infected monocytes, macrophages, or microglia that harbour the virus in the CNS. Experiments demonstrate that, in tissue culture, low picomolar concentrations of gp120 produce an early rise in neuronal intracellular calcium concen-tration and, subsequently, neuronal injury.

The effects of gp120 are dose dependent. The dose–response curve of gp120 induced neuronal injury has an inverted 'U' shape. Picomolar levels causing increases in intracellular calcium and subsequent neuronal injury, nanomolar concentrations of gp120 (10–1000 times more concentrated) are reported not to be toxic to neurons and may block NMDA-receptor-operated ion channels, so preventing NMDA-elicited increases in calcium influx.

These and other data suggest that both gp120 and glutamate-related molecules are necessary for neuronal cell dysfunction and damage. They probably act synergistically because neither one alone is sufficient to produce pathological effects at low concentrations. This mechanism of toxicity is essentially the same as that mediated by excessive stimulation of the NMDA subtype of excitatory amino acid receptors. Such increases in intracellular calcium are thought to represent a final common pathway for a diverse group of acute and chronic neurological insults (ranging from stroke to neurodegenerative dementias) that induce neuronal cell death (see Chapter 3).

It is probable that gp120 sensitizes neurons to the lethal effects of excitatory amino acids acting at the NMDA receptor (Fig. 6.15). It is not known whether these effects are primarily:

- direct;
- macrophage mediated; or
- astrocyte mediated.

Direct neuronal injury   Neuronal injury could be directly mediated by gp120 or by a fragment of gp120 that is shed by infected macrophages or microglia (see Fig. 16.15a). This mechanism would require a specific interaction between gp120 and the NMDA receptor to make the neuron sensitive to glutamate and thus cause a direct neurotoxic effect.

Macrophage-mediated neuronal injury   Human monocytes can secrete factors that cause neuronal degeneration. These cells possess the CD4 receptor which binds the HIV gp120 protein, and gp120 might induce secretion from macrophages even in the absence of active HIV infection. Infection of monocytes could increase their rates of secretion and, in addition, infected mono-cytes can also secrete the gp120 protein. Macrophages may proteolyse gp120 and release a fragment of the molecule that is neurotoxic (see Fig. 16.15c).

Some of the factors released by macrophages stimulate NMDA receptor-mediated neurotoxicity directly (because NMDA ant-agonists are known to block this form of neuronal damage). However, gp120-related neurotoxicity requires the activation of NMDA receptors by endogenous excitatory amino acids. Thus, gp120 acts synergistically to amplify the normal mechanism of excitation into one of excitotoxicity. It is possible that other, potentially toxic, factors released by macrophages have similar indirect actions on the NMDA receptor channel complex.

Fragments of gp120 bind to galactosyl ceramide, a molecule found on the surfce of oligodendrocytes. HIV might also infect this type of cell leading to the disruption of myelin formation and indirect neuronal injury.

HIV Related Neurotoxicity

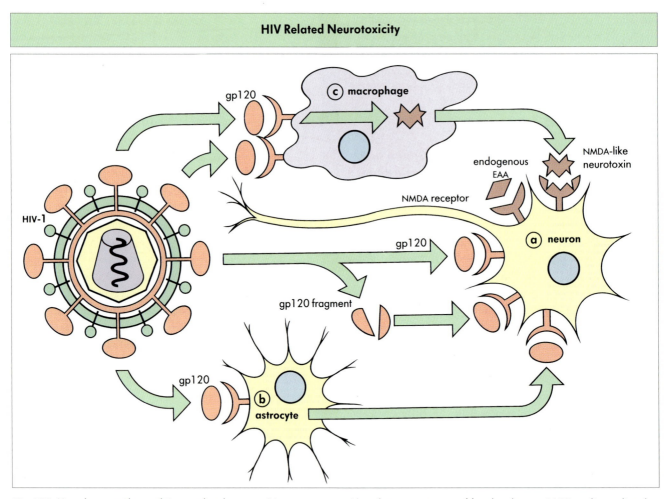

Fig. 6.15 Hypotheses used to explain HIV-related neurotoxicity.
(a) Direct neuronal injury: neurotoxicity may be directly mediated by
gp120 or a fragment of gp120; (b) Astrocyte-mediated neuronal
injury: gp120 or a gp120 fragment may bind to astrocytes, competing
with VIP for a receptor, possibly related to CD; (c) Microglia-mediated
neuronal injury: monocytoid cells (e.g. macrophages and microglia)
infected with HIV-1 may secrete toxic factors which lead to
neuronal destruction.

Astrocyte-mediated neuronal injury It is also possible that
gp120 or a gp120 fragment from infected macrophages or microglia binds to astrocytes. The gp120 glycoprotein or its fragment
could compete with vasoactive intestinal polypeptide (VIP), or
possibly peptide T, for a specific receptor site that might be
related to CD4 (competition could also occur for similar receptors
on neurons). VIP is thought to influence the release of neuronal
growth factors by astrocytes (e.g. protease nexin). By binding
competitively to such receptors, gp120 would interfere with this
and similar VIP-mediated processes (see Fig. 16.15b).

THERAPY

At least three approaches to therapy are under development
(Fig. 16.16):
- immunization with vaccines to HIV;
- inhibition of HIV replication; and
- blocking the neurotoxic effects of HIV protein (e.g. gp120) and
  the factors released by monocytes.

Vaccines
The genes coding for HIV-coat proteins have high mutation
rates. The resultant changes in protein structure make the development of effective vaccines very difficult.

Inhibiting replication
HIV is a retrovirus and requires the action of reverse transcriptase
for replication. The actions of this enzyme can be blocked. AIDS
patients are treated with AZT, a thymidine analogue that acts to
disrupt the action of reverse transcriptase. At present, this is the
only effective treatment for AIDS. Whilst it slows down or stops
the progression of the disease, AZT does not destroy the virus nor
eliminate its infectivity. AZT is toxic in some patients and in
higher concentrations (approximately 100-fold) it can block the
action of the normal cellular α-DNA transcriptase.

Inhibiting neurotoxicity
AIDS-related neuronal injury could be mediated by several
pathways that most likely originate from toxins released by
HIV-infected macrophages. There may be an intricate web of

neurotoxic factors interacting with macrophages (or microglia), astrocytes, and neurons. Even so, this complex network may become amenable to pharmacotherapy because of common final pathways of attack involving growth factors, NMDA receptors, and deleteriously high levels of intracellular calcium.

DIFFERENTIAL DIAGNOSIS

Known AIDS patients

Differentiating the cognitive and neurological effects of (potentially treatable) opportunistic infections, neoplasms and metabolic encephalopathies from those caused by the neurodegenerative effects of HIV are the main difficulties.

Common infections include cryptococcal meningitis, cytomegalovirus, herpes simplex, and cerebral toxoplasmosis. These can be detected with appropriate diagnostic tests. Electrolyte imbalance, kidney or liver disease can give rise to metabolic

encephalopathies, and can be determined by laboratory investigations. The clinical course of the cognitive deficits can be a useful diagnostic indicator. Abrupt onset of symptoms, rapid progression, and fluctuations in state of consciousness indicate opportunistic diseases.

CT and MRI can demonstrate the presence of space-occupying lesions (toxoplasmosis, fungal infections) or the cerebral atrophy and white matter abnormalities characteristic of HIV-1-associated cognitive and motor complex. However, when the dementia complex and opportunistic infections co-exist, differentiating between them on the basis of imaging may not be possible.

Unconfirmed AIDS patients

Differential diagnosis in HIV-seronegative patients is extremely difficult. Depending on the patient's age, possible diagnoses include multiple sclerosis and all the neuropsychiatric disorders. A thorough clinical history and a consideration of the patient's lifestyle in relation to known risk factors may prove useful.

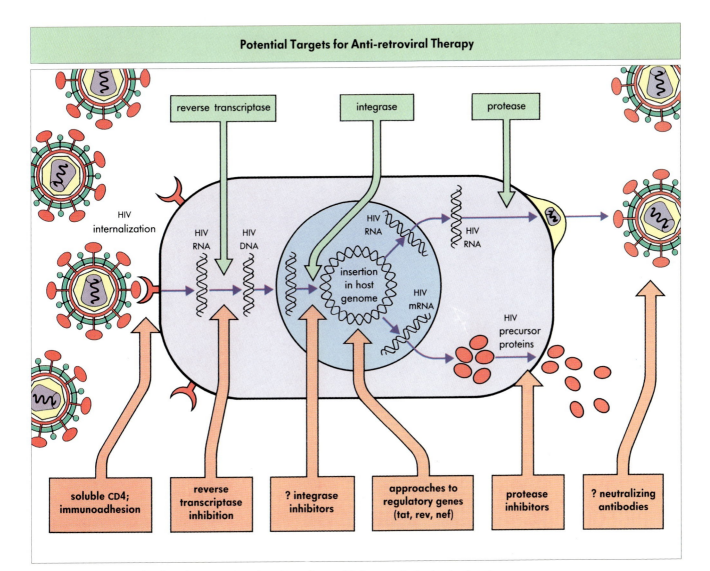

Fig. 6.16 Replication cycle of HIV, showing points where it may be possible to use antiretrovirus treatments.

SUMMARY

(i) HIV-associated cognitive and motor complex is a complication of HIV-1 infection of the CNS.

(ii) Approximately 10 per cent of AIDS patients develop a dementing syndrome.

(iii) The dementia is characterized by the presence of fine motor signs and symptoms and the absence of apraxia, aphasia, and agnosia.

(iv) The organic substrate of these symptoms is a result of a direct infection of the CNS.

(v) HIV-1 brain infection is characterized by the presence of HIV encephalitis and HIV leukodystrophy.

(vi) Dendritic damage with loss of spines is prominent and the post-synaptic pattern of damage may be an important feature.

(vii) HIV replication and neuronal damage are not co-localized.

(viii) Neuronal dysfunction and destruction is caused by direct neuronal injury, and by astrocyte-mediated and macrophage-mediated neuronal injury.

(ix) Effective therapy in AIDS is currently limited to blocking reverse transcriptase in order to inhibit viral replication.

7 Prion Disease

INTRODUCTION

Prion disease is a new nosological entity, derived from research which has uncovered a common molecular pathology underlying the disparate collection of syndromes previously known as the spongiform encephalopathies, unconventional viral infections, or transmissible dementias. These include the following neurodegenerative disorders:

- Creutzfeldt–Jakob disease (CJD);
- Gerstmann–Sträussler–Sheinker syndrome (GSS);
- Kuru.

Their collective name of spongiform encephalopathy derives from the characteristic vacuolar, spongy appearance of the brain seen at post-mortem. In 1959, the pathological similarities between CJD, kuru, and the sheep disease scrapie were first noted. Following these observations, essentially identical diseases (going by different names) are now recognized to occur in many species (Fig. 7.1). For 30 years these disorders have been the subject of research interest out of proportion to their apparent rarity because of a number of unique features. Most notably, the human forms have been shown to be transmissible by inoculation, both to other species, and also iatrogenically from person to person after transplantation, neurosurgery, and therapeutic procedures (e.g. treatment with human growth hormone). In addition, the human forms can also be inherited in an autosomal dominant fashion.

Prion disease shows an array of clinical presentations and neuropathological findings, apparently overlapping not only with each other but also with other neurodegenerative disorders. Until recently, there was no way unequivocally to separate one 'disease' from another, since neither the clinical nor neuropathological findings are pathognomonic. However, advances from molecular biology and immunocytochemistry have provided a means for a simpler and more rational grouping of these disorders based on their underlying features. These advances also suggest that the diseases may be commoner than hitherto suspected, increasing their potential clinical significance.

These diseases all have a common pathology which involves the conversion of a normal cell protein (prion protein – PrP) into an abnormal isoform (PrP^P). In view of the central and unifying role of prion protein, it has been suggested that the transmissible dementias be renamed the 'prion diseases' to reflect this. The invariable association of abnormal prion protein with the spongiform encephalopathies and with transmissibility provides a basis for categorizing these disorders.

Prion disease is a relatively rare neurodegenerative disorder with a variable age of onset. It can be inherited (autosomal dominant), sporadic (somatic mutation), or transmitted as summarized in Fig. 7.2. Typically, patients begin with minor motor signs, such as cerebellar ataxia, and progress to global dementia. Neurological signs are common. The pathology is usually characterized by the presence of an abnormal protease-

Prion Disease	
Humans	Creutzfeldt–Jakob disease (sporadic)
	Creutzfeldt–Jakob disease (familial)
	Gerstmann–Sträussler–Sheinker syndrome
	Kuru
	Atypical dementia
Sheep	Scrapie
Cow	Bovine spongiform encephalopathy
Cat	Feline spongiform encephalopathy
Mule, deer	Chronic wasting disease
Mink	Transmissible mink encephalopathy
Kudu	Transmissible encephalopathy
Nyala	Transmissible encephalopathy
Mice	Murine spongiform encephalopathy
Monkey	Transmissible encephalopathy

Fig. 7.1 Prion disease in humans and animals.

Types of Prion Disease in Humans		
Type	**Mechanism**	**Example**
Genetic	Mutation in germ line	Gerstmann–Sträussler–Sheinker syndrome
Sporadic	Mutation in somatic DNA	Creutzfeldt–Jakob disease
	Post-translational change in gene product	Sporadic CJD without apparent DNA mutation
Infectious	Iatrogenically induced	Growth-hormone related
	By contamination	Creutzfeldt–Jakob disease
	Cannibalism	Kuru

Fig. 7.2 Types of Prion disease.

resistant isoform of the cellular prion protein. The presence of the abnormal prion protein in the CNS is diagnostic.

Epidemiology

The true extent of Prion disease in the population is unknown at present. This is due to its recent emergence as a single nosological entity. A guide to the epidemiology of Prion disease can be obtained by looking at the figures for Creutzfeldt–Jakob disease. CJD is found all over the world and has a prevalence of one to two cases per million of the population. Higher rates than this have been recorded in some regions or populations, such as amongst Libyan Jews and in areas of central Slovakia, Hungary, and eastern England. It is now known that these high local rates are accounted for by large families with genetic lesions in the prion gene. Approximately equal numbers of men and women

are affected and around 10 per cent of cases are familial. The age at onset is usually between 55 and 75, with a peak frequency in the 60s (Fig. 7.3). Rare cases with onset as young as 16 or as old as 85 have been reported.

The disease is generally diagnosed using the criteria for CJD. However since the clinical phenotype is known to be very variable, these criteria mean that cases might be misdiagnosed, particularly in patients over 70.

CLINICAL FEATURES

Molecular biology offers the surest method of diagnosis. Detection of the abnormal isoform of prion protein in CNS tissue by immunological techniques (e.g. Western blots or inserts in the prion gene) are diagnostic (Figs 7.4 and 7.5).

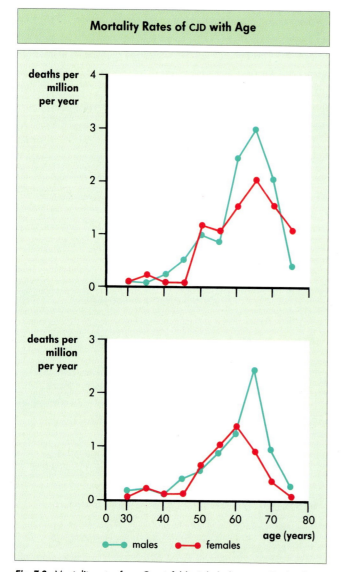

Fig. 7.3 Mortality rates from Creutzfeldt–Jakob disease in England and Wales: (a) 1980–1984; (b) 1970–1979. (Adapted from Will and Matthews, 1985.)

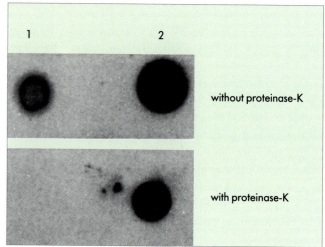

Fig. 7.4 Diagnostic testing for Prion disease using Western blotting. Blocks of protease-treated brain extract reveal the presence of PrP^p when immunostained (1 = control, 2 = CJD).

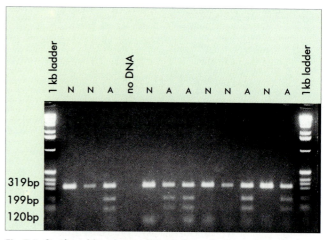

Fig. 7.5 Southern blot of gene defect in Prion disease. Additional bands are present in affected cases (A) which are not found in controls (N). By courtesy of Dr J. Collinge, London.

When such tests are not available or cannot be completed, diagnosis is based on the exclusion of similar conditions such as Huntington's chorea and Alzheimer's disease. In general the speed of disease progression is one of the best indicators. Confirmation of a clinical diagnosis by neuropathological examination is essential.

Course

It is not really possible to give a complete clinical description of Prion disease, for the recent discovery of familial cases with mutations within the prion gene has expanded (and continues to expand) our appreciation of the phenotype.

The presentation is variable, and ranges from an insidious onset typical of Alzheimer's disease to insomnia. Within families, the length of illness and the mode of presentation can differ widely. This is complemented by the huge variation observed in the neuropathology of the condition.

Despite the variability of the whole course of the disease, many of the patients, at one time or another, exhibit some of the symptoms which are found in the more circumscribed clinical descriptions of Creutzfeldt–Jakob disease. Therefore, a brief description of the core features of this syndrome will be given.

Typical Creutzfeldt–Jakob disease (CJD)

This syndrome was originally described in the early 1920s. It has since become apparent that, although CJD has a distinctive typical picture, it is only a variant of Prion disease. The main clinical features of the syndrome are: rapid progression, motor symptoms, dementia, and abnormal EEG activity.

A typical case of CJD is that of a presenile dementia, in the absence of a family history, occurring in the sixth decade and progressing rapidly to death within a year.

There is usually a brief prodromal stage, lasting a few weeks or months, characterized by feelings of fatigue, insomnia, anxiety, and depression. This develops into complaints of slowing of thought processes, impairment of memory, difficulty in concentrating, and, occasionally, behavioural disturbances. Patients may also present with giddiness, difficulties in balancing, and problems with walking.

Although a psychogenic disorder may be suspected initially, intellectual deterioration is relentless and neurological deficits appear. Neurological deficits can affect any system; they include cerebellar ataxias, spasticity of limbs with progressive paralysis, extrapyramidal rigidity, and tremor. Deficits in speech and vision also occur, with dysphasia, dysarthria, and cortical blindness. There are usually no other sensory changes. Myoclonic jerks are often seen and epileptic fits can occur.

Cognitive deficits appear; these progress over a period of weeks. The initial acute organic picture (clouding of consciousness or frank delirium) rapidly develops into a profound dementia with rigidity or spastic paralysis. A decorticate or decerebrate posture is often present, with repetitive myoclonic jerking. Deepening coma precedes death usually within two years.

Clinical Investigations

CT or MRI scans rarely show gross cortical atrophy or ventricular enlargement, except in the end stages or in cases with a long survival time. The speed of progression suggests the presence of an expanding intracranial mass, and CT and MRI provide useful negative data in this respect. The presence of a normal scan in a patient with a rapidly progressing dementia is useful in differential diagnosis.

Cerebrospinal fluid CSF is usually normal throughout the course of the illness.

Electro-encephalography Investigations with EEG often show marked abnormalities, which alter during the course of the disease:

- initially, diffuse or focal slowing;
- then, repetitive bilaterally synchronous sharp waves or slow spike and wave discharges;
- finally, synchronous triphasic sharp wave complexes (1–2 per second), superimposed on progressive suppression of cortical background activity.

These triphasic complexes seen late in the course of the disease have been regarded as diagnostic of the condition.

Biopsy Brain biopsy can be used to obtain material for neuropathological and immunocytochemical examination. Establishing the presence of the abnormal PrP^P isoform confirms the diagnosis. In general, the course is much more rapid than that of other primary degenerative diseases.

Clinical Variability

The emphasis on particular clinical features of marked severity in individual cases has led to many subtypes being recognized. Two examples are an ataxic form with prominent cerebellar signs, and a variety named after Heidenhain (1929) with severe occipital cortical involvement. However a close examination of these and other cases demonstrates that these variants lie within the broad spectrum of the disorder, so that much overlapping of pathological and clinical features is evident from case to case, and the continuation of subtypes in the clinical or pathological descriptions of the disorder appears to be unjustified.

Prion disease can be atypical in several ways. A familial form exists, accounting for 6–15 per cent of cases. These tend to be younger than sporadic cases but survive longer. Familial cases may also be less transmissible to primates (64 per cent of cases compared to over 90 per cent of sporadic CJD).

Gerstmann–Sträussler–Sheinker syndrome (GSS) is rarer than CJD, and is an autosomal dominant cerebellar disorder, in which dementia tends to be mild. Mean age of death is earlier than in CJD (around 50 years old) but the duration of illness is longer (four to five years). Most pathological features are similar to those of CJD, but amyloid plaques in the cortex and cerebellum (see below) are invariably present. Like CJD, the pathology of GSS may sometimes overlap with that of Alzheimer's disease and the clinical and pathological pictures of GSS and CJD merge into each other.

Kuru is another cerebellar ataxia, associated with tremor and dementia, which runs a fulminating course leading to incapacitation and death within a year. It is notable mainly for its historical importance in establishing the transmissibility of the spongiform encephalopathies. However, it is unlikely to be encountered outside the Fore tribe of New Guinea, and is reputed to have virtually disappeared since the ending of particular funeral rites.

ACCIDENTAL TRANSMISSION OF PRION DISEASES

Once the fundamental similarity between animal and human types of spongiform encephalopathy was appreciated, the experimental evidence for transmissibility of these disorders within and between species led to concern. Several points can be made.

The recent spread of Prion disease to cows and cats in the UK, and the experimental transmission to pigs – all species not previously known to be affected – underlines the potential of all animals who possess a prion gene to develop Prion disease when challenged with the abnormal isoform of the prion protein (PrP^P). However, it is important to put this risk into perspective. For example, the extensive scrapie research is reassuring: there is no epidemiological association between the prevalence of classically diagnosed CJD and that of scrapie, nor a clear association with 'high-risk' occupations such as pathology technicians and butchers, despite anecdotal reports and occasional findings to the contrary. The occurrence of CJD in a lifelong vegetarian may also provide comfort to meat-eaters. More importantly, experimental oral transmission is calculated to be 10^9 times less efficient than intracerebral inoculation (although 1g of infected tissue may be sufficient for transmission to animals) and often fails to produce disease at all.

Furthermore, the apparent spread of kuru via cannibalism may in fact have been due to the agent entering through cuts and mucous membranes during ritual ceremonies with affected corpses. Whilst a similar route of infection would not preclude bovine spongiform encephalopathy (the form of Prion disease found in cows) being a health risk, it would minimize the risk still further to all except those handling animals or their carcasses on a regular basis.

Patient Management in Relation to Risk of Infection

The related question of precautions required when managing cases of human Prion disease is easier to answer: Prion disease patients are not infectious and should be so treated. This is in keeping with the epidemiological data, which show no convincing evidence of person-to-person spread. However, since internal organs, blood, and cerebrospinal fluid all contain varying degrees of infectivity, venepuncture, lumbar puncture, and surgical procedures on patients with atypical dementia should be carried out with appropriate precautions; this also applies to handling of specimens and of equipment afterwards. Additionally, by virtue of the proven iatrogenic spread of CJD, no patient with dementia should be a donor of any kind (including blood).

The potential infectivity of tissues also has implications for their handling after death. Post-mortem permission and full neuropathological investigation (including PrP immunostaining) should always be sought in order to establish diagnosis, but the possibility of a transmissible dementia should be documented and the case discussed with the pathologist. It is unfortunate that, because of exaggerated fears of the infection risk, autopsies are rarely performed on atypical dementia cases. This is a major obstacle to pathological and epidemiological understanding of the spongiform encephalopathies.

Partly as a result of the low autopsy rate, and the tendency to certify 'Alzheimer's disease' as the cause of death for any dementia lacking tissue diagnosis, the true prevalence of the prion diseases (as opposed to classical CJD and GSS) is unknown. However, it is likely to be higher than the often quoted figure of 0.5 per million (corresponding to 30 cases per year in the UK and approximately 125 in the USA). For example, extrapolation from figures provided by a 'straw poll' of neuropathologists gave a theoretical range for these disorders of 2–12 per cent of all dementias, or 1500–9000 cases in the UK per year. Even if the latter range overestimates the true prevalence by a factor of ten, the prion diseases are still seriously underdiagnosed at present. Such uncertainties must be taken into account when interpreting epidemiological surveys or assessing apparent changes in disease incidence over the next few years.

DIAGNOSIS – DETECTION OF PrP

Reliable detection of PrP^P by immunostaining or other methods can define the diseases and can be used as a diagnostic test (see Fig. 7.4).

Within the rubric of the prion diseases, a subgrouping could be based on the origin of the PrP^P in terms of genetic, sporadic/ idiopathic or iatrogenic factors (see Fig. 7.2). The disease could then be classified further in terms of the specific molecular causes (e.g. the exact prion mutation) as such details become pathological features. At present, the identification of PrP^P can only be carried out on brain tissue either at biopsy or autopsy. However, genetic analysis is rapidly becoming a diagnostic tool at regional centres, and it is hoped that improvements in immunological techniques will allow a test to be developed for demonstration of PrP^P in serum.

The value of PrP testing over the conventional diagnostic approaches to possible transmissible dementias is illustrated by a recent extreme example, in which a familial CJD patient shared the prion gene mutation seen in other affected members of his family (Figs 7.6 and 7.7), yet at post-mortem the brain did not show significant pathology. Moreover, this patient had satisfied apparent. This approach supersedes the inevitably inconclusive debates as to the correct nomenclature for each clinicopathological variant, or the relationship between one syndrome and another.

The clinical overlap with other atypical dementias would remain a problem but could unequivocally be resolved by prion gene or protein analysis, irrespective of confounding clinical or pathological features. At present, the identification of PrP^P can only be carried out on brain tissue either at biopsy or autopsy. However, genetic analysis is rapidly becoming a diagnostic

Family Tree of Affected Pedigree

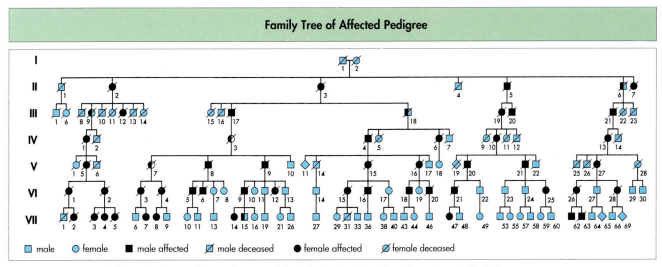

Fig. 7.6 Family tree of affected pedigree; the case histories of the individuals V 27 and VII 63 are given in Fig. 7.7.

Case Histories of V27 and VII63

V27 female. Born 1904. Born prematurely but had normal childhood. She married at age 19 and had three children. Several years later she separated from her husband. She moved away to seek work. Occasional letters to her father were described as strange with unusual handwriting. At age 38 she visited her sister who felt that she seemed different and anxious. At age 45 she was admitted to hospital with what was estimated to be a five-year history of progressive dementia. She was disorientated with gross memory impairment and loss of intellect. She was euphoric. She had marked chorea, ataxia, and extrapyramidal rigidity with pyramidal signs. A diagnosis of presenile dementia was made, and Huntington's disease or chorea following encephalitis were considered. Several months later, she was noted to be dysarthric and to have limb spasticity with an equivocal plantar reflex. A diagnosis of presenile dementia was made. The possibility of Creutzfeldt–Jakob disease was considered. Jerky movement of the upper limbs were noted. EEG was abnormal but without specific features. A repeat EEG eight months later was diffusely abnormal. She died at 46 from bronchopneumonia.

VII63 male. Born 1952. Both his mother and maternal grandmother had developed presenile dementia. He exhibited several antisocial personality traits during childhood, including

theft, fighting, and being verbally abusive. He left school aged 17 with no qualifications. His IQ was later assessed to be 100. He was referred to a psychiatrist at age 19 because of antisocial behaviour; at this stage he was working as an unskilled labourer. By the age of 21 he was married with one son. He became increasingly aggressive from his early 20s, in particular towards his wife. His loss of control was exacerbated by failure at simple tasks. He developed a criminal record for attempted burglary, and began to steal money openly and to borrow money he had no intention of returning. At this time he complained of loss of balance and was noted to have intermittently unsteady gait. Between two and three years later he became dysarthric with jerky, abrupt speech. On assessment at age 27, he showed obvious intellectual decline with memory loss and profound dyspraxia which resulted in complete dependency. The working diagnosis at this stage was presenile dementia; diagnoses of Alzheimer's disease and Huntinton's disease had been considered previously. By age 30 he had negligible abilities on verbal tasks and a severe memory deficit. He perseverated in verbal responses. In addition he was severely ataxic and began to develop clonic episodes. Later he developed generalized seizures. He became permanently hypertonic and unable to talk in his last months, and died at age 36 with bronchopneumonia.

Fig. 7.7 Case histories of V 27 and VII 63.

tool at regional centres, and it is hoped that improvements in immunological techniques will allow a test to be developed for demonstration of PrP^P in serum.

The value of PrP testing over the conventional diagnostic approaches to possible transmissible dementias is illustrated by a recent extreme example, in which a familial CJD patient shared the prion gene mutation seen in other affected members of his family (Figs 7.6 and 7.7), yet at post-mortem the brain did not show significant pathology. Moreover, this patient had satisfied clinical diagnostic criteria for AD. Subsequent PrP immunostaining confirmed the presence of PrP^P despite the lack of any other neuropathological features of a spongiform encephalopathy (Fig. 7.8). In this instance, therefore, conventional clinical and pathological criteria would have been inadequate to make the correct diagnosis. This case also illustrates the neuropathological variation that is associated with this group of disorders.

PrP analysis may also clarify the prion positivity (and thus potential transmissibility) of other disorders, such as amyotrophic lateral sclerosis with dementia and other atypical dementias, whose nosological and aetiological status is unclear. This molecular classification of prion diseases could take its place within a broader grouping of several disorders conceptualized on similar grounds according to the nature of their cerebral amyloidosis; it represents an important example of the shift towards classification of neuropsychiatric disorders according to their pathogenesis.

NEUROPATHOLOGY

Pathology

The degree of neuropathology varies from absent (using standard histological techniques) to severe. The morphology of the disease is affected by the type of gene defect (if familial), the patient's genotype, and the length of the illness.

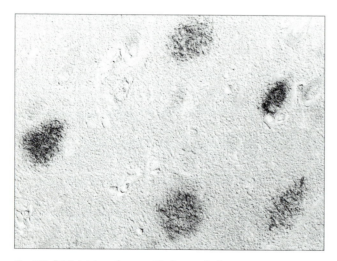

Fig. 7.8 PrP^P staining of neuropil in the cerebellum.

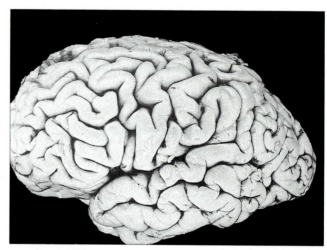

Fig. 7.9 Brain of a patient with Creutzfeldt–Jakob disease which is almost normal.

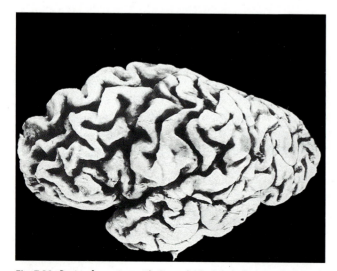

Fig. 7.10 Brain of a patient with Creutzfeldt–Jakob disease which is shrunken.

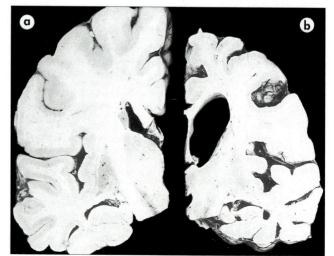

Fig. 7.11 Shrunken striatum and ventricular enlargement in Creutzfeldt–Jakob disease (b) compared to a control (a).

The macroscopic appearance of the brain may appear normal even in familial cases of long duration (Fig. 7.9). More typical cases show moderate or severe atrophy with obvious gyral atrophy and reductions in brain weight to as low as 850 g (Fig. 7.10). In such cases, ventricular enlargement is marked, and atrophy is often seen in the hippocampus, caudate, and thalamus (Fig. 7.11). In some cases, the brain stem also appears atrophic. In general, the loss in brain substance seems to be confined to the grey matter; the white matter is relatively unaffected. Meninges and blood vessels appear normal with no signs of inflammation.

Histopathology

In the light of recent advances, the histopathology of Prion disease is now known to encompass:
- spongiform change;
- neuronal loss;
- gliosis; and
- synaptic loss.

Spongiform change   Microscopic examination of the cortex in typical cases reveals the presence of numerous oval vacuoles in the neuropil. This typical appearance is called spongiform change (Fig. 7.12). The vacuoles are formed by disruptions in the membranes of neuronal and glial processes. Membranes thicken and split, and this process is one of the earliest pathological changes. The pathophysiology of this process is unknown, but it is probably related to the presence of prion protein within the cell membrane. The vacuoles usually range in size from 1 to 5 μm. However, vacuoles can appear to merge into each other, and larger structures measuring up to 50 μm can be seen. Lysosomes in affected terminals have been shown to contain PrPᵖ; this has led to the hypothesis that aberrant lysosomal function may be related to the process of vacuolization.

Vacuolation can be found in any cortical layer, and is often present in the grey matter of subcortical structures such as the thalamus, brain stem, and cerebellum. The distribution of pathology is often heterogeneous, and affected regions alternate with seemingly unaffected areas.

Neuronal loss   Loss of neurons is marked in most cases. The loss is greatest in cortical layers 3, 4, and 5, and in focal regions of the caudate and thalamus. The pattern of loss is variable, and ranges from the complete loss of neurons from large stretches of cortex, with a consequent collapse in the cortical structure, to irregular patches of cell loss. The factors that determine the vulnerability of cells to destruction are unknown. Careful examination can also reveal the presence of shrunken, palely staining atrophic remnants of neurons in the midst of apparently unaffected cells.

Neuronal loss tends to accentuate the overall appreciation of spongiform change. As such, it is a considerable aid to diagnosis. In cases with minimal cell loss or irregular foci of cell loss, diagnosis becomes much more difficult. This is particularly awkward in cases with psychiatric symptoms, and in cases with a long clinical course, in which cortical Lewy body dementia or frontal lobe dementia may be potential alternative diagnoses.

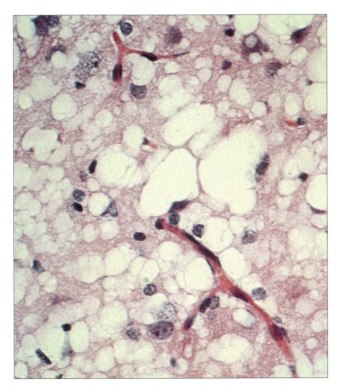

Fig. 7.12 Spongiform change (haematoxylin and eosin stain).

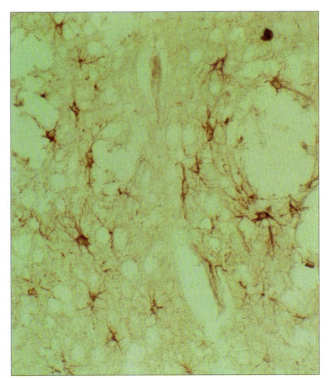

Fig. 7.13 Gliosis visualized by immunostaining of glial fibrillary acidic protein (GFAP).

Gliosis Loss of neurons is accompanied by massive activation of and proliferation of glial cells (Fig. 7.13). In severe cases, the neuronal component of cortical areas may well have disappeared and have been replaced by reactive glia. Vacuolation can be seen in the processes of glial cells in these regions.

Synaptic loss Electron microscopy has shown that axons and dendrites are damaged early during the disease. Quantitative studies to assess synaptic density in cases with obvious spongiform changes estimate synaptic loss to be about 30 per cent in the cortex. Synaptic loss of some 20 per cent has been shown even in atypical cases that lack obvious pathology at the light microscope level (see Figs 7.6 and 7.7).

Such studies (and previous work with the electron microscope) indicate that the progressive loss of pre-synaptic terminals underlies the appearance of dementia in Prion disease. The appearance of spongiform change and gliosis, although spectacular, is probably an epiphenomenon of the disease process and may not correlate with the occurrence of neurological deficits.

Other changes

Despite the transmissible nature of the disease, there is no evidence of an inflammatory response either within the brain or in the periphery. This is probably related to the fact that the protein involved is host coded.

Peripheral tissues (spleen, lungs, and gut) have been shown to be either the sites of conformational change of PrP_c into PrP^p, or to be the sites where the abnormal isoform can accumulate in low levels. However, no obvious pathology is seen in these regions.

Plaques About 15 per cent of Prion disease brains contain extracellular amyloid plaques, usually restricted to the cerebellum. These plaques are congophilic and show birefringence with polarized light. They have a 'halo' of reactive glial processes (Fig. 7.14). Although these plaques can be morphologically indistinguishable from the senile plaques of Alzheimer's disease (AD), immunocytochemistry has shown that they are formed from prion protein (rather than β-amyloid protein). This fact forms the basis of a method of diagnosing cases of Prion disease (Fig. 7.15).

Finally, differences in the distribution of plaques and other signs of pathology exist between Prion disease cases, and are counterparts of the clinical variation mentioned above.

Molecular Pathology

It is now probable that the spongiform encephalopathies occurring in various species, including the three human variants, are all caused by a single common agent. What is surprising is that increasing evidence points to the transmissible factor being a protein, called a prion (proteinaceous infectious agent). Conversely, although not completely excluded, evidence for the involvement of DNA or RNA in the infective process – as would be axiomatic for a conventional infection of any kind – is lacking. Initial indications that the causative agent might be unusual came from several sources (Fig. 7.16).

Research into kuru and scrapie has shown that the infectivity of affected brain tissue is not removed by procedures which are routinely used to destroy nucleic acids. Even traditional disinfectants and preservatives are often not effective – exemplified

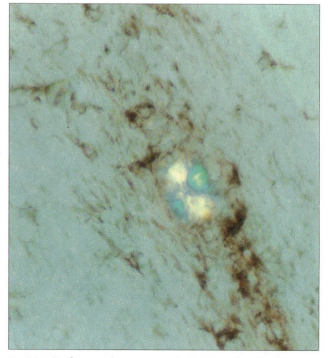

Fig. 7.14 Birefringent plaque, surrounded by reactive astrocytes.

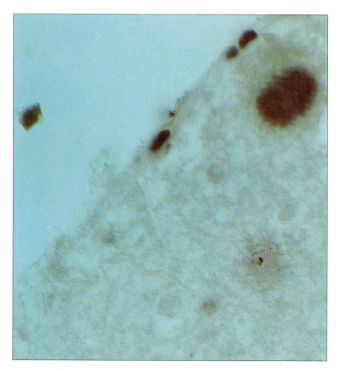

Fig. 7.15 Prion-positive plaque.

by the iatrogenic spread of CJD by intracranial EEG electrodes despite sterilization. The agent can also pass through fine-pored filters, showing that it is much smaller than most conventional infective agents such as viruses of the kinds which cause other neurodegenerative disorders. However, infectivity can be countered by proteolytic treatments, such as strong alkali or autoclaving; this suggests instead that proteins might be central to the process.

Cellular fractionation experiments have supported this view, since infectivity of different fractions generally coincides closely with the presence of the protease-resistant prion protein (PrP^P, see below). Importantly, several recent, independent techniques have also now failed to separate PrP^P from infectivity, or produced any evidence for the association of nucleic acid (or other non-PrP component) with infectivity.

Immunocytochemistry and immunoblotting have provided another indication of the central role of PrP in the transmissible dementias. Antibodies raised against the protease-resistant PrP^P found in scrapie-infected mouse or hamster brains cross-react with similar proteins seen in affected brains of other species, including CJD, GSS, and kuru in humans. This antigenic similarity is strong evidence for the unitary nature of the transmissible dementias across and within species, and emphasizes the central

role of this protein. In total, a large series of experiments have produced results consistent with the hypothesis that a protein – PrP^P – represents the infectious agent.

Molecular pathology of prion proteins

Making the connection between the tentative evidence that PrP^P might cause the diseases and the presence of PrP^P immunoreactivity as an established pathological feature of the transmissible dementias awaited the application of molecular biological techniques. These have determined the identity of the PrP which characterizes these disorders, and allowed major advances in understanding of its aetiological role. These findings have given significant support to the 'prion hypothesis' of the spongiform encephalopathies.

The prion hypothesis came of age in the mid-1980s when it was established that PrP is encoded by a normal cellular gene located on human chromosome 20. Other experiments showed that the PrP gene is expressed and its encoded protein synthesized by cells, including neurons and glia, throughout life. These data provided unequivocal evidence that PrP production is a normal event in a healthy brain. Therefore, any pathological potential of PrP must result from an alteration in some aspect of its sequence, expression, or properties.

Fig. 7.16 Summary of the evidence that prion protein causes Prion disease.

Evidence that the Abnormal Isoform of Prion Protein Causes Prion Disease

Biochemical co-purification of PrP 27–30 and scrapie infectivity demonstrated.

Concentration of PrP 27–30 is proportional to prion titre.

Kinetics of proteolytic digestion of PrP 27–30 and infectivity are coincident.

Immunoaffinity co-purification of PrP^P and infectivity and the use of PrP antisera to neutralize infectivity demonstrated.

PrP^P detected only in clones of cultured cells producing prion infectivity.

PrP amyloid plaques are specific for prion diseases of animals and humans.

Excellent correlation found between PrP^P in brain tissue and prion diseases in animals and humans.

Genetic linkage between mouse PrP gene and scrapie incubation times found. PrP gene of mice with long incubation times encodes amino acid substitutions at codons 108 and 189 compared to mice with short or intermediate incubation times.

Syrian hamster PrP transgene and PrP^P in the inoculum govern the 'species barrier', scrapie incubation times, neuropathology, and prion synthesis in mice.

Genetic linkage between HuPrP gene mutation at codon 102 and development of GSS demonstrated. Significant association between codon 200 point mutation or codon 53 insertion of six octarepeats and familial CJD found.

Mice expressing MoPrP transgenes with the point mutation of GSS spontaneously develop neurological dysfunction, spongiform change, and astrocytic gliosis.

Another important finding was that the prion gene in scrapie-affected animals had the same nucleotide sequence as in unaffected individuals, indicating that scrapie (at least in these cases) is not caused by a mutation. Moreover, prion gene expression is not increased during the disease, suggesting that the deposition of PrP^P in amyloid plaques which occurs in the disease is not simply the result of excessive production. Neither are variants of PrP likely to arise from differential processing of its messenger RNA, since the protein is encoded on a single exon. Further analysis of the gene sequence indicated PrP to be a 'housekeeping' gene, necessary for basic functioning of cells, in keeping with its marked conservation between organisms as diverse in evolution as fruitflies and humans. These data were also suggestive that PrP is a membrane protein, agreeing with the biochemical localization of PrP (and infectivity) to membranes. The cellular expression of the prion gene is summarized in Fig. 7.17.

These findings answered some perplexing questions, but raised several more. The normal presence of PrP provided an explanation for the lack of an immune response during disease, since the disease-producing form of the protein is not sufficiently different to be recognized as an antigen by the host. It also removed the requirement for PrP to be a self-replicating protein to account for its proposed infectivity; its infectious properties could now be explained (much more plausibly) in terms of a disruption of pre-existing cellular PrP metabolism (Fig. 7.18).

Prion gene mutations

Genetic linkage analysis has confirmed that prion mutations do occur in some familial cases and that they are tightly linked to disease. This data provides the strongest support yet for the prion hypothesis and also indicates that the aetiology of Prion disease is not homogeneous. The first mutation was described by

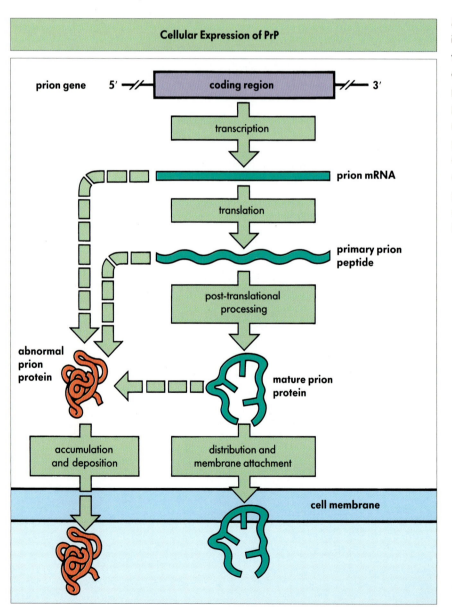

Cellular Expression of PrP

Fig. 7.17 The prion gene is transcribed into its complementary messenger RNA (mRNA), which migrates to the cytoplasm and serves as the template for translation into prion protein. In healthy cells, the encoded prion peptide undergoes post-translational modifications before attachment to the plasma membrane (solid arrows). In infected cells, one or more steps of this process are abnormal, resulting in deposition of the protein within and between cells (dashed arrows). (Adapted from Harrison and Roberts, 1991.)

Pathways of Abnormal PrP Formation

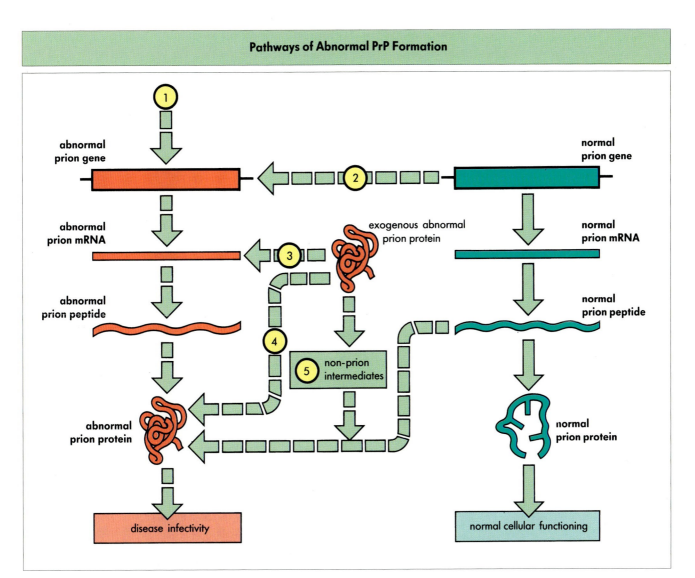

Fig. 7.18 Possible mechanisms for production of abnormal prions: (1) inherited abnormal prion gene; (2) spontaneous mutation of the prion gene; (3) reverse translation of abnormal prion mRNA; (4) autocatalysis of abnormal prion protein; (5) abnormal prion protein initiates its own production via non-prion intermediates. Process 1 could account for inherited cases, process 2 for sporadic cases, and processes 3–5 for cases acquired by infection. (Adapted from Harrison and Roberts, 1991.)

Pathogenic Mutations in Familial Prion Disease

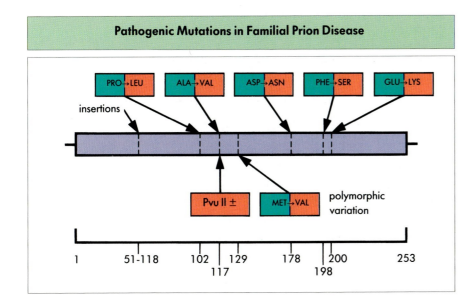

Fig. 7.19 The location and type of pathogenic mutations in the prion gene.

Owen and colleagues (1989), who found an insertion of an extra 144 base pairs at codon 52 in the prion gene in affected members of a family with CJD. Interestingly, the same insertion was then found in a case clinically diagnosed as familial AD, and has been identified in five (out of 101) cases of atypical dementias of various diagnoses but in which CJD and GSS had not been suspected.

Soon afterwards, Hsaio et al (1989) reported a pedigree of GSS in which the prion gene contained a single base mutation, leading to an amino acid substitution (at codon 102) of proline to leucine. This mutation was confirmed in other families with GSS, and an additional mutation at codon 189 (changing alanine to valine) was reported in another pedigree. The link between GSS and CJD was emphasized when the same group identified the codon 102 mutation in a familial CJD case. Further mutations have been identified (Fig. 7.19). It is assumed, though unproven, that these mutations are the direct cause of disease in these families. It is also assumed that such mutations are pathogenic by virtue of the encoded prion protein having altered properties which result in cellular dysfunction and ultimately neurological disorder (see below).

Further support for the central role of PrP in the transmissible dementias is provided by studies investigating factors which determine the incubation period of scrapie. It has long been known that the incubation time is affected both by the strain of the host and of the infectious agent. Various theories for the basis of this phenomenon had been advanced, but it became likely from linkage data that the scrapie incubation gene was either identical to the prion gene, or very tightly linked to it. Soon afterwards, it was demonstrated that the two genes are almost certainly the same, by showing that mice with long incubation times differed from those with short incubation times by variation in the prion gene sequence. Specifically, they varied in the amino acid coded for at either codon 108 or 189; the latter change was predicted to produce a significant effect on the extracellular part of PrP and its potential for post-translational modification.

These differences in the host-encoded PrP demonstrate another central role for the prion gene in the disease: not only does it encode the protein associated with infectivity, it also controls the incubation period for the disease. These findings were confirmed when it was shown that forms of the PrP encoded by these alleles affected incubation time, and that introducing different prion genes into transgenic mice resulted in different incubation periods and altered susceptibility to the infection and the pattern of pathology features.

A similar effect on incubation time has now been shown to occur in humans. In a large family with CJD and a 144bp insert in the prion gene, age of disease onset appears to be linked to valine or methionine homozygosity at codon 129. Patients who are VV at codon 129 have an early age of onset, and patients who are MM have a late age of onset (see Figs 7.6 and 7.19).

Together, these findings provide explanations for many aspects of these disorders for which nucleic acid in the infectious agent

had been assumed to be essential. It is now postulated that allelic heterogeneity within the prion gene, as this sequence variability is called, can explain differences in individual susceptibility to, and features of, prion-related diseases in humans. What is not clear is whether the mutations now known to be associated with cases of GSS and CJD are simply other allelic variants equivalent to those described in mice, or whether they have different relationships to the occurrence of disease. For example, the codon 200 mutation has now been discovered in some unaffected members of the previously described pedigree; it remains to be seen whether these individuals subsequently develop CJD, or whether this particular mutation is not invariably associated with disease. Further study of prion gene sequences in both humans and animals is needed to clarify these points.

Origin of PrP^P

The presence of PrP^P in Prion disease could arise in at least two different ways (see Fig. 7.18):
(i) the alterations in the prion gene structure would lead directly to the translation of a protein with an abnormal conformation;
(ii) other changes within the cell could alter the process of prion protein post-translational modification and lead to a subsequent alteration in the protein conformation.

Newly synthesized peptides often undergo post-translational processing and additions of various moieties before they can adopt their final conformation and position within the cell. Slight changes in any one of these steps, even when the primary amino-acid sequence specified by the gene is normal, can produce a protein with modified properties leading to alterations in its functioning and antigenicity of the type seen in the prion diseases.

Indeed, the main feature which distinguishes PrP from PrP^P is the resistance to proteolysis of the latter; this change in property is likely to be a correlate of such post-translational modifications. For example, a specific glycolipid must be added to the carboxy-terminal of PrP to permit its attachment to the cell membrane, whilst other data show that the membrane attachment and transmembrane transfer of PrP is altered in prion diseases, although the mechanisms are unclear.

Molecular Pathology of Prion Disease

There is uncertainty as to the molecular events by which the inheritance of an abnormal prion gene or acquisition of abnormal PrP results in the clinical and pathological stigmata of the spongiform encephalopathies. This question is relevant as to whether or not prions are the sole infectious agent. A number of mechanisms have been proposed. If PrP^P is indeed the cause, it could produce more of itself either by reverse translation (whereby a protein gives rise to its encoding messenger RNA), or by promoting synthesis of further aberrant PrP molecules through a variety of indirect pathways. Some of these possibilities are shown in Fig. 7.18. At present, there is no data to indicate which of these candidate cellular and molecular processes actually occur to explain how the inheritance of an abnormal prion gene, or contraction of infection results in production of pathology. One possibility currently under investigation to account for the acquired form is that PrP^P serves as a template for the catalytic conversion of normally produced PrP into more PrP^P.

EVIDENCE AGAINST THE PRION HYPOTHESIS

Some workers continue to argue strongly that PrP^P is not the infective agent, although its status as a defining characteristic of the transmissible dementias is no longer in question.

There are three main points against the prion hypothesis. Firstly, it remains possible that a small amount of nucleic acid (in a particle sometimes called a 'virino') could be present, intimately associated with PrP but experimentally inaccessible either by virtue of its smallness or some unusual property. It is suggested that this putative nucleic acid co-purifies with PrP, explaining the apparent but spurious infectivity of PrP itself. Certainly, several resistant viruses with unexpected properties have been discovered in recent years, including the retroviruses which can become incorporated in host genomes, potentially accounting for familial forms of diseases.

Secondly, it has been claimed that cellular fractionation experiments have in fact demonstrated infectivity in the absence of protein, precluding the latter as being either a necessary or sufficient infective agent. The more widely accepted contrary findings of others are attributed to experimental artefact during purification procedures.

Thirdly, others have shown infectivity of tissues apparently not expressing PrP, and the presence of PrP^P in tissues which are not infective.

However, the weight and diversity of evidence outlined here has led to a consensus which increasingly favours the aetiological role of PrP^P. Notably, the evidence from linkage, transgenic mice, and protein studies suggests strongly that expression of certain prion gene products, either through a mutation or through exogenous acquisition of abnormal PrP isoforms, is a necessary condition for the disease. This evidence markedly increases the likelihood that PrP^P is also sufficient to account for all the main features of these disorders, including transmissibility.

PRION DISEASE AND ALZHEIMER'S DISEASE – COMMON THEMES

There are a number of interesting similarities in the pathogenesis of Prion disease and Alzheimer's disease despite the fact that there is no evidence that AD is infectious. Both, for example, are characterized by the deposition of proteins which share the pleated conformation of amyloid, hence their generic name of cerebral amyloidoses. Although it is now clear that the individual proteins vary between these disorders (see Chapter 2), they are both membrane proteins encoded by cellular genes, expressed in normal brains and other tissues, and are central to the pathological features of their associated disease.

Moreover, pathology can result both from mutations of the encoding genes, and probably from abnormal processing of the gene product. As a consequence of either event, a change occurs in the localization and fate of the protein, a process thought to be closely involved in producing the clinicopathological picture. Since three further groups of neurological diseases are also caused by mutations affecting amyloidogenic proteins, it is possible that genes encoding such proteins might have a particular vulnerability to mutation (or propensity to aberrant expression); alternatively, perhaps a compensatory benefit is associated with such changes which prevents selection against these mutations.

Cerebral dysfunctions may be promoted by the loss of the normal functions of proteins with amyloid potential, and by the undesirable presence of the abnormal variants in an amyloid form.

Pathogenic theories of AD involving aberrant growth and plasticity processes have therefore been formulated. In this regard, it will be interesting to determine the biological actions of PrP – which are entirely unknown – since there is some evidence for the presence of similar developmental and regenerative processes occurring in Prion disease. Finally, neuron-to-neuron spread of disease may occur in both AD and prion diseases. For example, injection of scrapie into the eye results in a sequential appearance of pathology along visual pathways. It is thought that spread occurs by slow axonal transport (in anterograde and retrograde directions) and trans-synaptic transfer. Whether it is PrP itself which is distributed in this way is unknown. In AD, progression of disease along olfactory and corticocortical connections has been proposed. The transported substance in AD is also unknown; interestingly, β-APP has recently been shown to undergo axonal transport.

DIFFERENTIAL DIAGNOSIS

When the triad of presenile dementia, myoclonus, and abnormal EEG are present, clinical diagnosis is usually reliable and accurate; conversely, the absence of the last two features in advanced clinical cases virtually excludes Prion disease.

Unfortunately, these conditions are not always satisfied, and the occurrence of clinical variants can make definite diagnosis impossible in the absence of biopsy or post-mortem confirmation or the demonstration of experimental transmissibility. To compound the problem, the atypical clinical forms are less likely to show helpful EEGs. In some cases, therefore, the differential diagnosis includes all causes of dementia and ataxia.

On probability grounds, the commonest misdiagnosis is that of AD, especially for those cases of later onset (about a third have an onset between 60 and 70), and the 10–25 per cent which have a prolonged course over two years. Helpful differentiating features, apart from speed of the progression of illness, include cerebellar, pyramidal, or extra-pyramidal signs, and early visual disturbances, all of which are more common in Prion disease.

With the exception of the EEG, routine investigations are generally unhelpful in both conditions, although CT and MRI scans tend to remain normal in early Prion disease, whereas in AD cortical atrophy is common. The clinical overlap between Prion disease and AD is mirrored pathologically; AD can show spongiform changes, whilst Prion disease brains may contain Alzheimer-type senile plaques and neurofibrillary tangles, or show cell loss in the cholinergic basal nucleus.

Moreover, a third of familial AD cases are clinically indistinguishable from Prion disease, yet show unequivocal AD pathology and are not transmissible to animals. Other diseases which have been confused clinically with CJD include tumours, Huntington's chorea, supranuclear palsy, amyotrophic lateral sclerosis, Leigh's disease, corticostriate degeneration, and progressive multifocal leucoencephalopathy. Most of these diagnoses are more likely to be considered if motor or bizarre neurological symptoms are prominent relative to dementia, and such cases are often seen and managed by neurologists.

SUMMARY

(i) Prion disease is an uncommon neurological disease of man and other animals.

(ii) It has a variable spectrum of clinical symptoms and pathology and is often confused with other neurodegenerative disease.

(iii) Prion disease is the only neurological disease which is both inherited and transmissible.

(iv) Prion disease is probably due to the change in conformation of the cellular prion protein into an abnormal protease-resistant isoform (PrP^P). This may occur because of a genetic mutation or because of post-translational change in the gene product.

(v) The abnormal protein (PrP^P) results in the formation of vacuoles in neuronal membranes and the deposition of amyloid, and leads to cellular destruction.

(vi) The presence of alterations in the prion gene in a DNA sample, or the presence of the abnormal PrP^P isoform in CNS tissue is diagnostic of the disease.

8 Other Dementias

Dementia can be caused by a wide variety of other, generally rare conditions (Fig. 8.1); often the aetiology and pathophysiology are poorly defined. Examples from the various categories are discussed below.

PRIMARY NEURODEGENERATION

Pick's Disease

Pick's disease was first described in 1892 (before Alzheimer's disease, which occurs more frequently). The clinical syndrome and pattern of pathology indicate that Pick's disease is a distinct aetiological entity:

- the relative incidence in the USA of Pick's and Alzheimer's diseases varies from 1:3 (Minnesota) to 1:50 (New York);
- 20 per cent of cases are familial (gene unknown);
- characteristic neuropathology includes cortical Pick bodies; and
- the cause of Pick's disease is unknown.

Clinical course

Cases have been reported in patients as young as 20. Generally, onset of symptoms is between 50 and 60, and women are affected

Causes of Dementia			
Cerebral infection and inflammation	**Toxic/Metabolic**	**Neoplasm and hydrocephalus**	**Primary cerebral degenerations**
Encephalitis	Alcohol	Meningioma	Alzheimer's disease
Neurosyphilis	Hypothyroidism	Gliomas	Parkinson's disease
Multiple sclerosis	Wilson's disease	Parapituitary lesions	Huntington's disease
Whipple's disease	Hypoglycaemia		Pick's disease
Granulomatous diseases	Porphyria	Subdural haematoma	Cortical Lewy body disease
Prion disease	Drugs	Midbrain tumour	Motor neuron disease
Multifocal leucoencephalopathy	Heavy metals	Aqueduct stenosis	
AIDS dementia	Chronic uraemia or dialysis	Communicating hydrocephalus	
Systemic lupus erythematosis			
Storage diseases	**Congenital**	**Psychiatric**	**Vascular**
Adrenoleucodystrophy	Autism	Depressive pseudodementia	Multi-infarct dementia
Metachromic leucodystrophy	Down's syndrome	Hysterical pseudodementia	Binswanger's disease
Kupf's disease	Neurofibromatosis	Ganser's syndrome	Congophilic angiopathy
Cerebrotendinous xanthomatosis	Tuberous sclerosis		Cranial arteritis
	Inborn errors of metabolism		Other vasculitides

Fig. 8.1 Differential diagnosis of various causes of dementia.

more often than men. The distinctive clinical features on presentation are changes of character and social behaviour (indicative of frontal lobe damage), rather than impairment of memory and intellect. Drive becomes diminished, and loss of inhibition leads to grossly inappropriate social behaviour (e.g. stealing, alcoholism, sexual misadventures). As might be expected, insight is considerably impaired from the early stages of the disease. Marked changes in mood are also seen; euphoria or apathy predominate. In contrast to Alzheimer's disease, delusions and hallucinations are comparatively rare and epilepsy is usually absent.

As the disease progresses, language problems appear, with perseverative speech and reduced vocabulary. Apraxia and agnosia can also occur. Motor disorders are relatively uncommon. The language and behavioural difficulties are gradually subsumed by increasing impairments of intellect and memory. The final stages of the disease are marked by the disintegration of intellect and personality.

CT and MRI appearance can be so characteristic as to confirm a tentative clinical diagnosis (Fig. 8.2). In typical cases, marked atrophy affects the anterior portions of the frontal and temporal lobes, with considerable enlargement of the frontal horns; by contrast, the bodies of the lateral ventricles and the sulci over the parietal and occipital lobes are much less affected. Scans sometimes, however, resemble those seen in Huntington's chorea, especially when caudate atrophy is marked.

Neuropathology

The gross appearance of the brain is characteristic, as described above. In the frontal lobe the convexity or the orbital surface may be affected alone, and in the temporal lobe the posterior half of the superior temporal gyrus may stand out as relatively spared. The distribution of atrophy varies considerably from case to case, but major involvement of the parietal lobes is unusual and occipital or cerebellar atrophy extremely rare.

Microscopy shows neuronal loss from superficial layers of the cortex, accompanied by dense astrocytic proliferation and fibrous gliosis in the cortex and underlying white matter (Fig. 8.3). The affected neurons are swollen (balloon cells) and oval in shape. They show a loss of Nissl substance and have irregularly shaped argentophilic inclusions (Pick bodies), which displace the nucleus towards the periphery (Fig. 8.4).

Pick bodies are made up of filaments that show variable morphologies (straight, tubular, or paired helical). These filaments are composed of aberrantly processed or packaged neurofilaments and proteins such as β-crystallin (which also marks ballooned neurons). The use of monoclonal anti-neurofilament

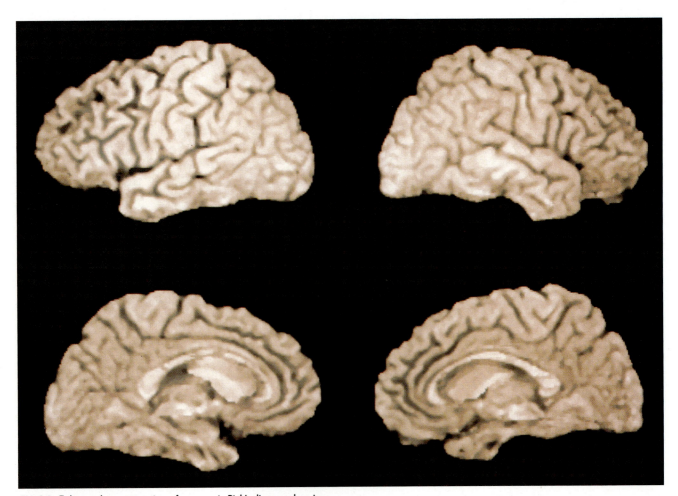

Fig. 8.2 Enhanced reconstruction of MRI scan in Pick's disease, showing localized frontal atrophy.

antibodies has shown that Pick bodies share antigenic determinants with both neurofilaments and neurofibrillary tangles (see Fig. 8.4). Neurofibrillary tangles and Pick bodies are both associated with identical phosphorylated neurofilament epitopes. Alzheimer's disease and Pick's disease may share a common molecular pathogenesis, which involves the disruption of cytoskeletal organization.

Eosinophilic inclusions (Hirano bodies) and granulovascular changes are often present. In most cases there are no senile plaques, neurofibrillary tangles, or cerebrovascular degeneration. The middle cortical layers may have a spongy appearance similar to that seen in Prion disease. Loss of myelin in the white matter of affected lobes is usually considerable.

Although these neuropathological features are diagnostic of Pick's disease, approximately half of clinically diagnosed cases

lack the distinctive pathology on biopsy or autopsy examination. These cases may represent variants or distinct diseases with similar clinical profiles.

Neurochemistry

Biochemical studies have failed to show the cholinergic brain deficits typical of Alzheimer's disease though muscarinic cholinergic binding sites may be reduced (Fig. 8.5).

Progressive Subcortical Gliosis

Pathological variants of Pick's disease exist (Pick's Disease Type II or progressive subcortical gliosis). It is possible that these variants have different aetiologies. Microscopical examination reveals severe gliosis in the subcortical white matter with only slight or moderate gliosis in the cortex. Glial proliferation is also marked in the subcortical nuclear masses, the brain stem and the ventral columns of the cord. Cortical neuronal loss is much less prominent and affected neurons tend to be shrunken rather than swollen.

Amyotrophic Lateral Sclerosis (ALS) with Dementia

Although typically ALS is not associated with cognitive impairments or dementia, about one third of patients perform poorly on tests of frontal lobe function, and about 5 per cent of patients

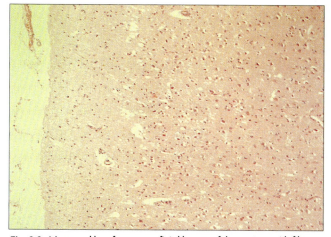

Fig. 8.3 Neuronal loss from superficial layers of the cortex, with fibrous gliosis, in Pick's disease.

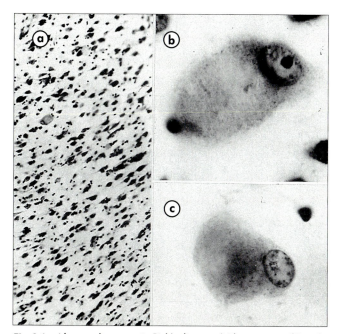

Fig. 8.4 Abnormal neurons in Pick's disease: (a) low power; (b) and (c) high power.

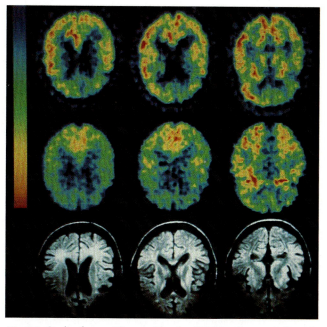

Fig. 8.5 Studies from a 62 year old male with Pick's disease confirmed by biopsy. Each column represents a brain level. The top row is an MRI showing prominent frontal and anterior temporal atrophy. The middle row is a SPECT scan of the distribution of muscarinic receptors labelled with I-123 QNB showing dramatic loss of muscarinic receptors mainly in the frontal cortex. The bottom row is a PET scan of glucose utilization with F^{18}DG as the tracer, again showing reduced metabolism mainly in the frontal cortex.

with typical sporadic ALS have an associated dementia, which may precede evidence of motor system degeneration. Dementia may be more common in familial ALS. Although the dementia of ALS may be non-specific, affecting most aspects of cognitive function, it is commonly of frontal lobe type, when it may be associated with frontotemporal atrophy. Typical Pick's disease pathology, with neocortical ballooned neurons and Pick bodies in the neocortex and hippocampus, is occasionally found, but more commonly the pathological changes include:

- neuron loss and spongy change in neocortical layers 2 and 3;
- gliosis in the cortical and subcortical grey matter and white matter; and
- neuronal loss in the subcortical structures, including the substantia nigra, thalamus, and amygdala.

Degeneration of large pyramidal neurons of the motor cortex and the corticospinal tract, and loss of brain stem and spinal motor neurons is indistinguishable from that seen in typical ALS. Immunocytochemistry with antibodies against ubiquitin have revealed ubiquitin-immunoreactive inclusions in the superficial layers of the frontal and temporal neocortex, and in the hippocampal dentate granule neurons of patients with dementia and ALS (Fig. 8.6). Unlike Pick bodies or the neurofibrillary tangles of Alzheimer's disease, the ubiquitin-immunoreactive inclusions in dementia with ALS are not argyrophilic, nor are they identified by antibodies against microtubule-associated protein tau, phosphorylated neurofilaments, or other cytoskeletal proteins. They are thus similar to ubiquitin-immunoreactive inclusions which

are present in the lower motor neurons of the cranial motor nuclei and spinal anterior horns.

The relationship between dementia with ALS and other forms of frontal-type dementia, including those cases with typical Pick's disease pathology, remains uncertain, but these syndromes are familial in at least 40 per cent of cases, often with a presumed autosomal-dominant mode of inheritance, and either dementia or ALS can occur in such families.

DEMENTIA OF FRONTAL LOBE TYPE

This type of dementia is characterized by frontotemporal lobar atrophy with progressive behavioural and cognitive dysfunction and mutism. Half the patients show a family history of a similar disorder in a first degree relative. Symmetrical frontal and temporal atrophy occurs due to the loss of large pyramidal neurons, spongiform change and gliosis. Pick bodies are not seen.

INFECTION AND INFLAMMATION

Systemic Lupus Erythematosus (SLE)

SLE is a connective tissue disorder which affects many organs, including the brain. It has a number of characteristics:

- it is more common in females (male:female ratio 1:9);

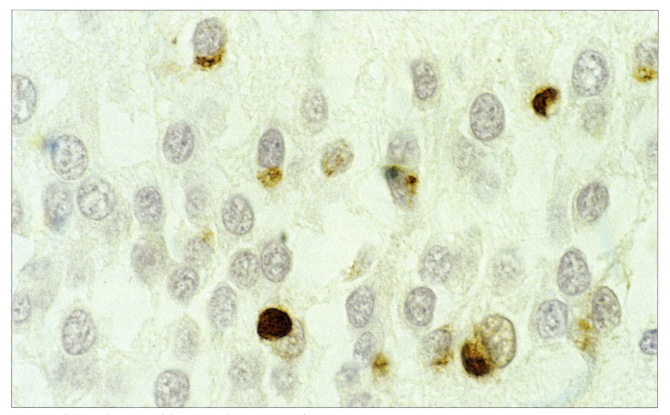

Fig. 8.6 Inclusions in hippocampal dentate granule neurons in ALS dementia.

- the mean age of onset is 30;
- it is a multisystem disease;
- the pathological process involves immune and inflammatory processes; and
- seizures and/or psychiatric symptoms including dementia are found in 60 per cent of patients.

Clinical course

Onset is usually insidious with muscle aching, fatigue, and low grade fever. Since SLE is a multisystem disease a wide range of symptoms is seen. Neuropsychiatric symptoms include acute and chronic organic reactions, schizophrenia-like psychoses, changes of personality, and neurotic reactions. Most symptoms are transient and often disappear within weeks, although relapses are common. Neurological findings encompass peripheral neuropathy, cranial nerve palsies, motor disorders, seizures, and aphasias. There is no characteristic pattern of neurological or psychiatric symptoms.

The clusters of symptoms which can appear together lead to considerable difficulties in diagnosis, particularly in the early stages of the disease. Patients with neurological symptoms can be misdiagnosed as suffering from multiple sclerosis or other multifocal disorders and psychotic symptoms can lead to a diagnosis of schizophrenia if the organic features are overlooked.

Chronic cerebral degeneration is uncommon but deterioration of memory and intellect can progress to a clinical state of dementia.

Pathology

Pathological features of the disease appear to be due to activation of the immune system with the resultant processes of localized inflammation leading to damage of arterioles and capillaries in the brain. The structural damage leads directly to the sequelae of cerebrovascular disease including microaneurysm, haemorrhage, and infarction; the symptoms suffered by the patient can often be related directly to the site and size of the lesion.

Imaging studies show areas of hyperattenuation (CT), hyperintensity (MRI), or hypometabolism (PET and SPECT).

Diagnosis

SLE is accompanied by leucopaenia and a raised erythrocyte sedimentation rate. Abnormalities in serum proteins are also common. Screening for the presence of DNA antibodies is a useful procedure. Treatment with steroids is often effective.

Hydrocephalus

Long-standing communicating hydrocephalus is often associated with the clinical triad of:
- dementia;
- gait disturbance; and
- urinary incontinence.

CSF pressure is usually within the normal range when a lumbar puncture is made. However, continuous monitoring of intracranial pressure can reveal A wave pressure surges (see Chapter 5), which can be particularly marked during sleep. As such, the commonly used term 'normal-pressure hydrocephalus' is probably a misnomer.

Reduction in CSF volume is one of the important mechanisms of spatial compensation within the skull. Blockage or disruption in the flow of CSF from the ventricular system to the cerebral subarachnoid space can supplement the rise in intracranial pressure that is caused by intracranial haematomas. Blockages can also be caused (as a long-term consequence of meningitis or head injury) by the formation of fibrous adhesions in the basal cisterns. In infants, hydrocephalus can occur as a result of congenital abnormalities.

CT and MRI scanning usually shows extensive ventricular enlargement. The pattern of ventricular enlargement can be used to determine the anatomical location of the blockage.

Hydrocephalus is amenable to therapy. Therefore, it is of considerable importance to distinguish hydrocephalus from primary degenerative brain diseases such as Prion disease, Alzheimer's disease, and cerebrovascular disease.

METABOLIC DEMENTIAS

Alcoholism and Dementia

The chronic amnestic syndrome (Korsakoff's syndrome) and the syndrome of subacute intellectual impairment (Wernicke's encephalopathy) associated with chronic alcohol abuse have been attributed to several different factors:
- neurotoxic effects of alcohol;
- vitamin B complex deficiency; and
- hepatic dysfunction.

The contribution of each factor to these syndromes is difficult to disentangle.

Clinical and neuropsychological deficits have been shown to improve in chronic alcoholics after a period of abstinence. The most marked improvement appears in the short term, and although less additional benefit is shown after longer periods of abstinence, there is some evidence that continued improvement may be possible. Difficulty sometimes occurs when attempting to decide whether improvement results from recovery from acute withdrawal symptoms, or whether from more specific diffuse brain damage.

The changes in the brain in chronic alcoholism have been extensively investigated in CT studies. Abnormalities are present in at least one half and possibly in as many as three quarters of patients with a history of chronic alcohol abuse. The manifestations include cortical atrophy and to a lesser extent ventricular enlargement. It is interesting to note that the CT studies reveal changes that are on the whole bilateral and reasonably symmetrical, in comparison to many of the neuropsychological assessments which have indicated a predominance of right hemisphere dysfunction. The widening of both the sulci and the Sylvian fissures, as seen on CT scans, has been shown to be negatively correlated with the duration of abstinence. These changes are potentially reversible, at least in part, after long periods of abstinence (more than six months). However, the CT scan appearance does not return completely to normal. PET and SPECT studies tend to show frontal cortical hypofunction.

Neuropathology

Neuropathological examination reveals petechial haemorrhages in the mamillary bodies and periaqueductal grey matter in acute cases. Chronic cases show localized atrophy of the mamillary bodies, mamillothalamic tract and dorsomedial nucleus of the thalamus. There is good evidence from scanning and neurological studies that abstention is of positive benefit to chronic alcoholics. The main treatment challenge is persuading them to abstain.

PSYCHIATRIC CAUSES

Pseudodementias

A number of psychiatric conditions can present with a clinical picture that resembles organic dementia. Such disorders can be descriptively labelled as pseudodementias. There are two main categories of such disorders:

- defined psychiatric syndromes (depressive pseudodementia, schizophrenia, mania, hysterical pseudodementia, Ganser syndrome); and
- factitious disorder (simulation).

Examination of patients suspected of having a pseudodementia requires both a detailed knowledge of the case history and information on the investigations undertaken in order to determine the presence or extent of degenerative disease. Obvious points, such as previous or coincident psychiatric illness or the presence of appropriate motivation, should also be borne in mind.

Defined Syndromes

The clinical manifestations of mood disorder (depression and mania) and schizophrenia can be confused with dementia, particularly in older patients. In many cases, differential diagnosis is made on previous history and the clinical course (see Chapters 14 and 15). In particular, variability in the level of cognitive deficits or inappropriate constellations of neurological deficits will raise suspicions of a pseudodementia.

Diagnostic pointers to an hysterical pseudodementia can be obtained by careful interview both of the patient and the relatives. The hysterical patient's responses to questions can be decisively or absurdly inaccurate and often seem to betray a knowledge of the purpose of the question. The purpose of distortion is often simplistic and obvious and may be related to the precipitating stressful situation. For example, when asked, 'what is the colour of grass', the hysterical patient may respond, 'blue'; or the hysterical patient may recognize all the hospital staff while appearing to be unable to recognize close family members. Pointing out such inconsistencies results in a puzzled or neutral response – *la belle indifférence*. Suggestibility is another feature that may help in making a diagnosis.

Factitious Disorders

Patients who are consciously simulating an organic disorder (malingering) are much more likely than hysterical patients to block ways of enquiring into their illness, and they co-operate poorly in subsequent investigations. There is often a clear indication of 'secondary gain'. However, fine diagnostic distinctions are often difficult to determine, and an impasse results in many cases. Even a confession of simulation does not always clarify the issue, as pressure causes some patients to confess even when there is ample evidence of organic or psychogenic causation.

Differential diagnosis between 'real' pseudodementia and factitious disorders is fraught with difficulty and should be made with caution. It is quite possible that the early stages of organic brain disease may cause a patient to react in such a fashion that a pseudodementia is suspected, and so there is always the possibility that a pseudodementia may, in reality, be a 'pseudo-pseudodementia' (Lishman, 1987).

In summary, such situations are difficult to resolve and a diagnosis of pseudodementia can only be made after the completion of all appropriate investigations, both physical and psychiatric.

DEMENTIA OF UNKNOWN AETIOLOGY

The nosological and aetiological problems raised by the patient who has a clear, clinically defined dementia yet has no characteristic lesion when subject to neuropathological examination are seldom discussed.

Experience shows that some 15 per cent of clinically defined cases of dementia in large neuropathological surveys defy the current strait-jacket of neuropathological diagnosis. Doubtless, some of these cases will be shown to be genetic or morphological variants of known disease. However, it is quite possible that some of these cases represent types of dementia which remain to be discovered and classified.

SUMMARY

(i) Dementia can be caused by a variety of other causes, including metabolic disturbances, generalized vascular disease, infections, and psychiatric conditions.

(ii) These known, 'other', causes account for less than 5 per cent of dementia cases.

(iii) Correct diagnosis is important because it is possible to treat some of these patients.

(iv) Approximately 15 per cent of patients with clinically diagnosed dementia have no definitive neuropathological diagnosis and the dementia is of unknown aetiology.

SECTION 2

Motor Disorders

While there are many disorders of the motor system, Parkinson's disease (PD) and parkinsonian syndromes, amyotrophic lateral sclerosis (ALS), and Huntington's disease represent the most common of these disabling disorders.

Idiopathic or Lewy body PD is the commonest form of akinetic-rigid syndrome. Although a number of clinical features point to the presence of Lewy body disease, clinical diagnosis is inaccurate in about 15 per cent of patients who have other forms of parkinsonism. As yet, there is no predictive test which will clearly identify patients with the Lewy body form of the disease.

A major advance in understanding of movement disorders was the discovery of dopamine depletion in the nigrostriatal system in PD, and the subsequent development of effective symptomatic treatment with laevodopa. More recently, the relationship between akinesia and rigidity on the one hand, and abnormal involuntary movements such as chorea on the other hand, has been clarified by experimental studies on the neurochemical anatomy and physiology of the basal ganglia (with the new interest in the pivotal function of the subthalamic nucleus) and realization of the importance of interactions between dopamine and excitatory and inhibitory amino acid neurotransmitters.

PD was long thought to be caused by an environmental factor, but it now seems more likely that genetic factors (for example, abnormalities of the cytochrome P450 debrisoquine hydroxylase enzyme) may interact with as yet unknown environmental factors to produce the disease state. Likewise, in ALS, a family history suggestive of an autosomal-dominant mode of inheritance can be elicited in about 5 per cent of patients and, in some families, linkage between the disease state and markers on chromosome 21 has been detected. Thus, for ALS, as for PD and indeed Alzheimer's disease, complex interactions between a gene and environment can be implicated.

Huntington's disease, on the other hand, is solely genetically determined, and is thought to have arisen as a single mutation event, perhaps in East Anglia, in the UK, several centuries ago. The identification of a link marker on chromosome 4 has facilitated genetic counselling. Much speculation has focused on the relationship between experimental excitotoxic lesions and the pathological changes in the neostriatum, but the molecular abnormality is unknown, and hence the mechanism of neuronal degeneration is not understood.

A key issue in these disorders is neuroprotection, but as yet we have no drug treatment which clearly prevents progression, despite hopes that the monoamine oxidase-B inhibitor selegiline (Eldepryl) might delay the progression of PD. Trials of agents protecting against free radical generation, and of potential neurotrophic substances, are possibilities for the near future, but a still vitally important part of care consists in counselling, support, and symptomatic relief.

9 Parkinson's Disease

DEFINITION OF PARKINSON'S DISEASE

Parkinson's disease (PD) is a progressive disorder of the nervous system characterized clinically by akinesia and bradykinesia, rigidity, rest tremor, postural and gait abnormalities, a therapeutic response to laevodopa, and the presence of Lewy bodies in pigmented neurons of the substantia nigra and other areas of the nervous system. The term parkinsonism is used to denote the clinical features (in whole or in part) of PD when they are due to other types of biochemical or pathological lesions (Fig. 9.1).

The characteristic clinical syndrome of PD was first highlighted by James Parkinson in *An Essay on the Shaking Palsy*, published in 1817, although there had been accounts of the condition before that time. James Parkinson, an east London apothecary, recognized the characteristic tremor, abnormality of posture, festinant (hurrying) gait, and the progressive nature of the disease.

THE BASAL GANGLIA

Anatomy

The basal ganglia comprise anatomically and functionally interconnected structures deep in the cerebral hemispheres, and include:

- the neostriatum (caudate and putamen);
- the pallidum (internal and external segments);
- the subthalamic nucleus; and
- the substantia nigra, which is composed of the dopamine-containing pars compacta, and the principally GABAergic neurons of the pars reticulata.

(Other deep structures such as the amygdala are sometimes included within the basal ganglia.)

Classification and Differential Diagnosis of Parkinsonism	
Idiopathic (primary or Lewy body) Parkinson's disease	**Parkinson-plus syndromes**
Symptomatic (secondary)	Progressive supranuclear palsy
Infectious and post-infectious Post-encephalitic (encephalitis lethargica) Other encephalitides Neuronal intranuclear hyaline inclusion disease	Multiple system atrophy Striatonigral degeneration Shy–Drager syndrome Olivo-ponto-cerebellar degeneration Parkinsonism with motor neuron disease (sporadic and familial forms)
Toxins Mn, CO, MPTP, cyanide, carbon disulphide, methanol	Cortico-basal degeneration
Drugs Dopamine receptor blockers Dopamine storage depleters	**Dementia syndromes** Parkinsonism–dementia–amyotrophic lateral sclerosis of western Pacific Creutzfeldt–Jakob disease Alzheimer's disease Normal-pressure hydrocephalus
Brain tumours	
Head trauma	**Hereditary disorders** Familial PD Wilson's disease Huntington's disease Neuroacanthocytosis Hallervorden–Spatz disease
Vascular	
Metabolic	

Fig. 9.1 Classification and differential diagnosis of parkinsonism.

The neostriatum receives inputs from all areas of the neocortex, and projects via the pallidal and nigral outflows to the thalamus, which in turn projects back to the neocortex (Fig. 9.2). The subthalamic nucleus forms a regulatory loop which receives inputs from the pallidum, and projects (via a glutamatergic pathway) back to it.

Not all basal ganglia outputs are processed through the thalamus. Branching efferents of the substantia nigra pars reticulata (SNR) project to the superior colliculus and the peduncular pontine nucleus, which in turn directly influence systems regulating eye movements and project to the brain stem reticular formation. Nevertheless, in primates, striatopallidothalamic circuits to the neocortex predominate over projections to the brain stem.

Neurochemical Anatomy of the Neostriatum

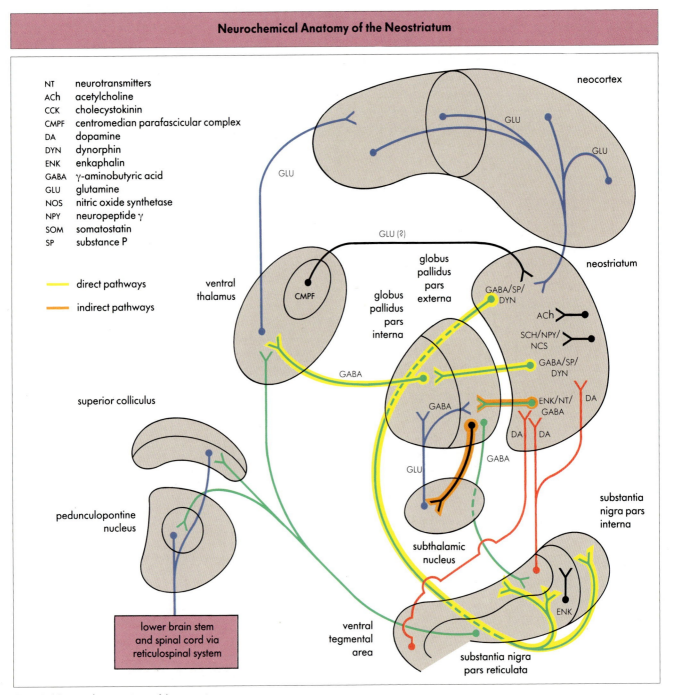

Fig. 9.2 Neuronal connections of the neostriatum.

Connectivity and Neurochemical Anatomy

Striatal Afferents

All areas of the neocortex project to the neostriatum in a topographically organized fashion. Corticostriate projections form mainly longitudinally arranged interdigitating arrays which have a patchlike structure relating to the compartmental organization of the neostriatum which was originally recognized on the basis of staining for acetylcholinesterase (ACHE) activity. ACHE-poor regions are called striosomes or patches, and the ACHE-rich areas comprise the matrix (Fig. 9.3). Striosomes comprise 10–20 per cent of the striatal volume, and their dimensions are similar to those of cortical columns. The deep and superficial cortical layers within a single area of cortex may project to the striosomal and matrix compartments respectively. As yet only very tentative conclusions can be drawn about the functional correlates of the striosome–matrix organization of the striatum.

The striatum also receives afferent projections from the substantia nigra pars compacta (SNC), and from the ventral tegmental area (VTA) of the brain stem (Fig. 9.4; see also Fig. 9.2); from the reticular nuclei of the thalamus (excitatory inputs, probably glutamatergic); from the dorsal raphe nucleus (serotoninergic); and scant inputs from the locus coeruleus (noradrenergic).

Greatest attention has focused on dopaminergic inputs to the striatum in view of their relevance to the pathophysiology of movement disorders. Projections from the reticular thalamus (centromedian–parafascicular complex) represent a major component of basal ganglia circuitry whose function is as yet little understood.

The organization of dopamine projections to the neostriatum

Neurons of the SNC project to the sensorimotor and 'association' components of the neostriatum, and neurons of VTA project mainly to the limbic neostriatum (see Figs 9.2 and 9.4). Within the SNC, more ventromedially placed neurons project largely to the putamen (i.e. the sensorimotor territory), whereas more dorsolaterally placed neurons project to those regions of the striatum which receive cortical inputs from the association areas. In Parkinson's disease, it is the ventrally placed SNC neurons which are preferentially (although not exclusively) affected by the disease process (see page 9.00). Dopaminergic terminals containing tyrosine hydroxylase form symmetrical synaptic contacts on the cell bodies, proximal dendritic shafts, and the necks of dendritic spines of neostriatal medium spiny neurons (MSNs), which account for about 90 per cent of all striatal neurons, and are the major projecting neurons of the striatum (Fig. 9.5). Dopamine may have either inhibitory or excitatory effects upon striatal MSNs. The inhibitory effects are targeted on GABA–ENK neurons which project to the external segment of the globus pallidus (GPE), and the excitatory effects act on GABA–substance P–dynorphin neurons projection to the internal pallidal segment (GPI) and substantia nigra pars reticularis (SNR). Some striatal output neurons project back to midbrain dopamine neurons, thus modifying dopamine-mediated neurotransmission in the striatum and SNC.

Striatal Output Systems

MSNs comprise 90 per cent of striatal output neurons. All MSNs probably utilize GABA as a neurotransmitter, but in some MSNs,

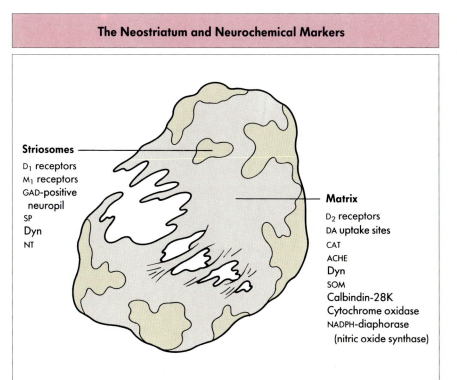

The Neostriatum and Neurochemical Markers

Striosomes

D_1 receptors
M_1 receptors
GAD-positive
  neuropil
SP
Dyn
NT

Matrix

D_2 receptors
DA uptake sites
CAT
ACHE
Dyn
SOM
Calbindin-28K
Cytochrome oxidase
NADPH-diaphorase
  (nitric oxide synthase)

Fig. 9.3 Preferential distribution of some neurochemical markers in striosome and matrix compartments of the neostriatum.

Basal Ganglia Pathways

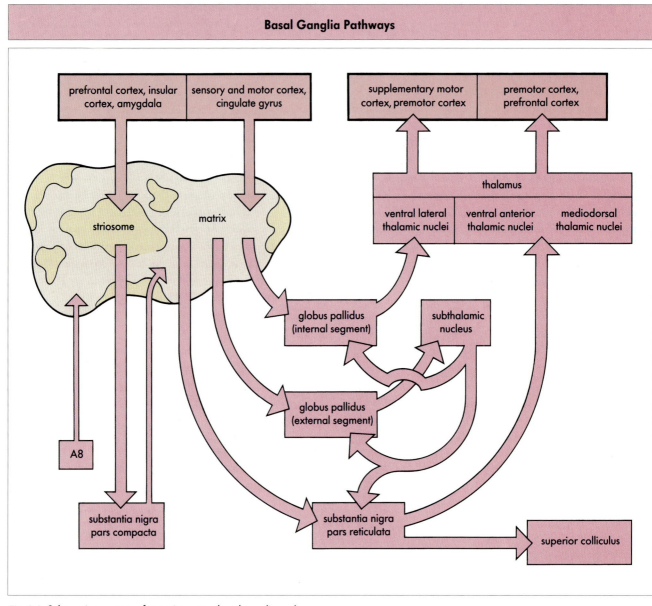

Fig. 9.4 Schematic summary of some important basal ganglia pathways.

Neostriatal Medium Spiny Neuron

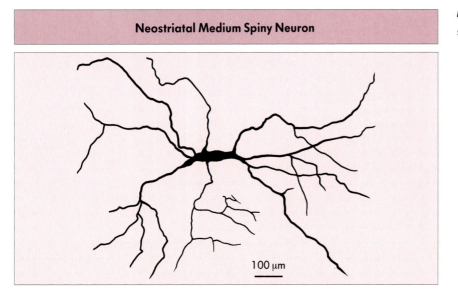

100 μm

Fig. 9.5 Drawing of a neostriatal medium spiny neuron.

GABA is co-localized with neuropeptides, such as substance P, neurotensin, dynorphin, and enkephalin (ENK). Some MSNs may utilize taurine as a neurotransmitter.

MSNs also receive inputs from striatal GABAergic and peptidergic neurons, from collaterals of other MSNs, and from cholinergic interneurons (Fig. 9.6). The major outflows of the basal ganglia (see Figs 9.2 and 9.4) pass to the globus pallidus and SNR. The subthalamic nucleus (STN) modifies striatopallidal outflow via an excitatory (glutamatergic) projection to both the internal and external pallidal segments, although it receives a GABAergic input only from GPE. GABAergic neurons in GPE and GPI, and in SNR, project to the ventro-anterior and ventrolateral nuclei of the thalamus, preserving the topographical organization of corticostriatal projections (see Fig. 9.4).

Most striatal neurons in resting animals are electrophysiologically silent, whereas neurons of the GPI and SNR are continuously active, with firing rates of up to 100 impulses per second. Increased firing of striatal cells inhibits GPI and SNR neurons, and thus disinhibits thalamic, collicular, and brain stem reticular formation neurons (Fig. 9.7a). Thus striatal outflow systems comprise a double inhibitory pathway which exerts strong synaptic inhibition over the thalamic, collicular and mesencephalic output targets of the basal ganglia.

In summary, a *direct striatofugal system* in which the action of dopamine is predominantly excitatory arises mainly from neurons in the putamen and projects directly to GPI and SNR, which in turn send topographically organized projections to specific thalamic nuclei. In addition, an *indirect striatofugal system* in which the action of dopamine is predominantly inhibitory, consists of a loop strategically placed to modify activity in the direct system, and comprising:

- GABA–ENK inputs from striatum to GPE;
- GABAergic neurons in GPE projecting to STN; and
- excitatory (probably glutamatergic) STN neurons projecting back upon both the pallidal segments.

Corticostriatal–thalamocortical circuits; the concept of parallel processing in the basal ganglia   Topographically and functionally distinctive relationships between different components of the corticostriatal projections may be preserved throughout striatopallidonigral outputs to the thalamus (Fig. 9.7b), although there is great capacity within the striatum, pallidus, and SN for integration as well as segregation of functions. Although all areas of cortex project to the striatum, the output systems project to the frontal and prefrontal areas implicated in motor planning, but not to the primary motor cortex or other cortical areas.

Pathophysiological Mechanisms in PD and Other Movement Disorders

In PD, and other akinetic–rigid syndromes, there is overactivity of projections from the striatum (chiefly putamen) to GPE, resulting in decreased activity of GPE output upon STN excitatory neurons (Fig. 9.8). The activity of STN neurons projecting upon both the pallidal segments is increased, the net result being increased firing of GABAergic projections from GPI, and hence suppression of neurons in the ventral thalamus.

In contrast, in hyperkinetic states (see Fig. 9.8) such as laevo-dopa-induced dyskinesia (see page 9.00), chorea (see chapter 12), and hemiballism, and perhaps in some forms of dystonic involuntary movements, there is decreased activity of the striatal neurons projecting to GPE, over-activity of pallidosubthalamic neurons, and decreased activity of subthalamopallidal neurons. The outcome is decreased activity of GABAergic neurons in GPI, and hence disinhibition of the ventral thalamus and thalamo-cortical circuits.

This concept is supported by observations that in monkeys with MPTP-induced parkinsonism, destructive lesions or injection of GABA agonists in the STN may relieve akinesia, presumably by reducing relative overactivity of the excitatory output from STN.

These schemes emphasize the key role of STN in the genesis of movement disorders, and suggest that new treatments may arise from manipulating both GABAergic and excitatory amino acid neurotransmission in the basal ganglia. They also throw light on the mechanism by which stereotactic surgical lesions of basal ganglia outflow pathways may relieve some of the symptoms of PD.

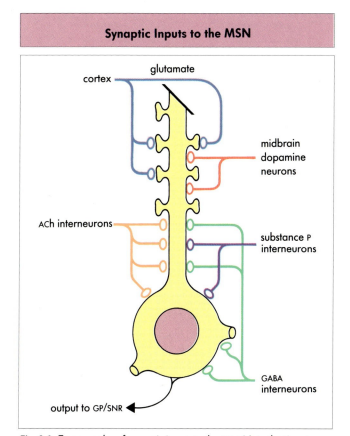

Synaptic Inputs to the MSN

Fig. 9.6 Topography of synaptic inputs to the MSN. Note that inputs from outside the striatum tend to terminate on more distal parts of the dendritic tree, while inputs from local neurons terminate more proximally. Inputs from large cholinergic interneurons terminate in an intermediate position.

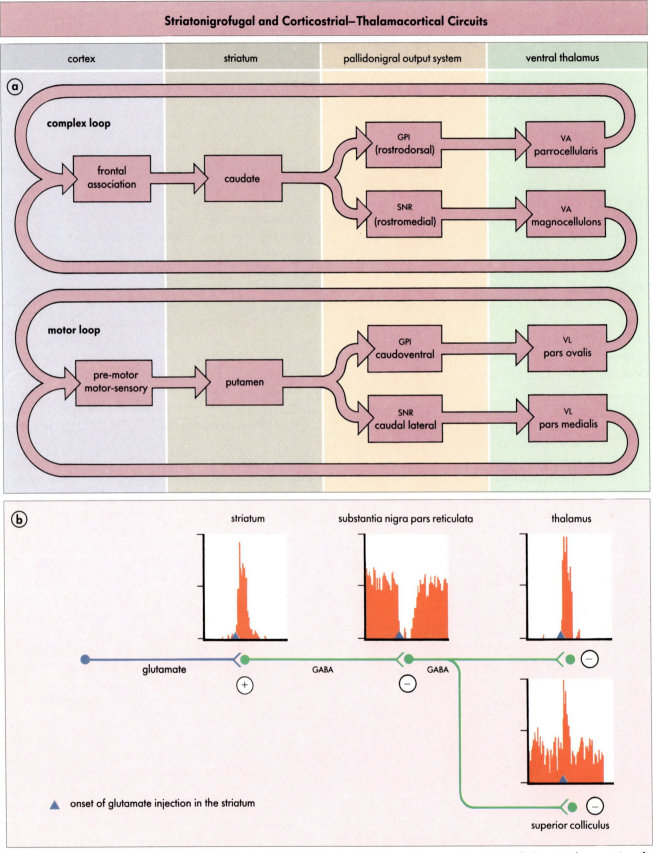

Fig. 9.7 (a) Organization of the striatonigrofugal pathways to the ventromedial thalamic nucleus and to the superior colliculus. The frequency histograms show the electrophysiological events underlying the disinhibitory influence of the striatum. (b) Suggested segregation of pathways from the association (complex loop) and sensorimotor (motor loop) areas through the basal ganglia and thalamus.

Basal Ganglia Interconnections in PD

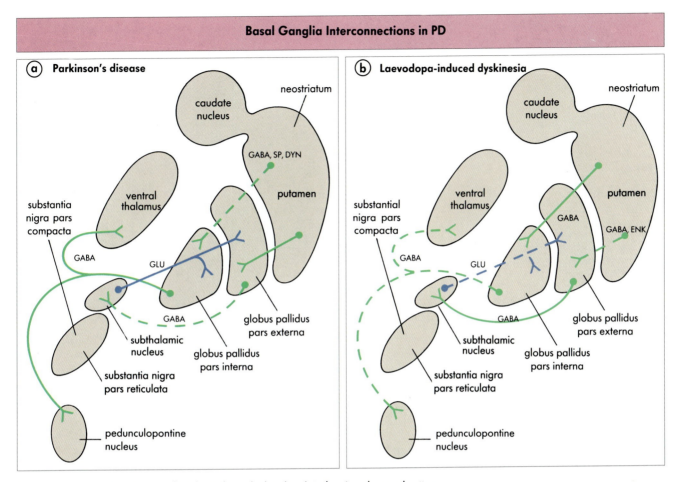

Fig. 9.8 Interconnections between basal ganglia and related nuclei, showing abnormal patterns of activity underlying motor symptoms of (a) PD and (b) laevodopa-induced dyskinesia.

SYMPTOMS AND SIGNS

The onset of PD is usually insidious, often with vague and non-specific symptoms, including aches and pains, and sensory symptoms including muscle pain, paraesthesiae, and cramps. Patients or their relatives may notice a general 'slowing up', affecting fine hand movements (handwriting often becomes smaller – micrographia), dexterity, and general mobility, so that dressing takes longer and the pace of walking decreases. When the symptoms are unilateral (hemiparkinsonism), the akinesia and rigidity may lead to the mistaken diagnosis of hemiparesis (Figs 9.9 and 9.10).

Some patients may present with gait and postural abnormalities. However, it is unusual for patients with Lewy body PD (idiopathic PD – IPD) to present with unsteadiness or falls, and this usually raises the possibility of parkinsonism due to other types of pathology such as multiple system atrophy, or progressive supranuclear palsy (see page 9.00). Other common clinical features include disturbances of mood (chiefly depression), excessive salivation and difficulty swallowing saliva, seborrhoea, and constipation.

The diagnosis of PD is often made as soon as the patient enters the room, since the facial appearance, posture, and gait are characteristic.

Tremor

About 80 per cent of patients with Lewy body PD (IPD) either present with tremor or develop tremor at some stage of their illness. Tremor often appears on one side of the body (usually in a hand, occasionally in a leg); most patients who present with unilateral tremor eventually develop tremor on the other side of the body. Typically, the tremor is present at rest, and may disappear as the patient makes a voluntary movement, although some patients exhibit both rest and action or postural tremor. However, in most cases, parkinsonism tremor, benign essential tremor, and tremor due to disease of the cerebellum or its connections are easily distinguished on clinical grounds (Fig. 9.11). Physiological recordings of tremor using surface or muscle electrodes may be helpful (see Fig. 9.10). Parkinsonian and other tremors generally increase in amplitude if the patient is anxious. Typically, the rest tremor of Lewy body PD has a frequency of 3–6Hz. In rare instances, rest and action tremor

Clinical Features of PD

Symptoms	Signs	Response to L-Dopa/PDI
Shaking, tremor	5–7 Hz rest tremor, often asymmetrical	+
Loss of dexterity, 'slowing up'	Akinesia, bradykinesia	++
Deteriorating hand-writing	Micrographia (akinesia and bradykinesia)	++
Difficulty initiating movements (walking, rising from chair, etc)	Akinesia	++
Stiffness	Rigidity of limbs and axial muscles	++
'Stooping'	Akinesia; postural changes	±
'Freezing'	Akinesia	++
Unsteadiness, imbalance	Impaired postural reflexes	–
Aches and pains	—	–
Constipation, bladder symptoms	—	–
Sexual dysfunction	—	–
Greasy skin	Seborrhoea	–
Less mental flexibility	Frontal lobe deficits	–
Memory impairment	Cognitive changes, dementia	–

Fig. 9.9 Symptoms and signs of PD, with their physiological correlates and response to treatment with L-dopa/PDI.

Parkinsonian and Essential Tremor

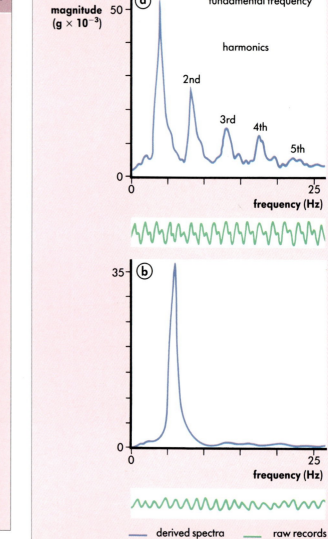

Fig. 9.10 EMGs from patients with (a) PD and (b) essential tremor.

Diagnostic Criteria for Idiopathic PD

Inclusion criteria	Exclusion criteria
At least two of the following present: tremor at rest rigidity akinesia/bradykinesia Unilateral or asymmetric involvement at onset Responsive to L-Dopa	Atypical features (e.g. rapid deterioration, strictly unilateral features of more than five years duration, prominent or early onset dementia, cerebellar signs, pyramidal signs, sensory deficits, disproportionate dysautonomia, significant supranuclear gaze palsies, oculogyric crises, prominent off-period dyskinesias) Secondary causes (e.g. Wilson's disease, drug-induced or post-encephalitic parkinsonism)

Fig. 9.11 Diagnostic criteria for PD.

may coexist, and a firm diagnosis of PD rests upon the demonstration of rigidity, akinesia and bradykinesia, postural and gait

Akinesia and Bradykinesia

Difficulty initiating fine and dexterous movements, poverty of movement, and slowness of movement, are characteristic and almost invariable clinical features of PD. Akinesia is strongly correlated with the degree of striatal dopamine deficiency, and usually responds well to laevodopa (see page 9.19). The physiological mechanisms underlying akinesia and bradykinesia are poorly understood, but the characteristic features of altered motor control in PD are summarized in Fig. 9.9.

Recordings in PD patients performing simple motor tasks show that the initial agonist EMG burst is smaller than required to move the limb through the appropriate angle, although additional bursts of EMG activity allow the action to be completed. This difficulty in scaling the EMG activity to the task contributes to, but does not wholly explain, parkinsonism akinesia and bradykinesia.

Sequential or simultaneous movements are markedly slowed in PD and there is an increase in the delay in executing these complex movements individually. This suggests that PD patients may have difficulty switching motor programs, or in running more than one motor program simultaneously.

In summary, parkinsonian patients can select muscles correctly for a simple motor task, activate muscles in the appropriate sequence, learn new motor tasks, use predictive information to anticipate changes in strategy, and use cues to correct errors. All this suggests that simple motor programs can be formulated and run relatively normally, but PD patients have difficulties producing strategies dependent upon planning for tasks which are self-directed. Activities which require sequential and complex movements are also impaired, suggesting a degradation of complex movements which may be related to a disturbance of the interactions between the motor cortex, the basal ganglia, and the premotor and prefrontal areas.

Rigidity

Stiffness is a common symptom in PD and on examination it is detected by increased resistance to passive movements of the limbs and trunk. It is termed 'lead-pipe' rigidity because, unlike spasticity, it persists through the whole range of passive movement about a joint. It may be associated with the cogwheel phenomenon. The pathophysiological basis of rigidity is poorly understood, and it correlates poorly with the degree of dopamine deficiency. Interruption of nigrostriatal dopamine pathways in the monkey does not lead to detectable increase in resistance to passive movements of the limbs, but a parkinsonian syndrome (including rigidity) can be produced by dopamine receptor blockade, by administration of dopamine-depleting drugs such as reserpine, or by the neurotoxin MPTP. Parkinsonian rigidity is increased by cholinergic drugs such as physostigmine, and reduced by anticholinergic or dopaminergic drugs and stereotactic lesions of striatal output pathways or ventrolateral thalamus.

Postural and Gait Abnormalities

Gait and postural abnormalities include a festinant (hurrying) gait, small steps with a tendency to shuffle, freezing (which is a manifestation of akinesia), and a liability to fall. Righting reflexes are impaired, as are anticipatory postural reflexes. Akinetic patients cannot compensate rapidly for sudden changes in their centre of gravity to prevent a fall. The flexed attitude ('simian posture') of the trunk of limbs, which may be asymmetrical, and the failure to swing the arms when walking reflect both akinesia and rigidity.

Psychiatric and Neuropsychological Changes in PD

Depression affects about 40 per cent of patients with PD. Usually it is mild and linked to motor disability, but severe depression may be difficult to detect in the patient with advanced disease, and may present as pseudodementia.

Neuropsychological abnormalities of the type found in frontal lobe damage can be detected in unmedicated patients with mild motor disability. Abnormalities of visuo-spatial memory and learning, and of attention, can also be detected, and such cognitive changes become more marked as the disease progresses. Comparison of PD and Alzheimer's disease patients reveals comparable deficits in pattern and spatial recognition, but patients with Alzheimer's disease show more severe impairments of delayed-response memory and conditional learning, and different types of deficits in matching-to-sample tests. Neuropsychological abnormalities may be due to impaired attention-switching, which would result in mental slowness (bradyphrenia). In this model, internally regulated tasks are less effective in activating the attention-shifting device than externally cued tasks.

It is still unclear whether dementia defined by DSM III criteria is more common in PD than would be expected in a suitable control population, although many studies have found dementia to occur in 20–50 per cent of PD patients. Alzheimer's disease pathology may be only marginally more common in PD brains compared to controls. Diffuse Lewy body disease accounts for only rare cases of dementia in patients with the typical presentation and course of PD.

EPIDEMIOLOGY AND PATHOGENESIS OF PD

Incidence and Prevalence Studies

PD occurs worldwide. The incidence in the USA may be increasing; this could be due to greater public awareness of the condition, and better case ascertainment. Incidence rates in the USA and Europe derived from surveys where case ascertainment has been the most thorough show figures close to 20 new cases per 100 000 per year (Fig. 9.12). Age-specific prevalence rates increase throughout the seventh, eighth and ninth decades, and in the USA and Europe range from 70–170. Lower prevalence rates of 44 cases per 100 000 have been found in urban populations in

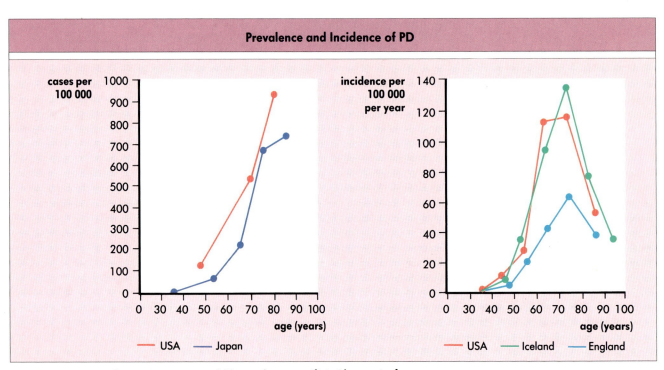

Fig. 9.12 (a) Age-specific prevalence rates; and (b) annual age- specific incidence rates for PD, from various studies.

the People's Republic of China. Suggestions that Parkinson's disease may be commoner amongst whites than blacks in the USA have not been confirmed in all studies, but there may be a lower prevalence of PD amongst rural west Africans, compared to rural American blacks. Some studies show an excess of men affected, but the male to female ratio is close to one.

The life expectancy for patients with untreated PD is reduced. The mortality of untreated patients is nearly two to three times that of non-parkinsonian controls, and although the mortality of patients (particularly those with younger age of onset) who receive laevodopa approaches that of controls, in some studies the ratio of observed to expected mortality ratios is increased.

Risk Factors in PD

No specific risk factor has been identified, other than age. Case control studies have detected an association between previous head trauma and PD, akin to the association between previous head trauma and Alzheimer's disease and amyotrophic lateral sclerosis. One of the most consistent epidemiological findings from case control studies is an inverse relationship between smoking and PD. Patients with PD show a lower frequency of smoking prior to disease onset compared to controls. This may reflect a pre-morbid personality type, a protective effect of smoking, or sensitivity to the pharmacological effects of smoking in predisposed individuals. However, smoking habits have changed dramatically over the last four or five decades, while the incidence and prevalence of PD has remained stable over many years, so smoking is unlikely to be protective.

Some studies, but not all, have suggested that there is an increased risk for PD for those who have lived in rural areas, or who have relied on well-water in childhood. Others have suggested that there is an increased exposure to herbicides, pesticides, and industrial toxins in those who develop PD. However, these findings have not been consistent.

Relationship Between PD and Encephalitis

Many thousands of cases of encephalitis lethargica occurred between 1916 and 1930, although rare sporadic instances of the clinical syndrome of encephalitis lethargica are still encountered. The illness was characterized by hypersomnolence, an akinetic–rigid state, and a bewildering variety of other movement disorders and neuropsychiatric abnormalities. Some patients who had apparently recovered from the acute illness developed parkinsonism within several years of the acute illness. Many of these patients were relatively young, and showed features which are not usually associated with typical Lewy body PD, namely cranial nerve palsies, oculogyric crises (Fig. 9.13), dystonia, chorea, and psychiatric abnormalities. Despite the distinctive nature of the post-encephalitic parkinsonian syndrome, it was proposed that virtually all parkinsonism might result from 'latent' damage to the basal ganglia by the virus assumed to have caused encephalitis lethargica. A cohort effect was predicted, with a steadily increasing age of onset of new cases, and finally a virtual disappearance of the PD by the early 1980s. This prediction has not been fulfilled, and the incidence and prevalence of PD has remained much the same in the 1980s as in the 1960s.

Attempts to identify viruses in the brain of patients dying with encephalitis lethargica using *in situ* hybridization and polymerase

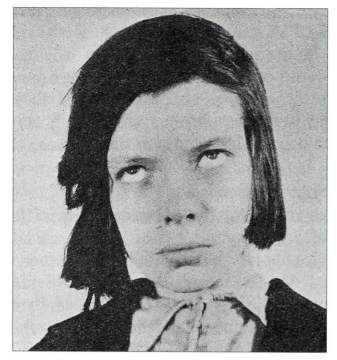

Fig. 9.13 Oculogyric crisis.

MPTP in Primates and PD in Humans		
Parameter	**PD**	**MPTP-induced parkinsonism**
Motor deficits		
Akinesia or bradykinesia	+++	+++
Rigidity	+++	++
Tremor	+++	++
Postural abnormalities	+++	++
Myoclonus	–	+
Exaggerated startle response	–	+
Dystonic posturing of head and trunk	–	+
Drug responsiveness		
L-Dopa	+++	+++
Dyskinesias	++	++
Wearing off	++	+
On–off	++	–
Pathology		
Substantia nigra	+++	+++
Ventral tegmental area	++	+
Locus coeruleus	+++	+
Substantia innominata	+++	–
Lewy bodies	+++	?
Biochemistry		
Dopamine depletion in:		
putamen	+++	+++
nucleus accumbens	++	+
Noradrenaline	++	+

Fig. 9.14 Comparison of the clinical effects of MPTP in primates and the characteristics of idiopathic PD in humans.

chain reaction have been unsuccessful, and attempts to link IPD to virus infection using serological techniques have also failed. The putative virus causing encephalitis lethargica has never been identified, despite the concurrence of the first cases of encephalitis lethargica with the great influenza pandemic of 1918–19. Finally, the pathology of post-encephalitic PD is distinct from that of idiopathic Lewy body PD (see page 9.00).

Parkinsonism and Neurotoxins

A parkinsonian syndrome results from poisoning with carbon monoxide, carbon disulphide, or cyanide. Manganese encephalopathy results in parkinsonism, with marked damage to the globus pallidus and relatively little destruction of the substantia nigra. A wide variety of neuroleptic agents cause parkinsonism which is usually reversible, although recovery may take months, and in rare instances parkinsonism may persist, apparently due to unmasking of underlying Lewy body PD.

MPTP and parkinsonism   MPTP (1-methyl-4-phenyl-1,2,3,6-tetrahydropyridine) is a neurotoxin which selectively destroys certain catecholamine-containing neurons. MPTP came to light following an epidemic of parkinsonism among young drug addicts, who had been exposed to varying amounts of MPTP, a by-product of the synthesis of the meperidine analogue MPPP (1-methyl-4-proprionoxypiperidine). Pathological studies in one patient revealed neuronal loss limited to the substantia nigra. Clinical, pharmacological, and biochemical changes in PD and MPTP-induced parkinsonism and non-human primates reveal remarkable similarities, although there are differences (Fig. 9.14). The mechanism of MPTP toxicity is summarized in Fig. 9.15.

MPTP reproduces classical parkinsonism in primates, but many rodents are resistant to the effects of MPTP, and primates often show some degree of recovery after repeated acute exposure to MPTP. In humans, MPTP may cause parkinsonism of varying severity, or subclinical damage to the substantia nigra which can be revealed by PET scanning with ^{18}F-dopa. However, the pathology of MPTP-induced parkinsonism in sub-human primates differs from that of IPD, since in the latter neuronal degeneration includes the cholinergic systems of the nucleus basalis of Meynert, the ventral tegmental area comprising neurons of the mesolimbic and mesocortical systems, noradrenergic neurons in the hypothalamus and brain stem, serotonergic neurons of the dorsal raphe nucleus, and peptidergic neurons at several sites.

There is no direct evidence that endogenous or exogenous MPTP-like substances cause IPD, but the mechanism of MPTP-induced neurotoxicity provides a valuable model for understanding selective neuronal damage in PD. In particular, MPP$^+$ interferes with mitochondrial respiration (see Fig. 9.15), which may also be a critical biochemical defect in IPD.

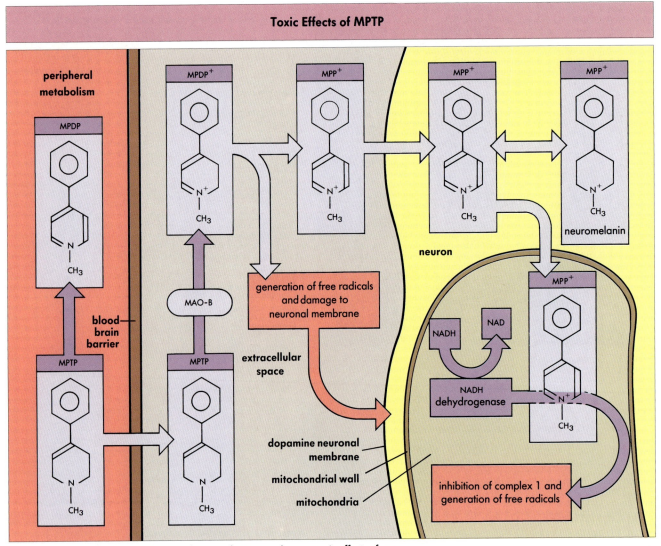

Fig. 9.15 The proposed metabolism, mechanism of action, and neurotoxic effects of MPTP (and MPP$^+$) to dopamine cells in substantia nigra.

Oxidative metabolism in PD The activity of mitochondrial complex 1 (and less consistently of complexes 2 and 3 and 4) is diminished in PD (Fig. 9.16). Complex 1 activity has also been found to be diminished in muscle biopsies and in platelets of some patients with PD. Deficiency of complex 1 is relatively specific for IPD. Immunochemical studies of the protein subunits of complex 1 have not yielded consistent abnormalities. Some complex 1 subunits are coded for by mitochondrial DNA, and there have been reports of an increase in deletions of mitochondrial DNA in IPD, but these occur also in the ageing brain.

Free radical formation There are several sources of free radical formation in PD. The auto-oxidation of dopamine to neuromelanin generates free radicals (Fig. 9.17). Amine-oxidation via MAO-B can produce hydrogen peroxide; and the substantia nigra of patients dying with PD contains an excess of iron but low amounts of the iron-binding protein ferritin, suggesting that unbound iron may be available for interaction with hydrogen peroxide to form ferric ions and hydroxyl radicals. There is

evidence supporting the selective damage of nigral neurons by free radicals (see Fig. 9.17).

Genetics and PD

If PD is due to endogenous or exogenous neurotoxins, then genetically determined differences in metabolism might render some individuals susceptible to such agents. One major detoxification system is the cytochrome P450 (CYP 2D6) debrisoquine hydroxylase system. Although initial reports of an excess of poor hydroxylators of debrisoquine amongst PD patients have not been confirmed, PD patients show a significant excess of the specific mutations in the CYP 2D6 gene which cause the poor metabolizer (PM) phenotype. The molecular basis of the PM defect has been identified as due to three distinct mutations in the CYP 2D6 gene, the most frequent mutation being a G to A transition at the intron 3-exon 4 junction, leading to a one base-pair frame shift, with premature termination of translation. This, and two other less frequent mutations, identify about 90

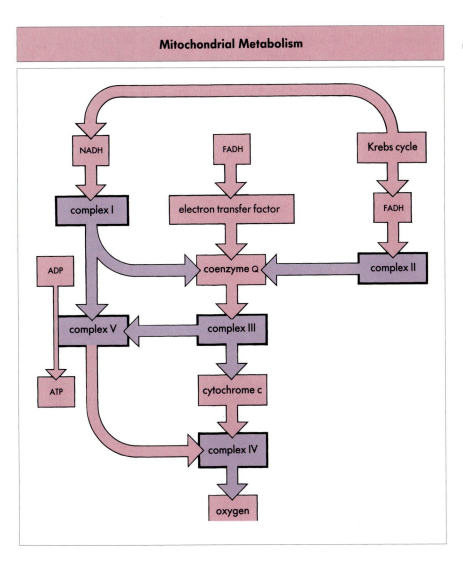

Fig. 9.16 Scheme of mitochondrial metabolism.

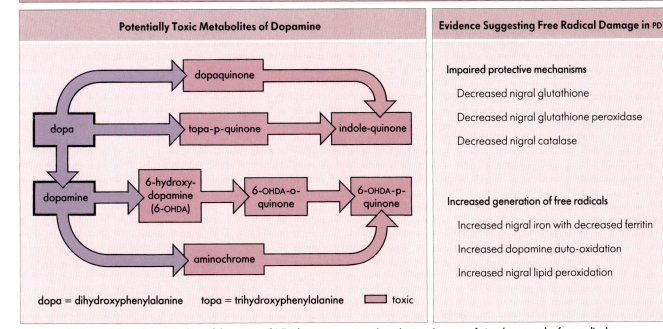

Fig. 9.17 (a) Potentially toxic metabolites of dopamine; (b) Evidence supporting the selective damage of nigral neurons by free radicals.

per cent of PM individuals. About 5 per cent of controls, and 12 per cent of parkinsonian patients can be genotyped as PMs, indicating a 2.5-fold higher risk for PD amongst individuals with these mutations.

Abnormalities of sulphur oxidation have been detected in PD, but also in Alzheimer's disease and in amyotrophic lateral sclerosis. Elevated plasma cysteine and low plasma sulphate levels likewise are not specific for PD, and may be an acquired rather than an inherited abnormality.

Twin studies have shown concordance rates of 2–12 per cent for monozygotic twins and of 0–5 per cent for dizygotic twins, depending on the criteria for diagnosis of PD. This has been interpreted to suggest that genetic factors are not important in the pathogenesis of PD.

However, several large kindreds have been described in whom Lewy body pathology was associated with a pattern of transmission suggesting autosomal-dominant inheritance (Fig. 9.18). Re-evaluation of data from the twin studies has suggested that they neither exclude nor prove a genetic contribution in PD. If a genetically determined abnormality of mitochondrial complex 1 were responsible for PD, inheritance would be Mendelian if a nuclear gene coded for the abnormal protein, and maternal if it were coded for by a mitochondrial gene. In the latter situation, no difference would be expected in concordance for PD in monozygotic and dizygotic twins. Maternal inheritance has been excluded in the large pedigrees which show probable autosomal-dominant transmission, but remains a possibility in other smaller kindreds. Re-evaluation of twin pairs may reveal evidence of presymptomatic PD in clinically unaffected twins, through alterations in striatal uptake of ^{18}F-dopa on PET scanning, together with long-term clinical and pathological follow-up.

Ageing and PD

There is no convincing evidence that PD results from a combination of an acute insult with the gradual neuronal attrition related to ageing. Some PET scan studies using ^{18}F-fluorodopa have shown a progressive decline in striatal dopamine uptake with age. There is a loss of about 5 per cent of cells per decade between the fifth and ninth decades in normal controls (Fig. 9.19), whereas cell loss in PD at the onset of symptoms is usually in the region of 60 per cent, and striatal dopamine loss in the region of 80 per cent (see page 9.00).

Furthermore, the distribution of age-related substantia nigra cell loss is different from that of PD. In the former situation, more heavily pigmented neurons of the dorsomedial substantia nigra are affected; in the latter, cell loss is most marked in the more lightly pigmented neurons of the ventrolateral substantia nigra (the ventral tier nuclei; see Fig. 9.19). Substantia nigra damage due to MPTP in non-human primates tends to affect the more heavily melanized parts of substantia nigra (i.e. the more dorsal areas). Thus the distribution of damage is not exactly equivalent to that seen in PD.

Finally, the substantia nigra in PD shows evidence of active neuronal degeneration associated with phagocytosing microglia which express HLA DR antigen. The evidence thus favours a progressive destructive process which continues until death, rather than the interaction between an acute (e.g. toxic) episode associated with chronic neuronal loss due to ageing.

PATHOLOGY OF PD

Nigral Degeneration, and the Significance of the Lewy Body

Macroscopically, the uncut brain and spinal cord appear normal, but cross sections of the brain stem reveal pallor of the substantia nigra and the locus coeruleus reflecting loss of neuromelanin-containing neurons (Fig. 9.20).

The pathological hallmarks of PD include:

- degeneration and loss of pigmented neurons of the substantia nigra (pars compacta); and
- the presence of Lewy bodies in the substantia nigra (Fig. 9.21).

Degeneration and Loss of Pigmented Neurons of the Substantia Nigra

Loss of nigral neurons usually exceeds 60 per cent in patients with symptoms of PD, and may be virtually complete in patients with a long history and advanced disease. Patients with diffuse

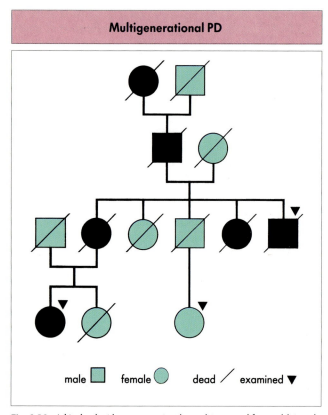

Multigenerational PD

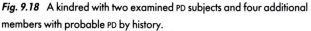

male ▢   female ◯   dead ╱   examined ▼

Fig. 9.18 A kindred with two examined PD subjects and four additional members with probable PD by history.

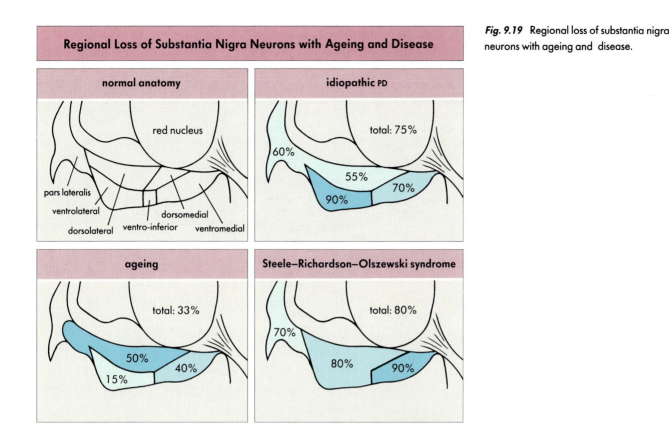

Regional Loss of Substantia Nigra Neurons with Ageing and Disease

normal anatomy

red nucleus

pars lateralis
ventrolateral
dorsolateral   ventro-inferior   dorsomedial   ventromedial

idiopathic PD

total: 75%
60%
55%
90%   70%

ageing

total: 33%
50%
15%   40%

Steele–Richardson–Olszewski syndrome

total: 80%
70%
80%   90%

Fig. 9.19 Regional loss of substantia nigra neurons with ageing and disease.

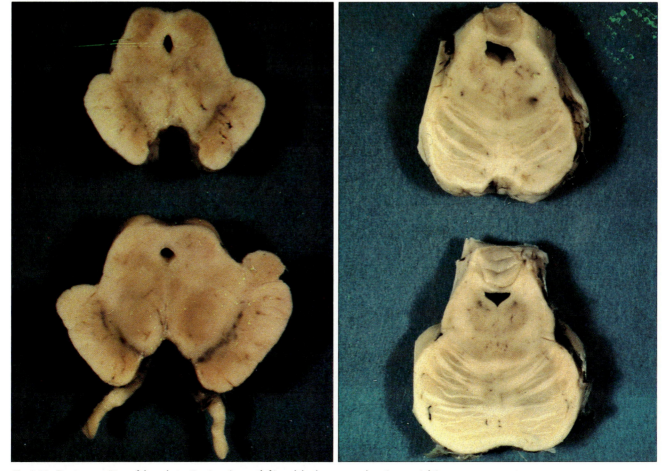

Fig. 9.20 Depigmentation of the substantia nigra (upper left) and the locus coeruleus (upper right) compared to normal (lower).

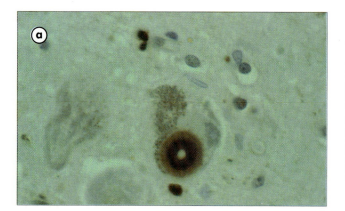

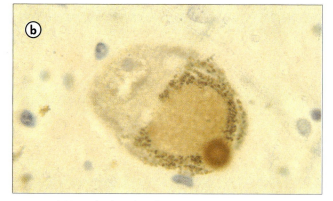

Fig. 9.21 (a) Lewy body in the substantia nigra pars compacta. (b) Pale body α-Lewy body (anti-ubiquitin) in a pigmented neuron of the substantia nigra.

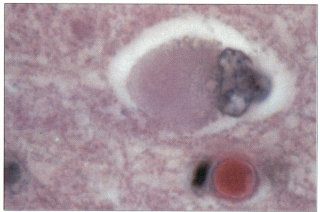

Fig. 9.22 Cortical Lewy body.

Molecular Components of Lewy Bodies					
Protein component	Inclusion				
	Brain stem Lewy body	Cortical Lewy body	Alzheimer's tangle	Pick body	GCIs (MSA)
Phosphorylated NFs	+	+	+	+	–
Tubulin	+	–	–	–	+
MAPs 1 & 2	+	–	+	–	–
Tau	–	–	++	++	+
Ubiquitin	+	+	+	+	+

Fig. 9.23 Components of Lewy bodies compared with other intraneuronal inclusions.

Lewy body disease, on the other hand, may show less marked nigral cell loss (see chapter 4).

The Presence of Lewy Bodies in the Substantia Nigra

The Lewy body is an intraneuronal inclusion body which is found in many parts of the central and peripheral nervous system in PD. Although Lewy bodies are characteristic of PD and are essential for a pathological diagnosis, they are seen in about 5 per cent of neurologically normal individuals over the age of 65 ('incidental Lewy body disease'). In conditions such as cortical-basal ganglionic degeneration, Hallevorden–Spatz disease, some familial olivopontocerebellar atrophies, juvenile hereditary Parkinsonian syndrome, and ataxia–telangiectasia, they may occur more frequently than can be accounted for by chance alone. In amyotrophic lateral sclerosis, Lewy body-like inclusions are usually restricted to brain stem and spinal motor neurons.

Lewy bodies are occasionally detected in other akinetic rigid syndromes such as multiple system atrophy, progressive supra-nuclear palsy, the parkinsonian–dementia complex of Guam, and Alzheimer's disease, but the association with these disorders may be coincidental. The relationship between Alzheimer's disease and diffuse (cortical) Lewy body disease in discussed in chapter 4.

The morphology of Lewy bodies differs in the various regions of the nervous system. Within the brain stem, they consist of a halo and body composed of radially arranged filamentous material of 5–10nm diameter, and an amorphous core composed of granular and amorphous material. Cortical Lewy bodies (Fig. 9.22) are more homogeneous, consisting of amorphous material containing randomly oriented filaments. Cortical Lewy bodies are present in most cases of typical PD (albeit in small numbers) usually in the medial temporal cortex. In diffuse Lewy body disease they are most abundant in the medial temporal cortex (but not in the hippocampus), and in the frontal and parietal cortex. Cortical Lewy bodies are usually found in the deeper cortical layers. They are most easily detected with ubiquitin antibodies.

Lewy bodies are composed of proteins, free fatty acids, sphingo-myelin, and polysaccharides. Immunocytochemical studies reveal that they contain elements of cytoskeletal and other neuronal proteins, including neurofilaments, tubulin, high molecular weight microtubule-associated proteins (MAPS) and ubiquitin (Fig. 9.23). Ubiquitin immunocytochemistry is particularly useful for revealing cortical Lewy bodies.

Another characteristic inclusion in PD is the pale or hyaline body (see Fig. 9.21) which is most readily found in pigmented neurons of the substantia nigra and locus coeruleus, and which is composed of straight filaments and labelled by antibodies against phosphorylated neurofilaments and ubiquitin. Pale bodies can be distinguished from the filamentous inclusions of progressive supranuclear palsy, cortical-basal ganglionic degeneration, and Pick's disease because they are non-agyrophilic and are not labelled by antibodies against microtubule-associated protein tau.

Extra-nigral Neuronal Loss in PD

Areas of cell loss in PD include the noradrenergic neurons of the locus coeruleus, the serotonin-containing neurons of the dorsal raphe nucleus, the cholinergic neurons of the basal forebrain cholinergic system, including the nucleus basalis of Meynert, and the pedunculopontine nucleus of the caudal midbrain. In the latter region there is also loss of substance P-containing neurons. In the cerebral cortex, somatostatin-containing neurons are probably lost, particularly in those patients with dementia, in whom the pathological changes of Alzheimer's disease may coexist. Cell loss in the intermediolateral columns of the spinal cord occurs in some patients.

NEUROCHEMICAL PATHOLOGY OF PD

Dopamine Systems

Ehringer and Hornykiewicz in 1960 first showed that striatal dopamine concentrations were decreased in PD. This reflects degeneration of the dopaminergic neurons of the substantia nigra pars compacta. Striatal dopamine deficiency is the distinctive biochemical feature of PD and other disorders which are associated with nigral degeneration. In PD, striatal dopamine

depletion is greatest in the putamen, and in the parolfactory gyrus (Fig. 9.24). Tissue dopamine concentrations are also decreased in the target areas of the mesocorticolimbic system. Dopamine levels are also reduced in the hypothalamus, in the locus coeruleus, and in the area postrema. Spinal cord dopamine levels are probably normal or slightly decreased. Dopamine depletion can be detected with PET scans using ^{18}F-dopa (Fig. 9.25). Dopamine depletion in parkinsonian syndromes such as multiple system atrophy, progressive supranuclear palsy, and corticobasal ganglia degeneration, tends to be distributed throughout the striatum, involving the caudate nucleus and putamen about equally (see Fig. 9.25).

There is evidence that the motor symptoms of PD appear when striatal dopamine levels are decreased by approximately 80 per cent, which corresponds to a 60–70 per cent loss of nigral dopamine neurons. The loss of the striatonigral dopamine system is accompanied by evidence of increased dopamine turnover in surviving neurons, reflected by an increased ratio of homovanillic

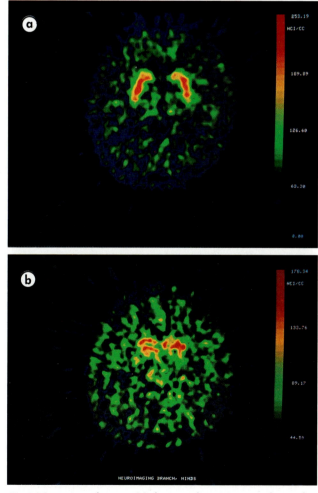

Fig. 9.25 PET scans showing F18-dopa uptake in (a) a normal control and (b) a patient with advanced (stage III) PD. In stage III disease, there is decreased uptake in the posterior putamen relative to the anterior putamen and caudate, as well as a generalized reduction in uptake, reflected in the decreased contrast between basal ganglia and the rest of the brain. (Courtesy of Robert Miletich MD, Bethseda, Maryland.)

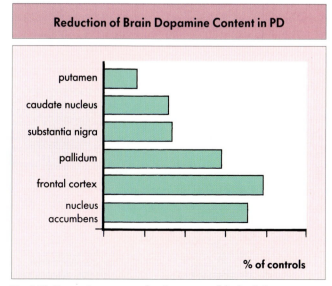

Fig. 9.24 Dopamine content of various areas of the brain in PD, expressed as percentage of that in controls.

PET Studies in Movement Disorders		
	Pre-synaptic dopaminergic system	Post-synaptic dopaminergic system
Parkinson's disease	Decrease; in the putamen more than the caudate nucleus	Normal, or increased in untreated patients
Huntington's disease	Normal	Decreased
Multiple system atrophy	Decreased in the putamen and caudate nucleus	Decreased
Steele–Richardson–Olszewski syndrome	Decreased in the putamen and caudate nucleus	Decreased

Fig. 9.26 Some main findings of PET studies in movement disorders.

acid (HVA) to dopamine in the striatum and other brain areas receiving dopamine input. Striatal dopamine receptor binding may be increased, compatible with denervation supersensitivity. This may be particularly marked in patients with untreated PD. PET studies with the D_2 receptor ligand raclopride indicate that increased receptor binding in untreated PD may return towards normal with laevodopa treatment (Fig. 9.26).

Dopamine deficiency in the striatum, and particularly in the putamen, is correlated with akinesia, but the correlation with tremor and rigidity is weaker. Asymmetrical onset is characteristic of PD, and striatal dopamine deficiency is greatest on the side opposite the more affected limbs, although dopamine depletion is almost always evident in both striata. The relationship between mesocorticolimbic dopamine deficiency and neuropsychiatric features of PD remains uncertain, but certain neuropsychological tests which are thought to reflect frontal lobe dysfunction are partially reversed by L-dopa therapy. The relationship between depression in PD and mesocorticolimbic dopamine levels is unclear.

Involvement of Other Neurochemical Systems

Noradrenergic systems originating in the locus coeruleus and the serotoninergic system originating in the dorsal raphe nucleus are affected in PD, with widespread decreases in cortical, subcortical, brain stem, and spinal cord noradrenaline levels; there are similarly widespread, although slightly less marked, decreases in brain serotonin. The clinical relevance of decreases in noradrenergic and serotonergic systems is not known, but deficiency of noradrenaline may contribute to 'freezing' episodes, which can sometimes be relieved by dihydroxyphenylserine, a noradrenaline precursor. Noradrenaline deficiency may also be related to depression, and to other cognitive impairments, although this remains unproven. Changes in central nervous system noradrenaline may also contribute to autonomic changes in PD. Serotonin deficiency may also contribute to depression and other neuropsychiatric changes, but manipulating serotonin function does not significantly alter motor deficits in PD.

Cholinergic systems in the basal forebrain undergo degeneration in PD. Decreased activity of the acetylcholine synthetic enzyme choline acetyltransferase (CAT) in several cortical areas reflects degeneration of cholinergic neurons in the basal forebrain (nucleus basalis of Meynert), and a modest decrease in cortical CAT activity is found even in patients without dementia, suggesting that loss of substantia in interneurons occurs relatively early in the disease process, and is present in virtually all patients. Cholinergic neurons in the septal nuclei and diagonal band of Broca, and in the peduncular pontine nucleus of the caudal midbrain also undergo degeneration, but cholinergic interneurons in the striatum are preserved. CAT activity in the cerebral cortex is particularly low in patients with PD and dementia, possibly reflecting the combination of PD and Alzheimer's disease pathology. The relationship between cortical cholinergic deficit and intellectual and cognitive impairments in PD remains uncertain, but it may explain the sensitivity of older parkinsonian patients to treatment with anticholinergic drugs. Muscarinic receptors are increased in the cerebral cortex but not the caudate nucleus of patients with PD, and changes in nicotinic receptor binding have also been observed.

DOPAMINE SYSTEMS THE TREATMENT OF PD

L-Dopa and Dopamine Metabolism

Pathways for dopamine synthesis and breakdown are shown in Fig. 9.27. Orally administered L-dopa is rapidly metabolized to dopamine by L-aromatic amino acid decarboxylase (dopa decarboxylase) in the gut, liver, and other tissues, leaving small amounts of L-dopa available to cross the blood–brain barrier, and provoking unwanted effects such as nausea. These difficulties are minimized by combining L-dopa with a peripheral decarboxylase inhibitor (PDI) such as benserazide or carbidopa (Fig. 9.28).

Within the brain, decarboxylation of L-dopa occurs in the synaptic terminals of dopaminergic nigrostriatal neurons, but also in other catecholamine neurons. Dopamine thus formed is presumed to be stored in surviving terminals. As the disease progresses, the capacity of the nigrostriatal system to generate and store dopamine from L-dopa probably diminishes, although surviving neurons may partially compensate by increased activity, reflected in higher levels of HVA and other dopamine metabolites compared to dopamine itself (Fig. 9.29).

Dopamine is metabolized to potentially toxic products (see Fig. 9.17), but there is no evidence that long-term use causes or accelerates cell death. Nevertheless, its use in PD is associated with well-defined but poorly understood complications.

L-Dopa Therapy and Complications

L-Dopa combined with a PDI (L-dopa/PDI) is the mainstay of drug therapy in PD. It is particularly effective in ameliorating akinesia and bradykinesia, but also improves rigidity and tremor.

Therapy with L-dopa/PDI is started when the patient has functionally significant disability. In the early stages of the disease L-dopa is often dramatically effective in reversing the symptoms and signs of PD. However, within three to five years of starting treatment, most patients develop complications, which include

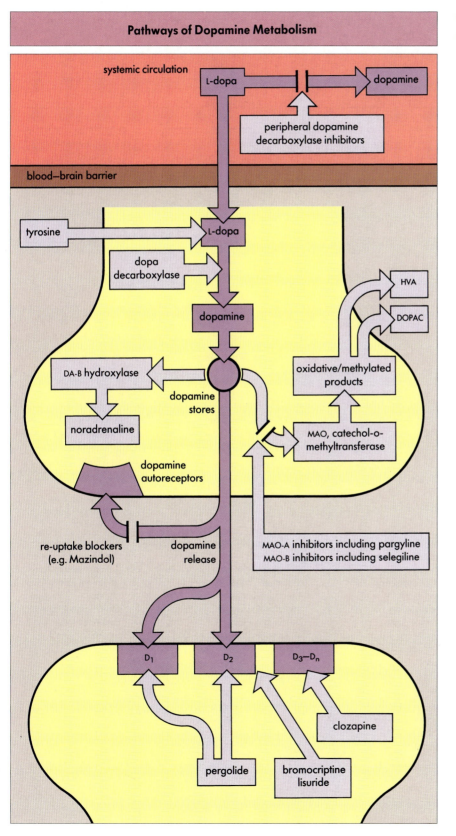

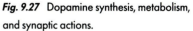

Fig. 9.27 Dopamine synthesis, metabolism, and synaptic actions.

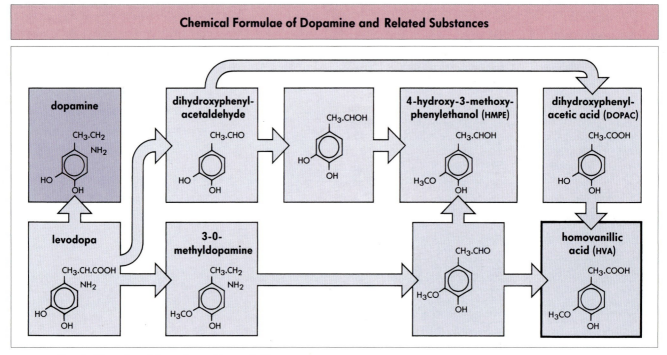

Fig. 9.28 Chemical formulae of dopamine and its metabolites.

Dopamine Agonist Agents in PD

Agent	Chemistry	Mode and site of action	Plasma half-life (hours)	Major unwanted effects	Usual daily dose (mg)	Indications
Apomorphine	Morphine analogue	Stimulator of D_1 and D_2 receptors	≈ 0.5	1. Vomiting and uraemia if used without domperidone	1–100	1. Increased flexibility of regime in active patients ('penject') 2. Treatment of fluctuations ('penject' or infusions) 3. Apomorphine 'challenge' text in atypical PD
Bromocriptine	Ergolene (lysergic and diethylamide derivative)	1. Activity depends on nigrostriatal DA system 2. May either stimulate or block presynaptic DA receptors 3. Mixed agonist/antagonist at post-synaptic D_1 non-adrenylcyclase-linked receptors 4. Blocks brain 5HT and NA receptors	≈ 5	1. Nausea, vomiting, hypotension 2. Neuropsychiatric symptoms (hallucinations, confusion, somnolence, psychosis) 3. Livedo reticularis 4. Retroperitoneal fibrosis 5. Exacerbation of peripheral vascular disease	10–100	1. Initial (low-dose) therapy with L-dopa/PDI 2. Treatment of 'late treatment failures' with L-dopa/PDI (wearing off, on–off phenomena, dyskinesias, nocturnal akinesia)
Lysuride	semi-synthetic ergolene	1. Stimulates post-synaptic DA receptors 2. Stimulates central 5HT receptors	≈ 2	As for Bromocriptine, *plus* increased appetite, and weight gain	1–5	As for Bromocriptine
Pergolide	synthetic ergolene	Stimulates D_1 and D_2 receptors	15–42	As for Bromocriptine and Lisuride	1–5	As for Bromocriptine and Lisuride

Fig. 9.29 Mode and site of action, plasma half-life, major side-effects, usual daily dosage, and indications for use of some of the main dopamine agonists.

end-of-dose deterioration, L-dopa induced dyskinesia, predictable and unpredictable variations in response to L-dopa ('on–off' phenomena), dystonic reactions, myoclonus, and neuropsychiatric complications such as confusion, hallucinations, depression, or psychotic symptoms.

Monoamine Oxidase B (MAO-B) Inhibition: Selegiline (L-Deprenyl)

Selegiline is a 'suicide' inhibitor of MAO-B, the enzyme that catalyses the oxidation of dopamine to HVA and other metabolites (see Fig. 9.27). Selegiline has an L-dopa-sparing effect, and when added to L-dopa/PDI, leads to improvements in disability scores of around 30 per cent. It is valuable in improving end-of-dose deterioration, and sometimes in reducing dose-reponse variations ('on–off' phenomena) although it is of little value in managing complex fluctuations later in the course of the disease. Selegiline protects against damage due to MPTP in the monkey (see page 9.11) by blocking conversion of MPTP to MPP$^+$. It may also block dopamine oxidation to products which may generate free radicals and might theoretically protect against cell death in PD. Clinical trials have suggested that selegiline delays the need for L-dopa/PDI therapy in newly diagnosed patients with PD, although there is no direct evidence that this effect is related to changes in the rate of neuronal death, and these studies probably underestimated the direct therapeutic effects of selegiline in previously untreated patients. Nevertheless, many clinicians would start patients on selegiline at the time of diagnosis.

Dopamine Agonists

Drugs which act directly on dopamine receptors include bromocriptine, lysuride, pergolide, and apomorphine (Fig. 9.30). The last is given by subcutaneous injection, either intermittently via a 'penject' in the same way of insulin, or by continuous infusion via a mini-pump. Because of its potent emetic effect it is used with domperidone, which blocks dopamine receptors in the area postrema, but does not cross the blood–brain barrier to block striatal dopamine receptors and thus does not exacerbate parkinsonian symptoms.

Dopamine agonists are best combined with L-dopa/PDI. Although dopamine agonists used alone as initial therapy may have similar anti-parkinsonian potency to L-dopa/PDI, they are not so well tolerated, and although patients rarely develop dyskinesia when treated with dopamine agonists alone, the overall benefits of this approach are marginal. Nevertheless, starting therapy with low dose L-dopa/PDI combined with a dopamine agonist is gaining acceptance in the light of evidence that this strategy may reduce or delay the appearance of L-dopa-induced dyskinesia.

Dopamine agonists are also helpful in controlling the late complications of L-dopa/PDI therapy. They have a longer duration of action than L-dopa, but more frequently cause unacceptable side-effects, including hypotension, nausea, hallucinations, confusion, and psychotic symptoms.

OTHER TREATMENTS

Other Drugs

The first effective drugs for PD were anticholinergic agents such as hyoscine and atropine. Later, synthetic agents including benzhexol, benztropine, and orphenadrine were introduced. These agents may improve tremor and rigidity, but have little effect upon akinesia. Thus they are useful in early tremor-predominant disease, but they should be avoided in elderly patients and in those with memory impairment.

Amantidine stimulates dopamine release and is sometimes used alone in early disease or in combination with L-dopa/PDI to improve end-of-dose deterioration.

Stereotaxic Surgery

Stereotaxic lesions of the basal ganglia outflow pathways (pallidotomy) or ventral thalamus (thalamotomy) can relieve tremor and rigidity, but have little effect upon akinesia and bradykinesia. Lesions of the ventral thalamus, and specifically the ventralis intermedialis nucleus, from which tremor bursts can be recorded electrophysiologically at the time of operation, are particularly effective in abolishing tremor in PD, and in ameliorating severe benign essential tremor. Lesions of the nucleus ventralis oralis which interrupt thalamopallidal outflows can reduce severe

Differential Diagnosis of Akinetic–Rigid Syndromes				
	MSA		SRO	CBD
	SND	OPCA		
Akinetic rigid syndrome (Parkinsonism)	+++	+	+++	+
Cerebellar signs	+	++	+	+
Supranuclear palsy	+	+	++	+
Axial dystonia	–	–	++	+
Limb dystonia	+	+	+	+
The 'alien limb' syndrome	–	–	–	+
Inspiratory stridor	+	+	–	–
Autonomic failure	+	+	–	–

MSA   multiple system atrophy
SND   striatonigral degeneration
OPCA   olivopontocerebellar atrophy
SRO   Steele–Richardson–Olszewski syndrome
CBD   cortical basal ganglionic degeneration

Fig. 9.30 Differential diagnosis of akinetic–rigid syndrome.

L-dopa-induced dyskinesia in the contralateral limbs in patients with juvenile-onset PD. Since the advent of L-dopa/PDI therapy, stereotaxic treatment of PD is rarely undertaken. Lesions of the lateral globus pallidus may reduce akinesia.

DIFFERENTIAL DIAGNOSIS

The clinical diagnosis of IPD can be made with reasonable but not complete confidence by following the criteria in Fig. 9.11. Causes of the parkinsonian syndrome are listed in Fig. 9.1. Pathological examination may prove the diagnosis wrong in 10–15 per cent of patients. The most common alternative pathological diagnoses are the various forms of multiple system atrophy (MSA), including the Shy–Drager syndrome, striatonigral degeneration (SND), olivopontocerebellar atrophy (OPCA), and Steele–Richardson–Olszewski (SRO) syndrome (also termed progressive supranuclear palsy). SRO syndrome and corticobasal ganglionic degeneration (CBD) and other rare forms of basal ganglia degeneration may present with an akinetic-rigid syndrome.

MSA almost certainly comprises a spectrum of disorders that share clinical and pathological features. Individual patients differ in their symptoms and signs according to which structures in the basal ganglia, brain stem and spinal cord bear the brunt of the disease process. Autonomic failure occurs in both the akinetic-rigid variant and the predominantly cerebellar variant (OPCA) of MSA, and is related to degeneration of intermediolateral cell columns of the spinal cord. Most MSA cases are sporadic, but familial forms of OPCA occur and usually show an autosomal dominant mode of inheritance. Deficiency of the enzyme glutamate dehydrogenase has been detected in some individuals and families with the OPCA form of MSA. It is not clear how this partial deficiency is related to disease expression or the mechanism of neuronal degeneration, although a disturbance of glutamate neurotransmission has been proposed.

Pathological changes common to all forms of MSA include loss of striatal, pallidal, nigral, brain stem, and cerebellar neurons with gliosis, and white matter degeneration with the presence of characteristic glial cell inclusions. In SRO, there is widespread neuronal loss, gliosis and neurofibrillary degeneration in the basal ganglia and brain stem. In CBD, neurofibrillary degeneration is found in the frontoparietal cortex associated with swollen neurons identical to those seen in Pick's disease.

MRI may help to distinguish between IPD and MSA. In MSA, altered signals can often be detected in the putamen, and atrophy of the cerebellum and brain stem may be prominent. In IPD, PET studies with ^{18}F-fluorodopa (F-dopa) show reduced uptake of tracer mainly in the putamen, but in MSA, F-dopa uptake is impaired throughout the striatum. Further, binding of ^{11}C-raclopride, a selective dopamine D_2 receptor ligand, is diminished in the striatum of patients with MSA and SRO, but not in those with untreated IPD. These differences reflect less selective degeneration of nigral dopamine neurons as well as extensive loss of striatal neurons and hence dopamine receptors in MSA and SRO compared to IPD.

Drug treatment of MSA and akinetic–rigid syndromes other than IPD is unsatisfactory. Occasionally patients improve with L-dopa, dopamine agonists, anticholinergics, or amantidine; antidepressants may be useful. Patients with MSA sometimes develop inspiratory stridor which may require tracheostomy. Urinary symptoms such as frequency may be treated with anticholinergic agents or may require intermittent catheterization or an in-dwelling device. Symptomatic postural hypotension may be helped by elastic support stockings, a 'G-suit', fludrocortisone, indomethacin, ergotamine, caffeine, DDAVP, head-up tilt at night, or atrial pacing. Support for patients and carers from therapists, doctors, and patient groups improves the quality of life.

SUMMARY AND CONCLUSIONS

IPD has provided a model for investigating the motor and cognitive functions of the basal ganglia, and knowledge gained from experimental studies in animals have provided insights into human movement disorders.

(i) The cause of IPD is unknown, though abnormalities of oxidative metabolism may underlie neuronal degeneration.

(ii) Interactions between genetic and environmental factors are probably important in triggering the neuronal degeneration.

(iii) There is no convincing evidence that the selective MAO-B inhibitor selegiline (eldepryl) retards or prevents neuronal degeneration, although it may alter symptom progression in the early stages of the disease.

(iv) Effective treatment with L-dopa is available for most patients. Unfortunately, some patients develop disabling complications of prolonged L-dopa therapy. The mechanisms underlying these unwanted effects of L-dopa are poorly understood. Dopamine agonist drugs may be helpful in this situation.

(v) Neural transplantation or implantation with fetal dopamine neurons, and eventually with neurons grown or modified *in vitro*, may become more widely applicable.

(vi) MRI and functional brain imaging have provided new insights into the pathophysiological mechanism of IPD and other movement disorders, and are increasingly important in diagnosis. Nevertheless, the diagnosis of IPD still depends on clinical judgement, as in the days of James Parkinson.

10 Huntington's Disease

DEFINITION

Huntington's disease is a genetically determined neurodegenerative disorder with autosomal-dominant inheritance, showing linkage to the short arm of chromosome 4. Clinically, the disease usually presents with chorea and cognitive impairments in middle age, although it can present in childhood. Characteristic caudate atrophy on CT or MRI is reflected pathologically by severe neuronal loss, gliosis, and atrophy of the neostriatum and pars reticulata of the substantia nigra.

CLINICAL FEATURES

Huntington's disease usually presents with the development of clumsiness due to choreiform movements in the fourth and fifth decades of life, although about 10 per cent of patients develop symptoms in childhood or adolescence, and a similar proportion may present in the sixth or even seventh decades. Chorea is a form of involuntary movements typified by brief muscle jerks that flit in random succession from area to area and affect virtually all muscle groups, including the facial muscles. Initially, the choreiform movements may be passed off as mannerisms, but gradually they become continuous and obtrusive, and eventually are associated with so much clumsiness that the patients cannot perform their work, and may be thrown off balance by violent jerks of the limb or trunk muscles. Facial grimacing can become very marked. Chorea affects the muscles of ventilation, and speech is often interrupted by jerky inspirations or expirations.

Cognitive impairment may be present when the patients present with chorea, or it may precede or follow by several years the involuntary movements.

In patients with onset in childhood or adolescence, the presentation is often with rigidity rather than chorea; these patients may show marked parkinsonism and dystonia, cerebellar ataxia, dysarthria, and abnormalities of eye movement. Epileptic seizures occur more often in the early onset cases than in the late onset ones. Patients with early onset Huntington's disease more often inherit the disease from their father (see page 10.00).

Cognitive impairment always develops at some stage of the disease, but the earliest change may be neuropsychiatric, with the development of depression, schizophrenia, or other psychotic disorders, and a high rate of interpersonal difficulties, marital breakdown, and conduct disorders (Fig. 10.1). Spouses and carers may note subtle but emotionally devastating changes in behaviour and character. Some patients appear to lose insight into the effects of their behaviour on others, but some retain in-

sight and become profoundly and sometimes suicidally depressed by the effects and prospects of the disease. Behavioural problems include promiscuity and alcoholism.

Assessment of functional disability

Shoulson (1982) has proposed a functional rating scale (Fig. 10.2). As the disease progresses, the severity of chorea may diminish, while dystonia, parkinsonism, and abnormal eye movements become more obvious. The latter comprise slow, horizontal saccades and abnormal optokinetic nystagmus.

As the disease progresses (with increasing disability due to rigidity, dystonia and dementia), institutional care is often necessary. The course of the disease is usually in the region of 10–15 years, but patients may survive for 20 years or more. The average age at death is 51–55 years.

INVESTIGATION AND DIFFERENTIAL DIAGNOSIS

The diagnosis of Huntington's disease is based on the characteristic clinical features in association with a family history that suggests an autosomal-dominant mode of inheritance. Because the psychiatric features of Huntington's disease may precede the more florid features of the disease, families often break up, with the result that offspring may not know of the disease in a parent. Not infrequently, the family history is concealed. Extramarital relationships yield affected children with no traceable family history.

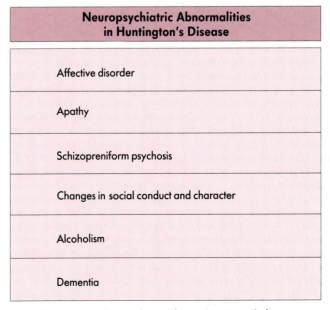

Neuropsychiatric Abnormalities in Huntington's Disease

Affective disorder

Apathy

Schizopreniform psychosis

Changes in social conduct and character

Alcoholism

Dementia

Fig. 10.1 Neuropsychiatric abnormalities in Huntington's disease.

(a)   Functional Rating Scale for Huntington's Disease

(a)   Engagement in occupation

3   *usual level*: full-time employment, actual or potential, with normal work expectations and satisfactory performance.

2   *lower level*: full- or part-time employment, actual or potential, with a lower than usual expectation or performance relative to patient's training and education.

1   *marginal level*: part-time, voluntary or salaried employment, actual or potential, with lower expectation and less than satisfactory work performance.

0   *unable*: totally unable to engage in employment.

(b)   Capacity to handle financial affairs

3   *full*: normal capacity to handle finances.

2   *requires slight assistance*: mildly impaired ability to handle financial affairs.

1   *requires major assistance*: moderately impaired ability to handle financial affairs such that patient comprehends nature and purpose of routine financial procedures but requires major assistance.

0   *unable*: patient is unable to comprehend the financial process and is unable to perform tasks related to routine financial procedures.

(c)   Capacity to manage domestic responsibilities

2   *full*: no impairment in performance of routine domestic tasks.

0   *unable*: marked impairment in function with marginal performance requiring major assistance.

1   *impaired*: moderate impairment in performance of routine domestic tasks such that patient requires some assistance in carrying out these tasks.

(d)   Capacity to perform activities of daily living

3   *full*: complete independence in eating, dressing and bathing activities.

2   *mildly impaired*: somewhat laboured performance in eating, in dressing, in bathing; requires only slight assistance.

1   *moderately impaired*: substantial difficulty in eating, in dressing and in bathing.

0   *severely impaired*: indicates patient requires total care in activities of daily living.

(e)   Care can be provided

2   *home*: patient living at home and family readily able to meet care needs.

1   *home or extended care facility*: patient may be living at home but care needs would be better provided at an extended care facility.

0   *total care facility only*: patient requires full-time skilled nursing care.

The total score is then calculated. Stage I is equal to a score of 11–13; stage II to a score of 7–10; III to a score of 3–6; IV, 1–2; and V, 0.

(b)   Profile of Functional Decline in Huntington's Disease

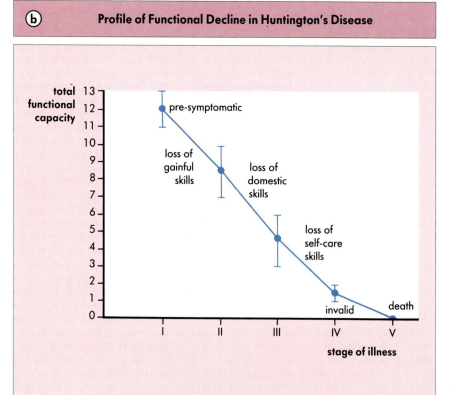

Fig. 10.2 (a) Functional rating scale for Huntington's disease; (b) graphic representation of the functional decline in Huntington's disease. (Reproduced courtesy of Shoulson I. Care of patients and families and patients with Huntington's disease. In *Movement Disorders*, Marsden CD, Fahn S, eds. New York: Butterworth Scientific, 1982.)

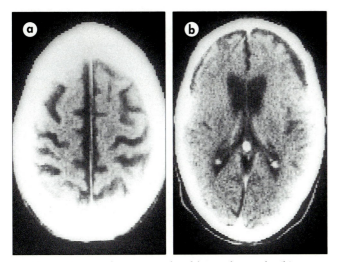

Fig. 10.3 (a) CT scan showing atrophy of the caudate nuclei; (b) CT scan showing cortical atrophy.

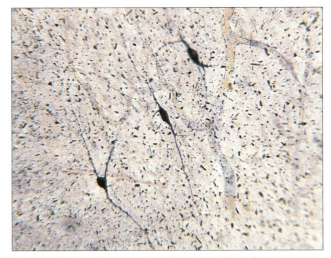

Fig. 10.4 Section of cortex, stained for nitric oxide synthase, in Huntington's disease.

The differential diagnosis includes:

- familial chorea without dementia;
- neuroacanthocytosis;
- benign familial chorea with myoclonus;
- paroxysmal dystonic choreoathetosis;
- spinocerebellar degenerations of the olivopontocerebellar type, in which choreoathetosis and dystonia occasionally occur;
- dentato-pallido-nigro-luysian atrophy; and
- Wilson's disease, particularly in young onset cases presenting with rigidity, dystonia and ataxia.

Investigations to exclude these conditions thus include a fresh wet film or a sample for scanning electron microscopy to detect acanthocytes; serum copper and caeruloplasmin levels, and 24-hour urine copper excretion estimations. Neuroimaging with CT and/or MRI is essential and may show caudate atrophy (Fig. 10.3), and neuropsychological evaluation is helpful. The EEG is usually normal in the early stages, and in the later stages tends to show non-specific changes. Analysis for prion gene mutations may be appropriate in some patients.

PATHOLOGY

Macroscopically, the brain shows varying degrees of atrophy and ventricular dilatation. There is marked atrophy and flattening of the caudate nucleus, and the putamen is shrunken to a lesser extent. There is also atrophy of the internal segment of the globus pallidus and the substantia nigra pars reticulata, although this may not be obvious macroscopically.

In the early stages of Huntington's disease, the brain may look macroscopically normal in patients who show obvious chorea and neuropsychiatric abnormalities (e.g. patients who come to autopsy following suicide).

Histopathological changes in the neostriatum include loss of neurons and gliosis. Neuronal loss is relatively selective, with marked depletion of median spiny neurons (MSNs – see Chapter

00), and relative preservation of cholinergic interneurons and medium-size aspiny neurons in which are co-localized neuropeptide Y, somatostatin, and NADPH-diaphorase (Fig. 10.4). NADPH-diaphorase is identical to nitric oxide synthase.

Neuronal degeneration begins in the tail of the caudate nucleus, and progresses in the medial to lateral gradient. It precedes degeneration in the putamen, which tends to proceed dorsolaterally, with relative preservation of the ventral putamen and nucleus accumbens. Loss of neurons is followed by progressive gliosis.

The most striking neurochemical abnormality in Huntington's disease is depletion of the GABA-synthetic enzyme glutamate decarboxylase (GAD), but acetylcholine, choline acetyltransferase (CAT) and neuropeptides such as enkephalin, substance P, dymorphism, and cholecystokinin are also depleted in the neostriatum. On the other hand, levels of dopamine, norepinepherine, somatostatin, neuropeptide Y, and neurotensin are normal or even slightly elevated. These changes parallel very closely the effects of experimental excitotoxic lesions of the neostriatum (Fig. 10.5).

The striatum can be divided into neurochemically distinguishable regions called striosomes and matrix (see Fig. 9.3). In Huntington's disease, the striosomes or patches are relatively spared compared to the acetylcholinesterase-rich compartment. Nevertheless, even within the matrix, NADPH-diaphorase and cholinergic interneurons are relatively spared. The GABA–enkephalin-utilizing MSNs projecting to the lateral segment of the globus pallidus are first to die, and since these neurons are part of an inhibitory circuit, their destruction probably results in disinhibition and involuntary movements (see Fig. 9.9). A key factor in the production of these involuntary movements is reduction in the activity of the subthalamic nucleus, which normally drives inhibitory GABAergic neurons of the medial pallidal segment and substantia nigra pars reticulata. The result is loss of GABAergic inhibitory input to the ventrolateral thalamus. Disinhibition of thalamocortical projections could be seen as preventing the filtering out of unwanted or superfluous components of consecutive motor programmes (see Fig. 9.9).

As the disease progresses, or in the juvenile form, the pattern of cell loss may fall equally upon GABA–substance P, and GABA–enkephalin MSNs, with the result that pallidothalamic inhibitory circuits become predominant, leading to rigidity and other features of parkinsonism, and perhaps at an earlier stage to slowing of saccadic eye movements (see Fig. 9.9).

Huntington's Disease and the Excitotoxic Hypothesis

There are similarities in the histological and neurochemical changes in Huntington's disease, and those that follow experimental excitotoxic lesions (see Fig. 10.5). Endogenous glutamate acting on NMDA receptors (see Chapter 00) in combination with some other factor determining tissue and cell selectivity might be to blame, but other endogenous excitotoxins, such as quinolinic acid, homocysteic acid, and even L-cysteic acid, have been implicated. Experimentally, quinolinic acid produces lesions very similar to those in Huntington's disease, with preservation of NADPH-diaphorase-staining neurons. Quinolinic acid is a glutamate agonist derived from tryptophan metabolism, and normally present in nanomolar concentrations in the brain. Its concentration increases with age, but it is unlikely that it reaches toxic levels in normal ageing, and no convincing excess of quinolinic acid has been detected in Huntington's disease brains postmortem. The biosynthetic enzyme for quinolinic acid (3-hydroxyanthranillic acid oxidase) is increased in Huntington's disease striatum, but this may be secondary to gliosis. Another possibility is that endogenous NMDA antagonists, such as kynurenic acid, may be deficient in Huntington's disease brain.

PET Studies in Huntington's Disease

Patients with symptomatic Huntington's disease show reduced glucose metabolism in the caudate nuclei. In some studies, impaired glucose metabolism has been detected in presymptomatic carriers of the Huntington's disease gene, even when there was no detectable caudate nucleus atrophy on CT scan. However, when PET is combined with presymptomatic testing using linked markers, not all presumed presymptomatic carriers have abnormal PET scans. To date, evidence from PET scans suggests that, although some patients in the early stages of the disease have abnormal scans, in others, glucose PET scans are normal. Thus, this technique has not been shown to provide a reliable method for detecting presymptomatic carriers of the gene.

PATHOGENESIS

Molecular Genetics

The mutation causing Huntington's disease probably arose as a single event many centuries ago, possibly in East Anglia, UK, and has subsequently become widely disseminated. Prevalence in the USA and the UK averages about 4–7 per 100 000. In some regions, such as Lake Marakaibo in Venezuela, it has been possible to trace a pedigree originating from a German sailor with the disease who landed in Venezuela in 1960–70. More than 10 000 living or dead individuals, including over 350 Huntington's disease patients, and over 4000 persons are at risk. Studies of this and other kindreds have shown that the Huntington's disease gene is fully penetrant. People who are homozygous for the Huntington's disease gene are phenotypically identical to heterozygotes. This implies that the gene defect relates to a 'gain of function' rather than a 'loss of function', perhaps relating to altered expression of a normal gene product. Although the Huntington's disease gene is always expressed if inherited, affected individuals within a pedigree often show striking pheno-

Factors Common to Huntington's Disease and Experimental Striatal Excitotoxin Lesions
Histology
preserved NADPH-diaphorase neurons
preserved parvalbumin neurons
preserved acetylcholinesterase (large) neurons
decreased enkephalin and substance P neurons
Neurochemistry
decreased GABA
decreased substance P
decreased enkephalin
decreased choline acetyltransferase
increased somatostatin
increased neuropeptide Y
increased neurotensin
preserved dopamine
increased serotonin
Receptors
decreased NMDA receptors
decreased opiate receptors
decreased muscarinic receptors
decreased GABA, benzodiazepine receptors
decreased serotonin receptors
decreased dopamine D_2 receptors

GABA	gamma aminobutyric acid	NMDA	N-methyl-D-aspartate

Fig. 10.5 Factors common to Huntington's disease and experimental striatal excitotoxin lesions. (Modified from Beal MF. *Ann Neurol* 1992; **32(2)**:119–130.)

typic variation. Presumably, this reflects the effect of modifying genes or environmental factors, although these do not seem to be relevant in the Venezuelan pedigree.

Inheritance of the mutation from the father results in an earlier onset of the disease, and juvenile onset Huntington's disease is almost always paternally inherited. Several hypotheses have been put forward to explain this effect. These hypotheses include transmission of a protective factor, such as a mitochondrial gene, from the mother; genomic imprinting; and position-effect variegation, in which the expression of a gene may be modified by its link to the centemere or telomere, or to heterochromatin.

Genetic linkage in Huntington's disease

The Huntington's disease gene is linked to a locus on the short arm of chromosome 4 (Fig. 10.6). Linkage was first established by Gusella and colleagues at Harvard in 1983, with a highly informative DNA probe G8, at locus D4S10, which was estimated to be approximately 4 million base pairs (4 cMs) away from the Huntington's disease gene. Further refinements of linkage have come from the identification of recombination events, and the development of a more detailed physical map of the chromosomal DNA in a region comprising about 6 million base pairs at the tip of chromosome 4. Yeast artificial chromosome (YAC) clones containing the telomeric region of 4P have been developed from individual homozygotes for the Huntington's disease gene, so this YAC clone should contain the mutant Huntington's disease locus.

Applications of genetic linkage in Huntington's disease Thus far, there is no evidence for more than one mutation in Huntington's disease, since many families throughout the world have been tested and show linkage between GH (D4S10) (Fig. 10.7). However, it remains a possibility that Huntington's disease is due to several mutations at the same locus, or even a mutation at another rare locus. Identification of linkage has provided the basis for genetic counselling, including prenatal prediction. The accuracy of prediction is limited by a very small possibility of recombination, reflecting uncertainty about the precise position of the Huntington's disease gene. Genetic counselling based on predictive tests should only be done at a centre with experience of genetic counselling after full discussion with, and preparation of, the individuals concerned. Bearing in mind the risk of depression and suicide in Huntington's disease, careful follow-up must be provided.

TREATMENT OF HUNTINGTON'S DISEASE

No drug is available to slow the progression or reverse the symptoms and signs of Huntington's disease. Symptomatic treatment of chorea can be achieved with drugs that deplete central catecholamines, such as tetrabenazine, but this may exacerbate depression. Similarly, neuroleptic drugs such as chlorpromazine, haloperidol, sulpiride, and the newer substituted benzamides

such as clozapine, will reduce chorea, but seldom lead to significant functional improvements, particularly since the involuntary movements are often more distressing to relatives and doctors than to patients. Isoniazid, which influences GABA levels in the CNS, has been claimed to be beneficial, although most rigorous clinical trials have not shown significant improvement. The cornerstone of management consists of personal and genetic counselling, support of families and immediate carers, establishing links with patient support groups, and treatment of depression, psychotic episodes, and epileptic seizures. A co-ordinated care strategy with a key worker approach, as for other disorders, is the key to better care here.

SUMMARY

(i) Although the gene for Huntington's disease has not yet been identified, genetic linkage analysis has provided sufficient information for presymptomatic diagnosis in many cases, and has indicated that a single locus (although not necessarily a single mutation) is involved in pathogenesis.

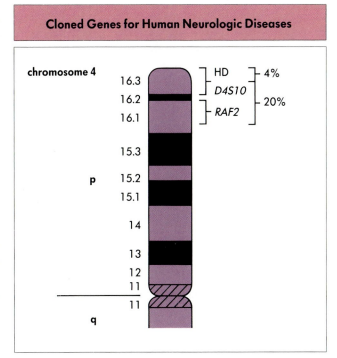

Cloned Genes for Human Neurologic Diseases

Fig. 10.6 Location of the Huntinton disease gene. The HD gene is located in the terminal 4p16.3 sub-band of the short arm of chromosome 4, a region corresponding to perhaps 0.2 per cent of the genome. The position of Huntington's disease was defined by tracing the degree of co-inheritance of the disease with the two mapped DNA markers, D4S10 and RAF2, which show 4 and 20 per cent recombination, respectively, with the disorder. (Reproduced courtesy of Gusella JF, Gilliam TC. DNA markers in dominant neurogenetic diseases. In: *Cloned Genes for Human Neurologic Diseases*, Rowland LP, ed. New York: Oxford University Press, 1989.)

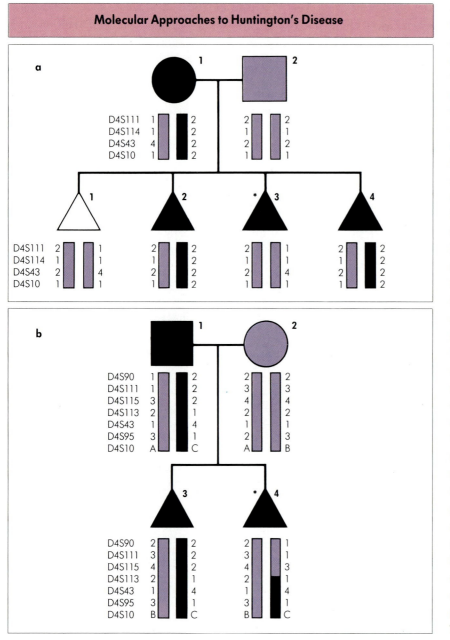

Molecular Approaches to Huntington's Disease

Fig. 10.7 (a) A recombination event placing the Huntington's disease gene in the telomeric candidate region. The genotype of the mother, who died of Huntington's disease, was reconstructed from the genotypes of the progeny shown and several additional unaffected offspring. The chromosome carrying the Huntington's disease gene is darkened. The alleles for specific marker loci from *D3S10 (G8)* to *D3S111 (P157)* are shown. The three progeny who are darkened triangles are affected. Progeny number 3, indicated by an asterisk, has the genotype of the mother's normal chromosome 4, but still has symptomatic Huntington's disease. This recombination event would suggest that the Huntington's disease gene is extremely telomeric, beyond the most distal marker tested.

(b) A recombination event placing the Huntington's disease gene in the proximal candidate region. In this family, progeny number 4 (indicated with an asterisk) has had a recombination event occur between *D3S113 (P62, P102)* and *D4S115 (P252)*. The alleles from *D4S115 (P252)* to the telomere are those that are associated with the chromosome 4 carrying the normal gene in this family. From *D3S113 (P62, P102)*, and proximally, the alleles are those that characterize the chromosome bearing the HD gene. (Reproduced courtesy of Wexler NS, Rose NS, Rose EA, Housman DE. Molecular approaches to hereditary diseases of the neurons system: Huntington's disease as a paradigm. *Ann Rev Neurosci* 1991; **14**:503–529.)

(ii) There is much circumstantial evidence to suggest that the pathological lesions in the neostriatum could be due to excitotoxicity, but no specific excitotoxin has been identified. If this proves true, agents that block glutamate receptors may prove helpful in preventing progression of the disease.

(iii) The diagnosis of Huntington's disease is usually relatively straightforward, but in those without known family history it is important to exclude Wilson's disease (particularly in the juvenile onset forms, which present with rigidity, dystonia, parkinsonism, and ataxia).

(iv) The neuropsychiatric aspects of Huntington's disease are important in management, since many patients develop depression, some become psychotic, and behavioural abnormalities including sexual misdemeanours and violent behaviour are frequent. Suicide is a major risk, and depression should be actively treated when it occurs.

(v) Genetic counselling forms an integral part of management, and presymptomatic and prenatal diagnosis is now possible in some kindreds.

11 Motor Neuron Disorders

DEFINITION OF AMYOTROPHIC LATERAL SCLEROSIS (ALS)

Amyotrophic lateral sclerosis (ALS) is a progressive disorder of unknown cause characterized by degeneration of cortical, brain stem, and spinal motor neurons. In its typical form there is clinical and neurophysiological evidence of upper and lower motor neuron involvement of the bulbar musculature and limbs. Suggested research diagnostic criteria for ALS are summarized in Fig. 11.1. The term motor neuron disease is often interchangeably with ALS, although there are a variety of different motor neuron disorders (Fig. 11.2).

Research Diagnostic Criteria for ALS		
1. The diagnosis of sporadic ALS requires the presence of:		**Clinical signs**
— lower motor neuron signs — upper motor neuron signs — progression.	**Definite**	— upper motor neuron and lower motor neuron signs in three regions (brain stem, cervical, lumbosacral), e.g. Charcot ALS
2. The diagnosis of sporadic ALS requires the absence of: — abnormal sensory signs — sphincter abnormalities — anterior visual system abnormalities — probable Parkinson's disease — significant autonomic nervous system abnormalities — probable Alzheimer's dementia — other causes of ALS-mimic syndrome.	**Probable**	— upper motor neuron and lower motor neuron signs in two different regions, and upper motor neuron signs rostral to the lower motor neuron signs, e.g. upper motor neuron bulbar, lower motor neuron spinal, upper motor neuron and lower motor neuron bulbar, lower motor neuron spinal, etc.
3. The diagnosis of sporadic ALS is supported by: — fasciculations in one or more regions (or) — abnormal pulmonary function tests (or) — abnormal muscle biopsy (or) — abnormal swallowing studies (or) — abnormal speech tests (or) — abnormal isokinetic/isometric strength tests.	**Possible**	— upper motor neuron and lower motor neuron in one region, or upper motor neuron in two or three regions, e.g. monomelic ALS, progressive bulbar palsy, primary lateral sclerosis.
	Suspected	— lower motor neuron in two or three regions or other motor syndromes, e.g. progressive muscular atrophy.

The diagnosis of definite, probable, possible and suspected sporadic ALS requires the grouping of clinical signs from 1 (above) in one or more regions (brainstem, cervical, thoracic, lumbosacral) of the central nervous system, progression, and the absence of clinical signs from 2.

Fig. 11.1 Research diagnostic criteria for ALS (based on the provisional criteria under consideration by the World Federation of Neurology).

Human Motor System Diseases	
Associated with specific mechanisms	
Congenital and familial	**Autosomal recessive inheritance**
	Spinal muscular — type 1
	atrophy (SMA) (acute infantile)
	type 2
	(intermediate)
	type 3
	(juvenile, chronic)
	type 4
	(adult onset, chronic)
	scapuloperoneal
	forms
	Hexosaminidase deficiency (Type B)
	Fazio–Londe disease
	North African and other forms of juvenile onset ALS
	Brown–Vialetto–Van Laere syndrome (juvenile onset pseudobulbar palsy)
	X-linked
	Bulbospinal neuronopathy (Kennedy's syndrome)
	Autosomal-dominant
	Familial ALS
	Familial ALS with frontal lobe-type dementia
Infective	Poliomyelitis
	HIV
	Spongiform encephalopathies ('prion' disorders)
	Syphilis
Associated with neurotoxins	Lead-induced motor neuropathy
	Neurolathyrism (related to ingestion of chickling pea lathyrus sativa: toxin – probably B-oxalyl-amino-L-alanine)
	'Mantakassa', 'Konzo' and related acute upper motor neurone syndromes (related to ingestion of untreated casava; toxin; probably cyanide)
Metabolic	Hyperparathyroidism
	Hyperthyroidism
Autoimmune	Motor neuropathy with anti-ganglioside antibodies
	Motor neuropathy with paraproteinaemia (? motor neuropathy associated with carcinoma)
Ischaemic myelopathy (radiation-induced)	Radiation-induced plexopathy
Idiopathic	
Sporadic ALS	
Western Pacific ALS-PD-dementia syndrome	
Monomelic motor neuron disease	
MND with dementia of frontal lobe type	
'Madras' type of motor neuron disease	
Other neurodegenerative disorders (e.g. MSA)	

Fig. 11.2 Motor system diseases in humans.

CLINICAL FEATURES OF ALS AND OTHER MOTOR NEURON DISORDERS

Characteristic clinical features include widespread fasciculations indicating anterior horn cell disease at multiple levels, wasting of the tongue (Fig. 11.3a) and limb muscles (Fig. 11.3b), and upper motor neuron signs reflecting degeneration of the cortico-spinal tracts. The clinical features of ALS and some other motor neuron disorders are summarized in Fig. 11.4.

The diagnosis of ALS is made on clinical grounds, supported by electrophysiological evidence of anterior horn cell damage (Fig. 11.5), and by the exclusion of conditions which may mimic ALS. About 20 per cent of ALS patients present with bulbar symptoms such as dysarthria and dysphagia (progressive bulbar palsy – PBP), but most of these patients eventually develop other features of ALS. About 10 per cent of patients show only lower motor neuron features (progressive muscular atrophy – PMA). Occasionally, only upper motor neuron signs are present (primary lateral sclerosis), but the relationship between progressive lateral sclerosis and ALS is uncertain.

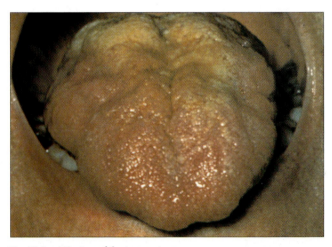

Fig. 11.3a Wasting of the tongue in ALS.

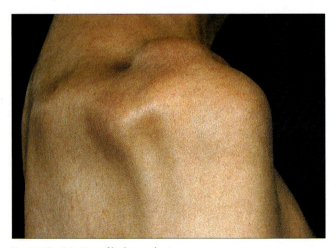

Fig. 11.3b Wasting of limb muscles in ALS.

Clinical Features of the Major Motor Neuron Disorders

	ALS	Type I (acute infantile)	SMA Type II	Types III & IV (juvenile chronic and adult onset)	Kennedy's syndrome (x-linked bulbospinal neuronopathy)
Familial/ genetic incidence & inheritance	5–10 per cent of all ALS. Autosomal dominant, with linkage to 21q in some kindreds.	Probably 100 per cent. Autosomal recessive. Linkage to 5q12–14.	Probably 100 per cent. Autosomal recessive. Linkage to 5q12–14.	Probably 100 per cent. Autosomal recessive. Linkage to 5q12–14.	100 per cent. Abnormal androgen receptor (Xq11–12).
Age at onset	Sporadic ≃ 60 FALS ≃ 50	In utero	Infancy	Childhood, rarely adulthood	Adolescence, early adult life
Sex ratio M:F	1.5:1 Sporadic ALS 1:1 FALS	1:1	1:1	1:1	Male
Duration	3–4 years (rarely up to 10 years)	Months; death in infancy	Death in childhood	May be prolonged	10–20 years
UMN signs	+ (≃ 80 per cent)	—	—	—*	—
LMN signs	+ (≃ 100 per cent)	+	+	+	+
Bulbar involvement	+ (≃ 80 per cent)	+/–	+/–	+/–	+
Dementia	5 per cent	—	—	—	—
Neuropathy	—	—	—	—	+ (↓ sensory action potential)
Other features	—	—	—	—	Gynaecomastia Hypogonadism Diabetes
	*rarely, extensor plantar responses are present.				

Fig. 11.4 Clinical features of the major motor neuron disorders.

Electrophysiological Abnormalities in ALS

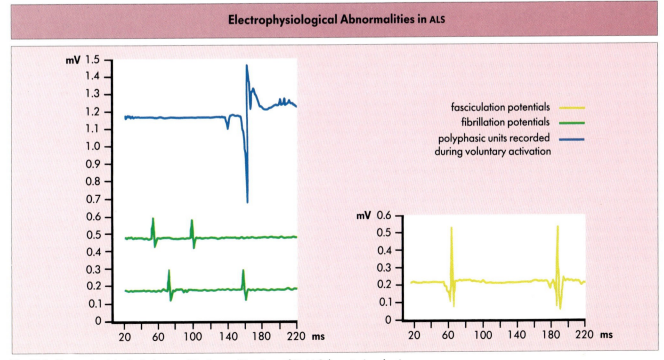

fasciculation potentials
fibrillation potentials
polyphasic units recorded during voluntary activation

Fig. 11.5 Electrophysiological abnormalities in ALS. (Courtesy of Dr M Schwartz, London.)

These clinical variants (with the exception of progressive lateral sclerosis) occur in both sporadic and familial ALS. Affected individuals within families showing an autosomal dominant mode of inheritance of ALS may show either upper and lower motor neuron signs (typical ALS) or only lower motor neuron signs. Typical ALS and its bulbar and lower motor neuron variants show essentially the same pathological features, although the severity of the pathological changes in a particular area differs from patient to patient.

A characteristic feature of ALS and its variants is inexorable progression leading to death within four to five years of onset. Occasionally, patients with well-documented ALS survive for 10 or more years without assisted ventilation. ALS patients have been kept alive with assisted ventilation for up to 10 years, but such patients eventually become 'locked-in' and unable to communicate except in very limited ways (e.g. by pupillary constriction and accommodation).

EPIDEMIOLOGY AND PATHOGENESIS

ALS is found worldwide. With the exception of foci of high incidence and prevalence in the Western Pacific the incidence, judged by standardized mortality rates, is relatively consistent throughout the world, although in some places mortality rates are lower than average (e.g. in Mexico). It is not clear whether this reflects real differences in incidence or artifacts of sampling. In the USA and Europe, the incidence varies between about 0.5 and 2 per 100 000 population, the average being around 1 per 100 000, with prevalence rates of 3–4 per 100 000. In the Western Pacific (the Mariana islands, the Kii peninsula of Japan, and certain parts of New Guinea) the mortality and prevalence rates of ALS are increased 10-fold over those in Europe and the USA. Local differences in mortality rates have been observed in some surveys, with increased rates most often occurring amongst rural populations and in agricultural or manual workers, although this trend is not consistent. There is no convincing evidence of biologically significant 'clustering' of ALS cases, although there are numerous anecdotes of case clusters within localities, work places, or communities. These clusters are probably attributable to chance.

On average the incidence of ALS has risen from 1 per 100 000 in the 1960–75 period to 1.4 per 100 000 in the 1975–85 period, an increase of about 40 per cent. This increase cannot be attributed entirely to improved case ascertainment. The incidence of sporadic ALS is higher in men than in women, with a male:female ratio of about 1.5:1, although the recent increases in mortality rates may be more marked in women than in men. Standardized mortality rates for ALS increase with age (Fig. 11.6). The mean age of onset of sporadic ALS is around 60, and the median duration of the disease is between three and four years. Most surveys find that age-specific mortality rates fall over the age of 70–75, but some indicate that rates continue to rise in the eighth and ninth decades.

Risk Factors

There is no evidence that race significantly alters the risk of ALS. A history of mechanical trauma is more common in ALS than in controls, and there may be a similar association with electrical trauma. Exposure to industrial solvents and agricultural toxins has been implicated as a cause of ALS, although no specific or consistent factors have been identified. As noted above, ALS may be more common in agricultural communities, but this trend probably pre-dates the large-scale use of pesticides and other agricultural chemicals. Although lead can cause motor neuropathy and an ALS-like syndrome there is no evidence that lead or other trace metals cause ALS. Nevertheless, a positive correlation between the occurrence of paralytic poliomyelitis and mortality from ALS 30–40 years later has been detected, but there is no evidence yet for a fall in ALS incidence or mortality in populations which have been immunized against poliomyelitis.

Genetic Factors and Motor Neuron Disorders

Between 5 and 10 per cent of patients with ALS have a family history of the disease. Inheritance is consistent with an autosomal-dominant pattern. The mean age of onset in familial ALS is about 50 (a decade earlier than in sporadic ALS), and men and women are equally affected. In most families the duration of the

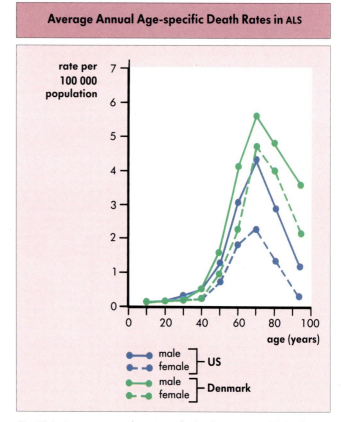

Average Annual Age-specific Death Rates in ALS

Fig. 11.6 Average annual age-specific death rates per 100 000 by sex in Denmark (1972–1977) and amongst whites in the USA (1959–1961). (Adapted from Kurtzke JF, *Advances in Neurology* **56**, Rowland LP, ed. New York: Raven Press, 1991.)

disease is about two years, somewhat shorter than the course in sporadic ALS, but some families have been recorded with early onset and a long course. In families with the slowly progressive form of familial motor neuron disease, the disorder tends to be of lower motor neuron type. Within families, most individuals show both upper and lower motor neuron signs but about 20 per cent of affected individuals show only lower motor neuron signs. As in sporadic ALS, bulbar symptoms are common. Indeed, the clinical and pathological features are very similar to those of sporadic ALS, although pathological changes may be more widespread in familial ALS, with more extensive involvement of the dorsal columns and spinocerebellar tracts than in sporadic ALS, and a more frequent association with dementia (see Chapter 8).

Linkage has been tentatively established between familial ALS and markers on chromosome 21q close to the APP locus (Fig. 11.7). However, there is genetic heterogeneity and it is not known precisely what proportion of families show linkage to chromosome 21.

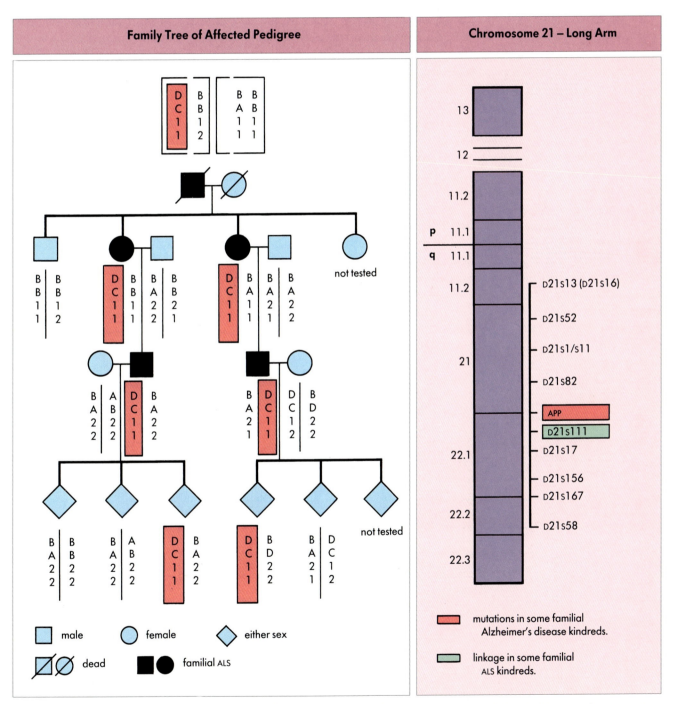

Fig. 11.7 (a) Cosegregation of chromosome 21 markers with familial ALS in one pedigree. Markers cosegregating with the disorder are boxed. The haplotype for each member is shown in the following order from top to bottom: D21S (A, B, C), D21S1/D21S11 (A, B, C, D), APP (allele: 1, 2) and D21S58 (allele 1:2). (Adapted from Siddique T *et al. New Eng J Med* 1991;**324**:1381.) (b) Ideogram of human chromosome 21 showing the order of 11 polymorphic markers located on the long arm of the chromosome.

Genetic linkage has been established between chromosome 5q 12–14 and spinal muscular atrophy (SMA). Another rare, X-linked form of SMA with juvenile or adult onset Kennedy's syndrome or X-linked bulbospinal neuronopathy is associated with a mutation of the androgen receptor (Fig. 11.8).

Neurotoxins and ALS

Toxicity resulting from altered metabolism or processing of endogenous excitotoxins such as L-glutamate has been proposed as a mechanism for neuronal damage in ALS and other multi-system disorders associated with anterior horn cell degeneration. Glutamate acts at several excitatory amino acid (EAA) receptor subtypes (see Chapters 16–17), and probably contributes to excitotoxic neuronal damage in cerebral ischaemia, trauma, epilepsy, and hypoglycaemia. Other EAAs (such as aspartate, L-cysteine, and L-homocysteic acid) and substances such as quinolinic acid may also act as endogenous excitotoxins. Naturally occurring excitotoxins such as B-oxalyl-amino-L-alanine (BOAA) have been implicated as the cause of the human upper motor neuron disorder neurolathyrism, and domoic acid, a potent kainic acid-like excitotoxin derived from algae and consumed with shellfish, was responsible for an outbreak of severe encephalopathy in Canada. For a while, it was thought that B-methyl-amino-L-alanine (BMAA), a weak excitotoxin acting at the NMDA receptor and present in flour from the cycad plant (*Cycas circinalis*), might be responsible for the Western Pacific form of ALS–PD dementia complex, but this now seems unlikely, since only minute amounts are present in washed cycad flour, which is used for cooking and for local application to wounds and sores. The use of cycad as food (or medication) is common to the major areas of high prevalence of ALS but the use of cycad is not restricted to these areas.

Experiments in which BMAA was fed to monkeys in large amounts were equivocal. Some animals developed clinical features reminiscent of the Western Pacific ALS–PD-dementia, and there was physiological evidence of damage to the corticospinal tracts, and pathological evidence of chromatolysis of cortical and spinal motor neurons, but the syndrome was reversible on stopping BMAA.

The role of endogenous excitotoxins in causing chronic neuro-degenerative disease is unproven. In olivo-ponto-cerebellar atrophy (OPCA), which is a form of multiple system atrophy, some patients show decreased activity of the enzyme glutamate dehydrogenase (GDH) which reversibly catalyzes the conversion of oxaloacetate to glutamate, the major EAA neurotransmitter in the CNS. The metabolism of glutamate is complex, and involves both glial and neuronal pools (see Chapters 16–17). A decrease in brain GDH could lead to an increase in glutamate at the synaptic cleft (and hence excitotoxic damage) if there were a failure to metabolize glutamate to glutamine in glia. However, measurements of GDH in ALS spinal cord show that activity of the enzyme is increased, and that there is a decrease in glutamate concentration. The latter change may reflect loss of nerve cells and terminals in the spinal cord, although glutamate levels are decreased in many brain regions and a generalized defect in glutamate metabolism and function has been suggested. Amino acids besides glutamate are altered in CSF and spinal cord in ALS (Fig. 11.9).

The finding of elevated L-cysteine and low inorganic sulphate levels in the plasma of ALS patients may indicate an alternative mechanism for excitotoxicity, since, in the presence of bicarbonate ion, L-cysteine is a weak excitotoxin acting on the NMDA receptor. Patients with Alzheimer's disease and Parkinson's disease also have high plasma cysteine levels and low plasma sulphate levels, so this change is not specific for ALS.

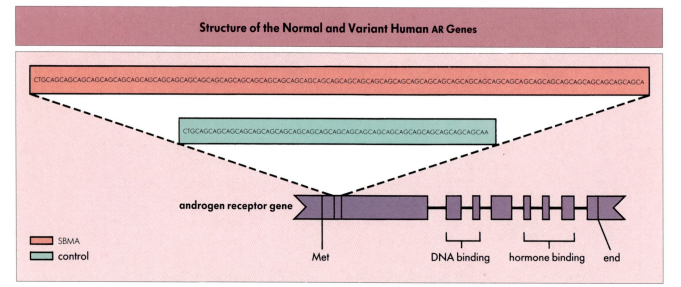

Fig. 11.8 Structure of the normal and variant human AR genes. Shown here are sequences of the CAG repeat in the first exon for a representative normal control and a Kennedy's syndrome patient. The patient's AR gene contains about twice as many CAGs as the control (44 compared with 21). (Adapted from La Spada *et al. Nature* 1991;**352**:77.)

Changes in Concentrations of some Amino Acids in ALS Spinal Cord and CSF		
	Spinal cord	**CSF**
glutamate	↓ 40–50%	↑ 100–200%
aspartate	↓ 30–60%	↑ 100%
glycine	no change or slight ↓	no change or ↑
taurine	↑ 40–50%, or no change	no change
GABA	no change, or slight ↓	no change
threonine	—	no change or ↑
serine	—	no change or ↑
alanine	—	no change or ↑
valine	—	no change or ↑
isoleucine	—	no change or ↑
leucine	—	no change or ↑

Fig. 11.9 Changes in concentrations of some amino acids in ALS spinal cord and CSF.

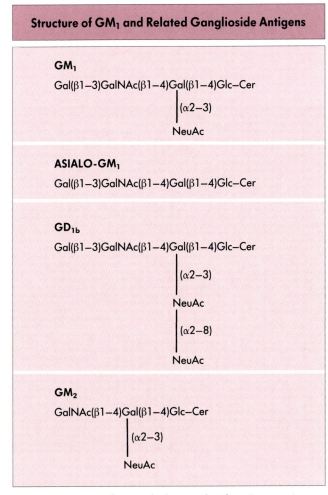

Fig. 11.10 Structure of GM$_1$ and other ganglioside antigens against which antibodies may be directed in motor neuron disorders.

Autoimmunity

Paraproteinaemia is more common in ALS than would be expected, and high titres of IgM auto-antibodies directed against gangliosides have been found in some patients with the clinical picture of progressive muscular atrophy (lower motor neuron disease), associated with motor neuropathy with electrophysiological evidence of conduction block, or with sensorimotor neuropathy. Low titres of anti-ganglioside antibodies are found in typical ALS and in a wide variety of neurological disorders, in patients with autoimmune disorders, and in normal individuals. Anti-ganglioside antibodies associated with progressive lower motor neuron disorders are present in high titres; these may be monoclonal or polyclonal, are often of λ light-chain type, and are usually directed against the Gal(β1–3)GalNAc epitope which is a component of several gangliosides including GM$_1$ and GD$_{1b}$ (Fig. 11.10). Some patients with high titre anti-ganglioside antibodies and lower motor neuron syndromes have improved clinically with immunosuppressive therapy, but in most ALS patients low titres of anti-ganglioside antibodies are unlikely to have pathogenic significance.

Defect in DNA Repair

A defect in DNA repair has been proposed as an underlying cause, leading to decreased transcription and protein synthesis. Motor neuron RNA content measured by microspectrophotometry is decreased, but total spinal cord mRNA and the mRNA coding for the neurofilament light chain subunit are present at normal levels, so there is no definite evidence for a generalized decrease in protein synthesis in ALS spinal cord.

PATHOLOGY

The brain in ALS is usually macroscopically normal, although rarely there is focal atrophy of the precentral gyri. More commonly, focal atrophy involves the frontal, cingulate, and anterior parietal cortex (Fig. 11.11a–d). Patients with ALS and dementia of frontal lobe type (see Chapter 8) may show severe frontotemporal atrophy of the type seen in Pick's disease. The spinal cord in ALS shows atrophy of the anterior (motor) nerve roots (Fig. 11.12), and the fresh cut surface may reveal collapse and discoloration of the ventral grey matter.

Characteristic histopathological lesions of ALS include:
- degeneration and loss of spinal cord anterior horn motor neurons;
- degeneration of the corticospinal tracts, which is best demonstrated in the thoracic spinal cord (Fig. 11.13), but which can be traced through the medullary pyramids, the cerebral peduncle, and the posterior limb of the internal capsule, to fibres underlying the primary sensory and motor cortex; and
- degeneration of giant motor neurons (Betz cells) of the primary motor cortex.

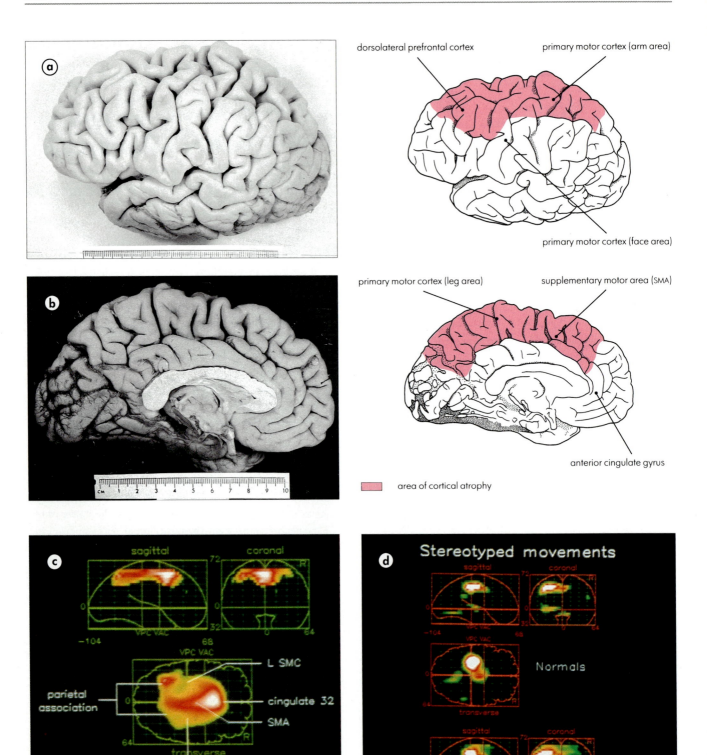

Fig. 11.11 Photographs of the brain from the (a) lateral and (b) medial side. Statistical parametric maps derived from C^{15}O$_2$ PET scans. Changes in regional cerebral blood flow (rCBF) in normals and in patients with ALS. (c) *Decreases* (coloured areas) in resting rCBF in ALS patients compared to normals. Motor and premotor areas (including SMA) show abnormalities. (d) Activation studies showing *increases* in rCBF associated with movements of the right arm. ALS patients show more extensive activation of the contralateral motor cortex than do normals, and activation of the ipsilateral motor cortex, which does not normally occur.

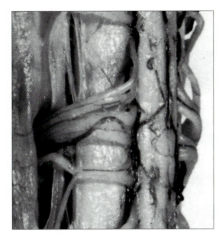

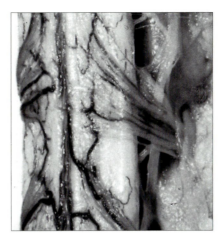

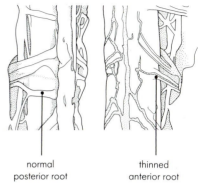

Fig. 11.12 Atrophy of the anterior nerve roots in ALS.

normal
posterior root

thinned
anterior root

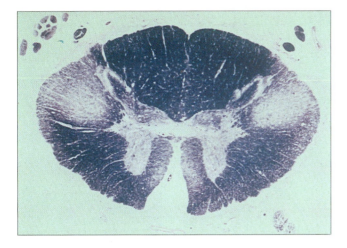

Fig. 11.13 Degeneration of corticospinal tracts in the thoracic spinal cord in ALS.

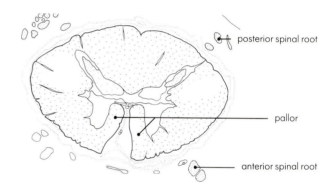

posterior spinal root

pallor

anterior spinal root

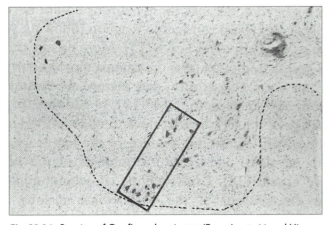

Fig. 11.14 Sparing of Onuf's nucleus in ALS. (From Iwata M and Hirano A. *Ann Neurol* 1978;4:245.)

This last feature is present in most cases with upper motor neuron signs, but is often absent in patients with only lower motor neuron signs. Studies using the Marchi technique for degenerating fibres indicate that cortical involvement extends beyond the confines of the primary motor cortex.

There may be variable involvement of the posterior columns, Clarke's column, and the spinocerebellar pathways in both familial and sporadic forms of the disease. In addition, patients maintained on ventilatory support for many years show more widespread pathological changes, with evidence of extensive degeneration in the posterior columns, spinocerebellar pathways, substantia nigra, and other subcortical areas.

Selective vulnerability

The nuclei of the 3rd, 4th and 6th cranial nerves are selectively spared in ALS, although there may be mild involvement of the oculomotor nucleus in some cases. Sparing of the nucleus of Onufruwicz (also referred to as Onuf's nucleus), situated in the ventral part of the anterior horn in the second sacral segment of the spinal cord, is also a striking feature of ALS (Fig. 11.14), but is also a feature of SMA and paralytic poliomyelitis. The neurons of Onuf's nucleus innervate the striated muscles of the external anal and urethral sphincters. They receive synaptic inputs typical of other somatic motor neurons, although Onuf's nucleus neurons also have extensive connections with the autonomic nervous system and are surrounded by peptidergic fibres which are preserved in ALS. Like oculomotor neurons, Onuf's nucleus neurons may receive little if any corticospinal tract input. It has been suggested that this relative lack of glutamatergic inputs may be related to selective sparing. However, such sparing is relative, and varying degrees of involvement of these nuclei have been observed.

Cellular and Molecular Pathology

As in Alzheimer's and Parkinson's disease, degenerating neurons in motor neuron disease contain characteristic cytoplasmic inclusions; in particular, the Bunina body is virtually specific for ALS (Fig. 11.15a). It is present in anterior horn cells and brain stem somatic motor neurons, although Bunina bodies have occasionally been described in cells of Clarke's column, medullary reticular formation, and pyramidal neurons of the motor cortex. Bunina bodies are found in 80 per cent or more of ALS cases. Lewy body-like inclusions (Fig. 11.15b) are found in anterior horns of about 20 per cent of patients. ALS has been reported in association with dementia and diffuse Lewy body disease, but brain stem Lewy bodies of the type seen in Parkinson's disease are not found in typical ALS.

Surviving anterior horn motor neurons in ALS are often shrunken, and may lose their Nissl substance, becoming achromasic. True chromatolysis is relatively rare. Dendritic atrophy may be an early change. Silver impregnation techniques may reveal accumulations of argyrophilic neurofilaments and, more recently, antibodies directed against neurofilament proteins have confirmed that a proportion of surviving motor neurons contain bundles of neurofilaments which may be abnormally phosphorylated. Antibodies directed against phosphorylated neurofilament epitopes stain motor neuron cell bodies only weakly, but they strongly label axons, since neurofilament proteins become increasingly phosphorylated as they are transported from the cell body into the axons (Fig. 11.16). In ALS, some surviving motor neurons show perikaryal labelling by antibodies directed against phosphorylated neurofilament epitopes, but this is not a specific change, and increased perikaryal labelling by such antibodies is seen in a variety of disorders associated with damage to motor axons, including axon section, spinal cord ischaemia, and degenerative disorders such as SMA (Fig. 11.17). Accumulations of neurofilaments within proximal axons of motor neurons are termed spheroids (Fig. 11.18). Anterior horn spheroids are larger and more abundant in ALS than in controls, but they are not a specific feature of ALS. Thus there is no evidence that ALS is caused by a primary disorder of neurofilament phosphorylation or metabolism, although changes in the phosphorylation status of neurofilaments may contribute to abnormalities of axonal transport in ALS.

Although Lewy body-like inclusions are occasionally labelled by antibodies directed against neurofilament proteins, antibodies against neurofilaments and other cytoskeletal proteins do not

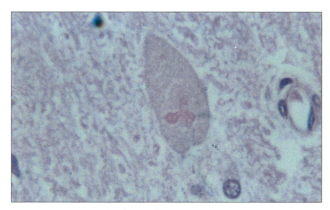

Fig. 11.15a A Bunina body in a degenerating neuron in ALS.

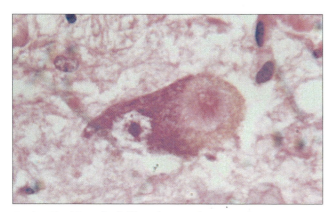

Fig. 11.15b A Lewy body-like inclusion in the anterior horn in ALS.

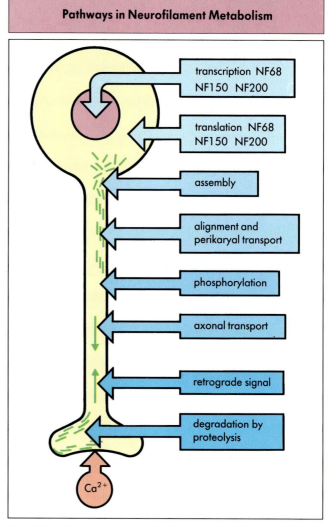

Pathways in Neurofilament Metabolism

transcription NF68 NF150 NF200

translation NF68 NF150 NF200

assembly

alignment and perikaryal transport

phosphorylation

axonal transport

retrograde signal

degradation by proteolysis

Ca²⁺

Fig. 11.16 Schematic diagram of pathways in neurofilament metabolism.

detect the most characteristic inclusion of ALS, the Bunina body. However, antibodies against ubiquitin have revealed characteristic inclusions which are not detected by other techniques. These ubiquitin immunoreactive inclusions take the form either of dense aggregates (Fig. 11.19), some of which correspond to Lewy body-like inclusions, or bundles and strings ('skeins') of filamentous-appearing material (Fig. 11.20) which ultrastructurally consists of fine filamentous structures ranging from 5–20 nm in diameter, and which are associated with fine granules.

Ubiquitin immunoreactive inclusions are found in 5–30 per cent of surviving brain stem and spinal cord motor neurons, but are only rarely found in cortical motor neurons. They are virtually specific for ALS.

Ubiquitin is a protein with a molecular weight of 8500. It has many functions, but particular attention has focused on its role in the non-lysosomal breakdown of short-lived or abnormal protein (Fig. 11.21). Ubiquitin becomes conjugated to such proteins, which are then targeted for proteolysis. Ubiquitin is a component of many types of inclusion bodies, including neurofibrillary tangles in Alzheimer's disease, and Lewy bodies in Parkinson's disease, and its presence probably denotes alterations in the target proteins which make them resistant to proteolysis.

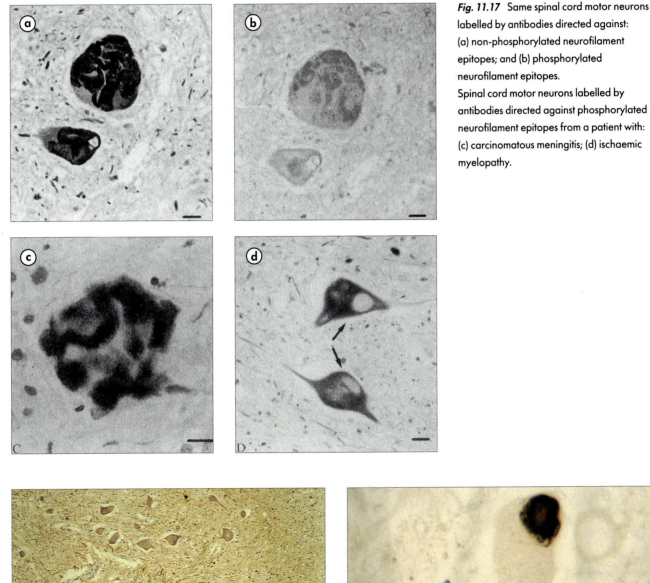

Fig. 11.17 Same spinal cord motor neurons labelled by antibodies directed against: (a) non-phosphorylated neurofilament epitopes; and (b) phosphorylated neurofilament epitopes.
Spinal cord motor neurons labelled by antibodies directed against phosphorylated neurofilament epitopes from a patient with: (c) carcinomatous meningitis; (d) ischaemic myelopathy.

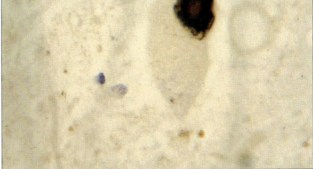

Fig. 11.18 Accumulation of neurofilaments within proximal axons of motor neurons in ALS.

Fig. 11.19 Dense aggregates of ubiquitin immunoreactive inclusion in a motor neuron in ALS.

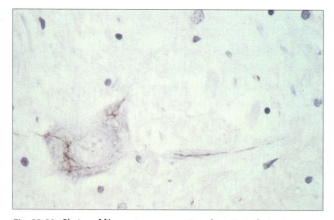

Fig. 11.20 Skeins of filamentous-appearing ubiquitin inclusion in a motor neuron in ALS.

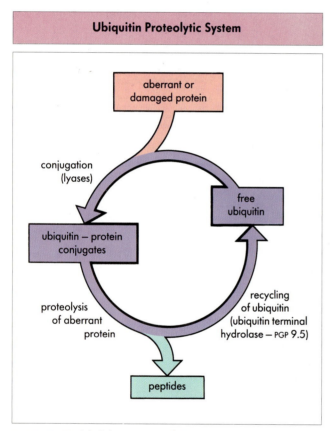

Fig. 11.21 Model of ubiquitin proteolytic system.

TREATMENT

There is no drug therapy which will modify the course of ALS, but much can be done to improve quality of life and to relieve symptoms. Information and counselling is of major importance, as is contact with local and national support groups. A team approach to management is desirable, involving a neurologist, physiotherapist, speech therapist, occupational therapist, social worker, ALS counsellor, and in some instances a psychologist or psychiatrist. The care team should have links with a respiratory unit, since occasionally patients develop distressing respiratory symptoms relatively early in the course of the disease, and assisted ventilation such as CPAP (continuous positive airway pressure) or a cuirasse ventilator may be helpful. In other patients who have widespread and advanced disease, relief of dyspnoea with small doses of oral morphine may be more appropriate, particularly in the setting of hospice care. A link with a gastroenterological team is also desirable, because endoscopic gastrostomy may be needed for patients with severe bulbar symptoms. The care team should also include expertise in neurological rehabilitation, with access to the full range of aids and appliances for disabled living.

DIFFERENTIAL DIAGNOSIS

Slowly progressive syndromes of LMN degeneration such as late onset (juvenile chronic) spinal muscular atrophy (SMA type III; Kugelberg–Welander disease) and X-linked bulbospinal neuronopathy (Kennedy's syndrome) may be difficult to differentiate from the lower motor neuron forms of ALS. Similarly, motor neuropathies associated with high titres of anti-ganglioside antibodies may mimic lower motor neuron forms of ALS. It should also be appreciated that anterior horn cell degeneration may be seen in association with other multisystem atrophies such as Shy–Drager syndrome, and with spongiform encephalopathies such as Creutzfeldt–Jakob disease.

Provided that care is taken to distinguish SMA and motor neuropathy from lower motor neuron forms of ALS, it is best to regard ALS, PBP, and PMA as part of the same clinical syndrome pending full understanding of the molecular basis of ALS and other motor system disorders.

SUMMARY

(i)   The cause of sporadic ALS is unknown.

(ii)   Risk factors include age, male sex, and possibly previous trauma.

(iii)   Pathologically the disease is characterized by degeneration of upper and lower motor neurons, the latter frequently containing ubiquitin-immunoreactive inclusions which have not yet been associated with any cytoskeletal protein.

(iv)   There is no effective drug therapy which will alter the rate of disease progression, but much can be done to relieve symptoms and improve quality of life.

(v)   Familial ALS has been tentatively linked to markers of chromosome 21, but is probably genetically heterogenous.

(vi)   A mutation of the androgen receptor has been identified in a rare form of SMA (Kennedy's syndrome), and the clinical variants of autosomal recessive SMA show linkage to chromosome 5q.

(vii)   Rapid advances in understanding of the molecular basis, and perhaps treatment, of motor neuron disorders are likely to be forthcoming.

SECTION 3

Epilepsy

Epilepsy is one of the commonest neurological disorders. It has been calculated that almost 5 per cent of the population will suffer from an epileptic episode at some time in their lives and that as many as 0.5 per cent (1:200) will have epilepsy.

The brain functions via massive interconnections between neurons. These interconnections are the physiological substrate of the extensive serial and parallel processing of both sensory and motor information. Many of these connections are excitatory, and thus have the potential of generating aberrant or epileptiform activity. Isolated events of this kind that involve small numbers of neurons have no great clinical import. However, large assemblies of neurons that show abnormal or uncontrolled synchronous patterns of excitation can give rise to epileptic seizures and a range of clinically significant phenomena: stereotyped and involuntary alterations in behaviour; transient losses of awareness; psychiatric disturbances; and convulsions and loss of consciousness.

Aetiology   Epileptic activity can arise from abnormalities in brain structure or as a consequence of brain damage. As a result, many factors and processes are involved in the aetiology of epilepsy. In many patients, aetiology is multifactorial, and a clear identification of a single causative factor is impossible. In addition, many epilepsies appear to have no identified cause (cryptogenic epilepsy). In one large cohort of patients studied in the UK (National General Practice Study of Epilepsy – NGPSE), the aetiology of the epilepsy after diagnosis was identified as: unknown in 70 per cent; cerebrovascular in 15 per cent; cerebral tumour in 6 per cent; alcohol related in 6 per cent; post-traumatic in 2 per cent; and other identified causes in 1 per cent.

Seizures that arise only as a result of toxic or metabolic disorders (e.g. hypoglycaemia) are not generally classified as epilepsy.

Onset   The incidence of epilepsy is greatest in children under 10. Thereafter, rates decline through adulthood before rising again in patients over 60. Males are affected more often than females.

Degree of disability   The true extent of disability occurring as a direct result of epilepsy is difficult to determine. It has been estimated that, of patients diagnosed as epileptic in the USA, approximately 33 per cent have fewer than one seizure a year; 33 per cent have between one and 12 seizures a year; 26 per cent have more than one seizure a month; and 8 per cent have more than one seizure a week.

In addition, some 60 per cent of all patients have concomitant behavioural disturbances, neurological problems, or cognitive deficits. Despite the widespread availability of anti-epileptic drug therapy, patients with active epilepsy are often untreated. In one community survey (Tonbridge, UK), some 40 per cent of those with active epilepsy were not receiving treatment on the day of the survey. The proportion of untreated patients is even greater in developing countries and has been estimated at 80 per cent in Ecuador and 94 per cent in the Philippines and Pakistan.

Classification of epilepsy   Epilepsy can be classified into a number of types based on the pattern of seizure activity, age, aetiology, localization, and EEG changes. This type of classification often conveys useful aetiological and prognostic information. Seizures are classified into four main groups: localization-related (local, focal, partial); generalized; undetermined; and special syndromes.

Localization-related (partial) epilepsy   In partial epilepsy, seizure activity begins in a circumscribed brain region, and either remains confined to this location or spreads to other brain regions (as a secondary phenomenon) during the progress of the seizure. Localization-related seizures are seen in 60 per cent of epilepsy patients and can be classified into idiopathic and symptomatic categories. In addition, such seizures are often categorized as simple partial (preservation of consciousness) or complex partial (altered consciousness).

Generalized epilepsy   Generalized seizures (as the term suggests) involve large areas of the brain from the outset, and seizure activity is present on EEG recordings from all brain areas simultaneously. They are seen in about 40 per cent of patients and can be divided into a number of subtypes.

Undetermined   These types of seizure may have characteristics of both the previous categories, or else the clinical documentation may be incomplete.

Special syndromes   This category includes epileptic attacks that are closely related to particular parameters, such as age (febrile convulsions) or situations.

The classification of epilepsy can be an inexact science, as many types of seizures share pathological and physiological characteristics. Comprehensive schemes for taxonomy are of recent origin (e.g. the scheme above was devised in 1989). As a result, detailed information on the aetiology, course, pathology, and physiology for each of the different categories of epilepsy is not available. This paucity of information will be resolved in time. In the light of this, we will consider the common themes present in most types of epilepsies, and then consider specific issues related to the best-defined categories.

12 Epilepsy: Pathophysiology and Classification

DEFINITION

Epilepsy is an episodic disorder of the nervous system that arises from the excessively synchronous and sustained discharge of a group of neurons.

An epileptic seizure is a brief and usually unprovoked stereotyped disturbance of behaviour, emotion, motor function, or sensation that on clinical evidence results from cortical neuronal discharge.

Epilepsy can only be diagnosed when seizures have recurred in an apparently spontaneous fashion.

EPIDEMIOLOGY

The lifetime prevalence of epilepsy (i.e. the total number of people in a population who have ever had epilepsy) has been estimated to be up to 5 per cent (WHO estimate). This is to say that as many as one in 20 of the population will have an epileptic seizure (excluding a febrile convulsion) during their lives. It is thought that some 0.5 per cent of the population will develop epilepsy.

Epilepsy is the commonest serious neurological condition: the prevalence rate is 10 times that of multiple sclerosis and 100 times that of motor neuron disease.

Determining an accurate figure for the extent of epilepsy within the population is difficult, despite the many studies that have reported on the incidence and prevalence of epilepsy. Definitions of epilepsy, methods of collecting cases and criteria for diagnosis vary widely between studies. A recent survey of the literature (Shorvon, 1990) reported incidence rates of 20–70 per 100 000 per year (range 11–134 per 100 000 per year), and point prevalence rates of 4–100 per 1000 in the general population (range 1.5–30 per 1000) are reported. Both incidence and prevalence vary with age (Fig. 12.1). Rates:
- are greatest in early childhood;
- decline between the ages of five and 60; and
- rise again in elderly people.

The incidence of epileptic disorders increases steeply after the age of 60. Epidemiological studies indicate typical incidence rates of 12 per 100 000 at ages 40–59, increasing to 80 per 100 000 in those over 60; and prevalence rates of 7.3 per 1000 in 40–59 year olds, increasing to 10.2 per 1000 for those over 60. Some 25 per cent of the total number of patients with epilepsy in the community are over 60.

Epilepsy rates differ according to sex, socio-economic class, race, and geographical location. Males are affected more often than females and rates of epilepsy are higher in lower socio-economic groups. US mortality data suggest that the prevalence of epilepsy may be significantly higher in blacks than in whites.

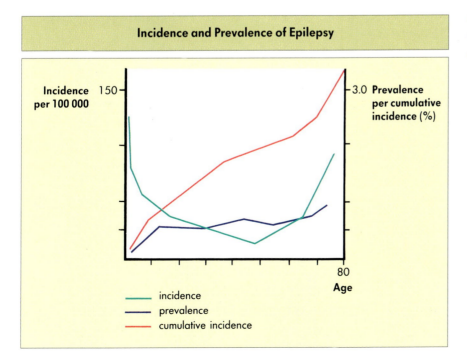

Incidence and Prevalence of Epilepsy

Incidence per 100 000   150

3.0   Prevalence per cumulative incidence (%)

80   **Age**

— incidence
— prevalence
— cumulative incidence

Fig. 12.1 Age-specific cumulative incidence and prevalence rates of epilepsy in Rochester, Minnesota for the period 1935–1974.

These factors are probably interrelated to a certain extent, in that males are more likely than females to have neurodevelopmental abnormalities and to experience neurological difficulties as a result of birth trauma, and low socioeconomic class is related to increased rates of birth difficulties.

Marked differences in prevalence rates in particular sub-groups of patients can often be related to aetiology. Young adult males show higher rates, and this has been related to rates of head injury and subsequent risk of post-traumatic epilepsy in this group (see Chapter 5). Increased rates are also seen in certain geographical regions. In many cases, these increases are related to CNS infections endemic to the region (e.g. neurocysticercosis, schistosomiasis, and malaria are common causes of epilepsy in Latin America).

AETIOLOGY

Virtually any event that can alter brain structure or disturb the electrical functions of the brain can give rise to epilepsy.

Unknown causes
In up to 70 per cent of people with epilepsy, no specific cause can be determined.

Genetic causes
Epilepsy can be familial, and such a pattern of disease indicates a genetic cause. Clear autosomal-dominant inheritance of an epileptic disorder is rare. The complicated pattern of inheritance in familial epilepsy is thought to be due to the combined effects of incomplete penetrance or to the synergistic effect of several different genes.

There are almost 150 rare genetic disorders which have epilepsy as a common feature:

- approximately 25 autosomal-dominant conditions (e.g. tuberous sclerosis, acute intermittent porphyria, neurofibromatosis);
- some 100 types of autosomal-recessive phenotypes (e.g. Krabbe's disease, Batten's disease); and
- chromosome X-linked disorders (e.g. Aicardi syndrome).

These known genetic disorders account for less than 1 per cent of all epilepsies; tuberous sclerosis is commonest.

Genetic influences are thought to be involved in familial primary generalized epilepsies that have an onset between five and 25 years of age; these are often characterized by a clinical picture that encompasses:

- generalized grand mal, absence, and/or myoclonic seizures;
- 3 Hz spike and wave EEG pattern;
- photosensitivity;
- a diurnal seizure pattern; and
- a particular clinical course, depending upon age.

Linkage between chromosomal markers and several epileptic syndromes has been reported (e.g. juvenile myoclonus syndrome and a marker on chromosome 6). However, the genes responsible for these conditions have yet to be identified. Epilepsy can also occur in association with a wide range of chromosomal defects.

Congenital malformations
Congenital malformations, such as porencephaly, microgyria, cortical dysplasia, and arteriovenous malformations (e.g. Sturge–Weber syndrome), are common causes of epilepsy. Historically, these types of defect were thought to be present in a minority of cases, but improved imaging and pathological methods indicate that abnormalities in brain (particularly cortical) structure are much commoner and more important than previously documented.

Birth trauma
Global anoxia during birth can lead to massive brain damage, and results in spasticity, mental retardation, and seizures.

Birth trauma can also lead to focal anoxia and subsequent ischaemic brain damage. The hippocampus is the region of the brain most affected by this type of damage, and this pattern of pathology has been related to the subsequent development of temporal lobe epilepsy (Ammon's horn sclerosis). The extent of this phenomenon and its significance is a matter of dispute.

Neurological disorders and neurodegenerative disease
Long-standing neurological disorders can often lead to the onset of seizures and the development of epilepsy. Clinical examinations should always include direct questions about birth trauma, developmental milestones, severe head injury, and the possibility of central nervous system infection.

Epilepsy can occur as a complication of almost any neurodegenerative condition, because of the destruction and alteration of brain substance that accompanies such disease processes. Epilepsy arising from such causes is generally seen in older patients. Elderly patients (those over 60) with seizures should undergo thorough investigation to determine whether they have a neurodegenerative disease.

Head trauma
Epilepsy is a common long-term consequence of the brain damage caused by head trauma (see Chapter 5). Penetrating head trauma is associated with a significantly higher risk of subsequent epilepsy (40 per cent) than is non-penetrating head trauma (15 per cent) (Fig. 12.2).

Alcohol and drug abuse
Epileptic seizures can occur in patients undergoing alcohol or drug withdrawal programmes. Administration of amphetamines, glutamate receptor agonists (e.g. phencyclidine derivatives), and occasionally tricyclic antidepressants can precipitate seizures.

Metabolic disorders
Reductions in blood glucose and altered electrolyte balance can precipitate seizures. Seizures can occur in infants as a result of disorders such as galactosaemia and pyridoxine deficiency.

CLINICAL COURSE

Effective drug therapy for the treatment of seizures has been available for almost 100 years, beginning with the introduction of bromides in 1900. As a result, no modern long-term follow-up studies of untreated patients has been undertaken. Despite this lack of information, it has long been accepted wisdom that epilepsy (even when patients are treated) has a poor prognosis because of the chronic nature of the illness. However, the prevalence and incidence figures indicate that, in most cases, epilepsy lasts for about 10 years and then remits. This is both an encouraging epidemiological feature of the disease and a cause for clinical concern because of the difficulties in deciding when to stop drug therapy.

Single seizures and epilepsy

A distinction between epilepsy and single seizures is commonly made. However, several studies have shown that recurrence of seizure activity within weeks or months after a first seizure is the norm. A consensus figure based on the data from these studies indicates that, following a seizure of any kind, there is a second seizure in 75 per cent of patients. Since the occurrence of a second seizure is usual, a distinction between single seizure and epilepsy seems pointless, as well as being a potential source of anxiety to patients.

Despite the high rate of seizure recurrence, epidemiological evidence and clinical practice indicate that, in most cases, the period of epilepsy is brief and the total number of seizures is low.

Once a definite diagnosis of epilepsy is accepted, the patient must be counselled about the effects of the disorder on driving, employment, schooling, and leisure activities, and advice must be given about treatment and prognosis.

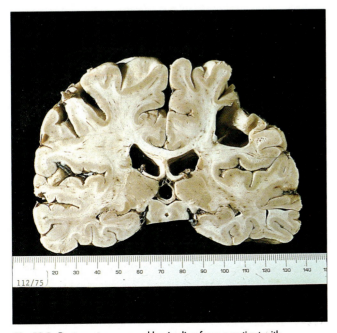

Fig. 12.2 Post-mortem coronal brain slice from a patient with generalized epilepsy secondary to trauma in the parietal lobe.

Outcome

Long-term outcome following diagnosis has been reported in two separate studies which retrospectively examined the course of epilepsy in patients in the USA (Rochester) and UK (Tonbridge). Broadly similar results were seen in each study. These can be interpreted to give the following pattern:

- 45 per cent were in remission after one year;
- 60 per cent were in remission after five years;
- 20 per cent remit and then relapse; and
- 20 per cent continued to have seizures.

Both studies showed that those entering remission tended to do so early in the course of the disease, and that the probability of remission declines the longer the epilepsy remained active.

These epidemiological studies indicate that at least two subgroups of patients exist:

- in one, epilepsy is mild and of short duration;
- in the other, epilepsy is chronic and seizures continue indefinitely despite treatment.

Different clinical features may exist in each group. Reliable documentation of such features would enable patients to be assigned to a good or poor prognosis group, and might ease the problems associated with the management of drug therapy.

Good prognosis

Patients with a good prognosis (mild epilepsy, early remission) are those with:

- seizures precipitated by alcohol or drugs, or by metabolic disturbance;
- benign syndromes (e.g. benign rolandic epilepsy);
- rare generalized seizures; and
- adult-onset idiopathic seizures.

Poor prognosis

Patients with the poorest prognosis are those with:

- early onset seizures;
- partial or mixed seizure types;
- severe epileptic syndromes (e.g. Lennox–Gastaut syndrome, West syndrome);
- progressive neurological disorders (e.g. cerebral tumour, progressive myoclonus epilepsy);
- evidence of diffuse cerebral disorder (often with intellectual or behavioural disturbance); and
- a long period of active epilepsy.

Drug therapy and prognosis

It is a common belief that drug therapy should be instigated as soon as possible, with a view to both inhibiting the seizure activity and suppressing the evolution of sporadic seizures into a chronic epileptic condition. This pattern of clinical response is based on the facts that:

- seizures are controlled in over 60 per cent of new patients;
- remission rates decline with increasing chronicity of seizures;
- chronic epilepsy is often refractory to treatment.

However, this pattern of response can lead to a monolithic approach to treatment. High doses of anti-epileptic drugs are administered to most patients over extended periods of time, with all the attendant difficulties associated with side effects.

The rationale for such an approach to treatment may be flawed. Clinical studies indicate that patients tend to fall into two groups and follow one of two courses: a mild disorder with early remission, or a more chronic course with the emergence of treatment-refractory seizures. In the light of this, drug therapy should be tailored to approximate the expected prognosis (good or poor) of the patient. Such an approach may reduce the risk of side effects in patients who may well be expected to remit as a matter of course.

Social problems, psychiatric disorder, and suicide

Epilepsy, particularly chronic epilepsy, can cause considerable social difficulties for patients. Difficulties in finding and maintaining employment are common: up to 10 per cent of patients are incapable of working and a further 10 per cent may only be able to cope with part-time employment. This degree of social dislocation cannot be explained entirely by the physical effects of fits. Social stigma, the patient's own lack of confidence, and psychiatric difficulties all contribute.

The extent and degree of psychiatric difficulties experienced by patients with epilepsy varies with the epileptic syndrome. Surveys of patients indicate that some 30 per cent of patients have a degree of psychiatric disorder (most often a neurotic disability or personality disorder), but this proportion is much greater (about 60 per cent) in patients with particular syndromes such as temporal lobe epilepsy. The age of the patient also has a marked effect; behavioural or psychiatric disorders occur more often in patients whose seizures started during childhood.

Rates of suicide and attempted suicide are five times higher in patients with epilepsy than in the general population. Rates in patients with temporal lobe epilepsy are some 20 times greater than in the general population. Males show higher rates than females.

PROPORTION OF SEIZURE CATEGORIES

The proportions of types of seizures vary enormously from study to study. This variability almost certainly reflects the sophistication of the medical investigations used to ascertain seizure types in the patient population (e.g. basic clinical interview versus neurological workup, ambulatory EEG, and subsequent PET and MRI scans). With these confounding factors in mind, an overview of the literature suggests that of the prevalent cases of epilepsy:

- 25 per cent are complex partial seizures;
- 35 per cent are secondary generalized seizures;
- 30 per cent are primary generalized tonic–clonic seizures;
- 5 per cent are simple partial seizures; and
- 5 per cent are generalized absence and myoclonic seizures.

INVESTIGATIONS

Electroencephalography (EEG)

Physiology EEG involves the detection, amplification, and display of the brain's electrical activity. This is commonly achieved by attaching a series of electrodes to the scalp. The resulting activity is displayed either as a trace or, increasingly (after processing the input with appropriate software), as a 'map' of brain activity (Fig. 12.3).

Only a portion of the electrical activity of the cortex is detected by EEG. This is the portion generated by pyramidal neurons. The reasons for this lies in the structural organization of the cortex. Pyramidal neurons are oriented parallel to each other with their dendrites perpendicular to the cortical surface. Therefore, synaptic potentials are recorded with little attenuation. Synaptic potentials are slower than action potentials; as a result they can summate. Most other neurons and glial cells are oriented in a variety of ways in relation to each other and the cortical surface. Thus, signals generated by these neurons attenuate and contribute little to the overall EEG pattern.

In summary, EEG patterns largely represent the changing synaptic potential of cortical pyramidal neurons.

Clinical utility EEGs require careful interpretation, as up to 15 per cent of non-epileptic patients have aberrant EEG patterns. This proportion of aberrant patterns is greater in patients over 65 years of age. However, most of this 'noise' can be removed by applying rigid criteria for the definition of focal, generalized spike, or polyspike abnormalities. Routine EEG investigation will reveal abnormalities in about 50 per cent of epileptic patients. EEG provides valuable information that may:

- confirm the clinical diagnosis;
- aid the classification of epilepsy; and
- increase the suspicion of an underlying structural lesion.

Epilepsy is ultimately a clinical diagnosis that can be confirmed but not made by EEG investigation.

EEG can be used to refine a clinical diagnosis; e.g. in a patient with seizures and brief periods of absence but no aura, a diagnosis of complex partial seizures (rather than typical absence seizure) would be supported by the presence of focal spike activity. Focal slow wave δ activity can suggest the presence of a structural lesion and give an indication as to its localization.

Imaging

CT scanning

CT abnormalities are found in less than 10 per cent of patients that present with a first seizure or early in the course of their epilepsy. Atrophic abnormalities are the commonest pathology. Surveys of patients with established epilepsy show that 60–80 per cent may have abnormal CT scans; again the majority of these abnormalities are atrophic in nature. Tumours can be identified in about 10 per cent of patients. CT scan abnormalities are very strongly predicted by:

- the presence of focal rather than generalized seizures;
- focal neurological signs; and
- focal EEG abnormalities.

CT abnormalities are found in over 70 per cent of patients with all three indicators. CT scans are particularly sensitive at identifying calcified lesions (e.g. meningioma, arteriovenous malformations).

MRI scanning

MRI is particularly useful for identifying minor pathology in the middle or posterior cranial fossae of the skull, where visualization using CT is difficult. In addition, in T2-weighted scan sequences, areas of high signal intensity consistent with Ammon's horn sclerosis may be seen in the region of the medial temporal lobe. Congenital abnormalities, including regions of cortical dysplasia and most focal pathologies, are also well visualized with MRI.

SPECT and PET

Both of these imaging techniques are useful for demonstrating the changes in blood flow, and PET can demonstrate abnormalities of glucose and oxygen metabolism that take place during or after seizure activity (Fig. 12.4). Hypermetabolism can be detected within the seizure focus during the seizure, whereas a more extensive hypometabolic zone with reduced activity is seen interictally.

Both of these techniques offer increasingly sophisticated ways of studying the dynamics of seizure activity and of localizing the origin of the seizure. Exactly how the changes in blood flow and metabolism correlate with EEG activity and pathological lesions is still being investigated, as is the question of whether these methods can replace intra-operative EEG monitoring as a means of localizing the seizure focus for surgical excision.

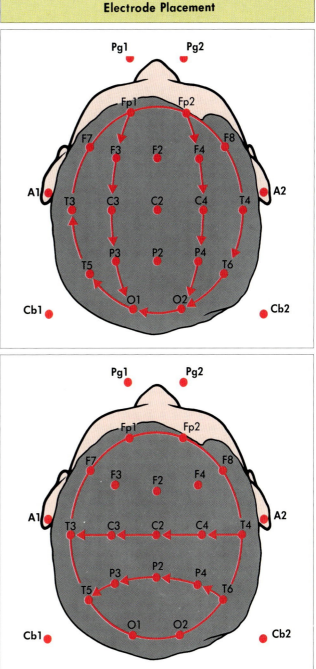

Electrode Placement

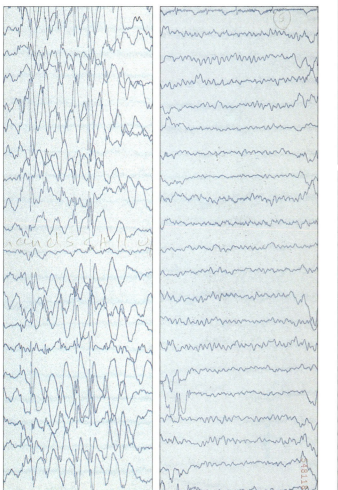

Fig. 12.3 Two sections from an EEG of a nine-year-old girl with absence seizures. Diagram shows electrode placement on the skull.

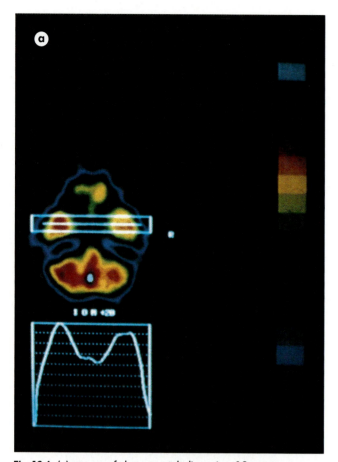

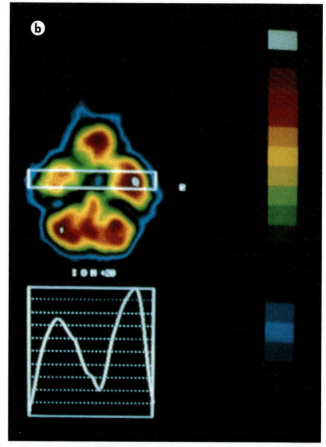

Fig. 12.4 (a) PET scan of glucose metabolism using F18DG as tracer through the posterior fossa, showing a focal decrease in activity in the right temporal lobe in a patient with complex partial epilepsy of temporal lobe origin. (Courtesy of William Theodore MD, Bethesda, Maryland.) (b) PET scan of glucose metabolism using F18DG of the same patient showing focal hyperfunction in the right temporal and orbital frontal lobe during a clinical seizure.

DIAGNOSIS

The type of epilepsy affecting patients is rarely categorized completely by a simple description of a single seizure type. The course of the disease is variable, often involving different kinds of seizures and, in childhood epilepsies, a shifting focus. To overcome the deficiencies inherent in describing epilepsy purely in terms of seizure type, epilepsy is categorized into a series of syndromes on the basis of the main seizure type (generalized or partial) and other relevant factors (Fig. 12.5):

• aetiology;
• anatomy;
• pathology;
• age of onset;
• precipitating factors;
• severity;
• chronicity;
• circadian cycle; and
• prognosis.

These factors can be related to each other and used to generate a series of syndromes. The syndromes can then be used to provide a more complete description of the patient's clinical condition. The advantages of a syndromal diagnosis are greater accuracy in estimating chronicity, improved prediction of prognosis, rational basis for treatment, and awareness of other factors that might be important for clinical management but that have not yet been uncovered (e.g. precipitation of seizures by sleep deprivation).

Many epileptic syndromes are age related, and age of seizure onset often provides a useful pointer to the correct diagnosis.

Age of Onset

The age at which seizure activity becomes established is associated with particular clinical symptoms and risks (see Chapter 13). These arise largely from the effects of seizure activity on the developing brain.

Febrile convulsions

The increase in body temperature that occurs as a response to systemic infection can induce convulsions (febrile convulsions) in children. This type of convulsion is much commoner than

International Classification of Epilepsies and Epileptic Syndromes and Related Seizure Disorders

Localization-related (local, focal, partial) epilepsies and syndromes

idiopathic (with age-related onset)
    benign childhood epilepsy with centrotemporal spike
    childhood epilepsy with occipital paroxysms
    primary reading epilepsy
symptomatic
    chronic progressive epilepsia partialis continua
    syndromes characterized by seizures with specific modes of
    precipitation
        temporal lobe epilepsies
        frontal lobe epilepsies
        parietal lobe epilepsies
        occipital lobe epilepsies
cryptogenic

Generalized epilepsies and syndromes

idiopathic (with age-related onset)
    benign neonatal familial convulsions
    benign neonatal convulsions
    benign myoclonic epilepsy in infancy
    childhood absence epilepsy
    juvenile absence epilepsy
    juvenile myoclonic epilepsy
    epilepsy with grand mal seizures (GTCS) on awakening
    other generalized idiopathic epilepsies
    epilepsies with seizures precipitated by specific modes of
    activation
cryptogenic or symptomatic
    West syndrome
    Lennox–Gestaut syndrome
    epilepsy with myoclonic–astatic seizures
    epilepsy with myoclonic absence
symptomatic
    non-specific aetiology
        early myoclonic encephalopathy
        early infantile epileptic encephalopathy with suppression
        burst
        other symptomatic generalized epilepsies
    specific syndromes
        epileptic seizures complicating other disease states

Epilepsies and syndromes undetermined whether focal or generalized

with both generalized and focal seizures
    neonatal seizures
    severe myoclonic epilepsy of infancy
    epilepsy with continuous spike waves during slow-wave
    sleep
    acquired epileptic aphasia
    other undetermined epilepsies
without unequivocal generalized or focal features

Special syndromes

situation-related seizures
febrile convulsions
isolated seizures or isolated status epilepticus
seizures occurring only with acute metabolic or toxic events

Fig. 12.5 International classification of epilepsies and epileptic syndromes and related seizure disorders, excluding the localization-related epilepsies and syndromes.

epilepsy. In a large American study, 2.5 per cent of children under the age of five experienced at least one febrile seizure. About 10 per cent of children that experience febrile convulsions will have further episodes of seizure activity in the absence of a raised body temperature.

Febrile convulsions require careful management since approximately 5 per cent of children will have a period of status epilepticus.

Status epilepticus

Status epilepticus has been described as 'a seizure lasting more than 30 minutes or several distinct episodes without restoration of consciousness' (Brodie, 1990).

Sustained seizure activity causes considerable disruption to the physiology of neurons and can result in permanent damage. The risk of neuronal damage and the difficulty of controlling the seizure increases with the duration of the seizure activity. Sustained generalized tonic–clonic seizures require prompt treatment. Commonly, this consists of intravenous benzodiazepine to suppress the seizure, followed by an infusion with an anticonvulsant (e.g. phenytoin) to prevent the recurrence of seizure activity.

Patients will require careful monitoring, because benzodiazopines can depress respiration, and phenytoin can cause cardiac arrhythmias. Hypoglycaemia and hypoxia may also occur and require remedial action. Status epilepticus can be caused by a wide range of factors (Fig. 12.6): non-compliance with anti-epileptic drug therapy and drug withdrawal are common causes. If such factors are not readily apparent, then intensive investigations should be made to determine the cause.

Localization-related seizures can also give rise to convulsive status (epilepsia partialis continua). Status of this type can be resistant to anti-epileptic drugs and responds best to high doses of corticosteroids.

Causes of Tonic–Clonic Status

Presenting *de novo*	Background of epilepsy
Cerebrovascular disease	Poor anticonvulsant compliance
Meningoencephalitis	Recent dose reduction or discontinuation
Acute head injury	
Cerebral tumour	Alcohol withdrawal
Brain abscess	Pseudostatus
Metabolic disorder, e.g. renal failure, hypoglycaemia, hepatic encephalopathy hyponatraemia, post cardiac arrest,	
Drug overdose, e.g. tricyclic antidepressant, phenothiazine, theophylline, isoniazid, cocaine	
Inflammatory arteritis, e.g. systemic lupus erythematosus	

Fig. 12.6 Causes of tonic–clonic status.

There are several diagnostic pitfalls associated with status epilepticus. Two common ones are:

- pseudostatus; and
- non-convulsive status.

  Pseudostatus is a possibility if the patient shows:

- aberrant motor activity;
- an on–off pattern of seizure activity;
- a poor response to treatment; or
- long periods of fits with no metabolic consequences.

The difficulties of pseudostatus arise from treatment given to patients in the erroneous belief that the patient is in status epilepticus.

Non-convulsive status epilepticus may be suspected in patients that present with:

- long-term clouding of consciousness;
- orofacial dyskinetic movements; or
- partial or generalized seizure (absence).

Mortality figures vary depending on the underlying cause of the status and on the duration of seizures before therapeutic intervention. These factors also influence the neurological outcome.

Status epilepticus in children   About one fifth of children with epilepsy have at least one episode of generalized tonic–clonic status, and status occurs in about 5 per cent of children with febrile seizures. Children are more likely than adults to have permanent neurological damage – e.g. about one third of children in one series were left with considerable problems, such as hemiparesis, diplegia, microcephaly, and mental retardation. Because of these complications and the risk of death, rapid therapy is needed, not only in true status (lasting over 30 minutes) but also in any child who continues to fit for more than five minutes. Status is seldom due to an underlying lesion in children (unlike adults). Non-tonic–clonic status may occur in children, and some forms – e.g. simple partial status – are difficult to treat.

NEUROPATHOLOGY

The neuropathology associated with epileptic seizures is described according to its general morphology rather than its association with any particular seizure type. In pathological terms, epilepsy is divided into three categories:

- symptomatic, in which identified pathology (e.g. tumour) is considered to give rise to seizure activity (this is also called secondary epilepsy);
- idiopathic, cryptogenic, or primary, in which no clearly identified pathology is found (but brain structure may not be normal); and
- special forms of epilepsy.

  As noted above, most patients with epilepsy have no identified pathological lesion.

Symptomatic Epilepsy

Epilepsy occurs in association with many underlying abnormalities: developmental defects (Fig. 12.7); vascular lesions (Fig. 12.8) such as venous thromboses and subdural haematomas; primary or secondary neoplasia; traumatic lesions; microbial or viral infections; parasitic disorders such as toxoplasmosis, cerebral malaria, and cysticercosis; and degenerative disorders, ranging from lesions induced by perinatal asphyxia to Huntington's chorea. These conditions do not necessarily cause epilepsy and may be only coincidentally present. However, they may show a temporal and spatial relation to the onset of seizures, and surgical removal of the affected areas may be followed by the disappearance of seizures – features that are often taken to imply a causal role. In these cases, the pathological features are those of the primary neuropsychiatric disease or neurological condition.

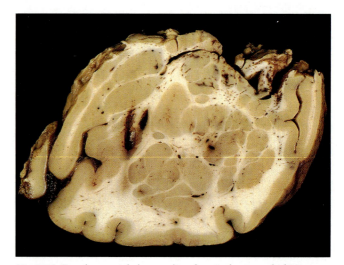

Fig. 12.7   Developmental abnormality of cortical grey and white matter in the temporal lobe; from a patient with generalized epilepsy.

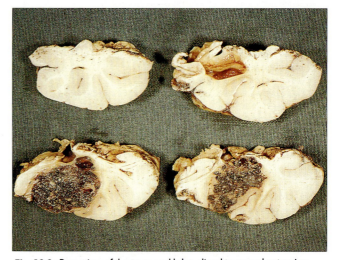

Fig. 12.8   Resection of the temporal lobe, sliced to reveal extensive arterovenous malformations.

Idiopathic Epilepsy

In general, there is no clearly defined pathology in idiopathic epilepsy. Pathologies that may be regarded as pathognomonic of epilepsy are:

- Ammon's horn sclerosis due to febrile convulsions;
- ischaemic damage due to status epilepticus; and
- microdysgenesis.

Ammon's horn sclerosis

Anoxia during birth or brain ischaemia induced by febrile convulsions can cause a specific pattern of neuronal loss in the hippocampus. The loss of neurons is particularly marked in the CA1 region and the endfolium (Fig. 12.9). In patients with intractable seizures, there is often a history of febrile convulsions in early childhood. It is thought that prolonged convulsions (lasting over 30 minutes) of this kind cause focal ischaemic damage in the hippocampus and a permanent loss of neurons. Damage of this type in the hippocampus or temporal lobe is a common necropsy finding in institutionalized patients with epilepsy, and is the most frequent pathological abnormality seen after surgical resection of the temporal lobe to alleviate intractable seizures (Fig. 12.10).

The pathological effects of recurrent or prolonged seizures during the course of chronic epilepsy is a subject of dispute. Seizures have been reported to accelerate the decline in neuronal number thought to occur during ageing (Fig. 12.11), but the magnitude of the effect is probably small. It has been well established that extensive neuronal loss occurs as a result of status epilepticus.

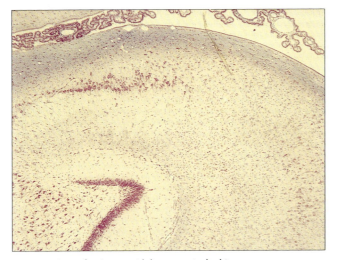

Fig. 12.9 Loss of CA1 pyramidal neurons in the hippocampus (haematoxylin and eosin).

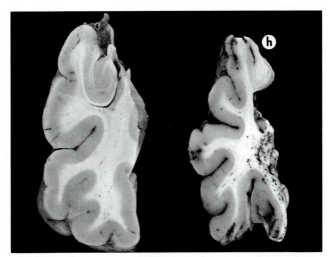

Fig. 12.10 Temporal lobe atrophy, especially marked in the hippocampus (h), in a resected specimen from a temporal lobectomy (left). A normal hippocampus (right).

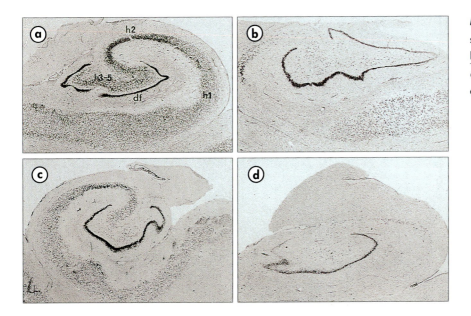

Fig. 12.11 Varying degrees of Ammon's horn sclerosis. (a) Normal hippocampus; (b) cell loss in a CA1 lesion; (c) cell loss in a CA1 and CA3/4 lesion; (d) cell loss in all regions, with consequent marked atrophy.

As an aside, it is worth noting that typical Ammon's horn sclerosis is an infrequent finding in children that undergo resection before the age of 10. This observation has strengthened the viewpoint that Ammon's horn sclerosis is a consequence of chronic seizure activity or extended periods of status epilepticus in adults rather than an early pathological process in children that leads to chronic epilepsy.

Ischaemic damage due to status epilepticus

The pathological consequence of sustained status epilepticus in children are:

- generalized damage involving the neocortex, hippocampus, thalamus, and cerebellum (Fig. 12.12);
- cerebral hemiatrophy with hemiparesis and possibly hemiconvulsions (Fig. 12.13); and
- ischaemic damage to the temporal lobe (Fig. 12.14) (e.g. Ammon's horn sclerosis) and subsequent temporal lobe epilepsy.

The damage caused by status epilepticus in the adult brain is less marked. However, even in adults, status epilepticus can be followed by acute degenerative changes that affect neurons in the hippocampus (especially the endfolium and the CA1 zone) and the cortex.

Disordered cortical cytoarchitecture

The absence of obvious pathology in up to 70 per cent of patients has been discussed above. It is possible that this feature of the pathology of epilepsy is a result of inadequate pathological investigation. Increasingly, studies report the presence of disordered cortical cytoarchitecture in regions of cortex that have been resected during surgery to alleviate chronic epilepsy. Such morphological abnormalities (graphically described as 'architectural follies') have been labelled as hamartomas, cortical dystopias, microdysgenesis, and focal cortical dysplasia (Fig. 12.15). Thes types of lesions appear as clusters of abnormally large neurons in the cortex, as disordered regions of cortical

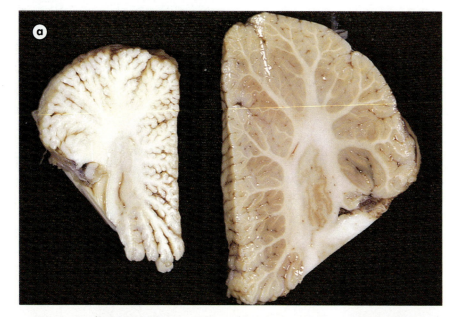

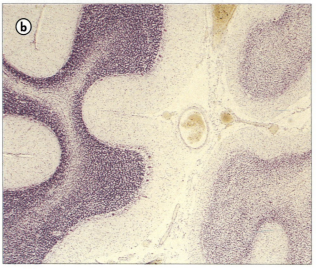

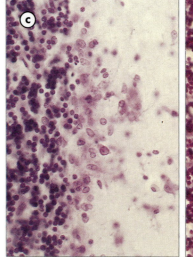

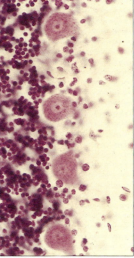

Fig. 12.12 Cerebellar damage in a five-year-old child, caused by status epilepticus. (a) Damage to the cerebellum visible at the gross level (left); normal cerebellum (right); (b) focal loss of granule cells in the folia of the cerebellum; (c) loss of Purkinje cells in the cerebellum (left); normal cerebellum (right).

lamination, or as dystopic groups of neurons in the subcortical white matter (Fig. 12.16). The site and extent of these lesions is variable, and to date there has been no close match between syndrome and pathology. These types of cortical abnormalities are thought to occur during the neurogenesis of the fetal cortex in the second half of pregnancy.

Fig. 12.13 Marked neuronal loss and atrophy with cortical gliosis throughout the cortical ribbon, after seizures (top); normal cortex (bottom) (haematoxylin and eosin).

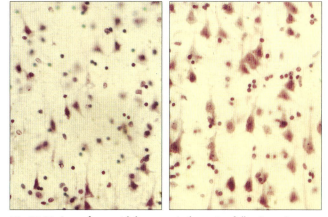

Fig. 12.14 Loss of pyramidal neurons in the cortex following seizures (left); normal cortex (right) (haematoxylin and eosin).

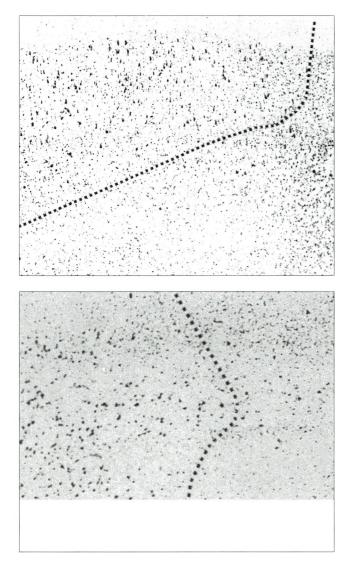

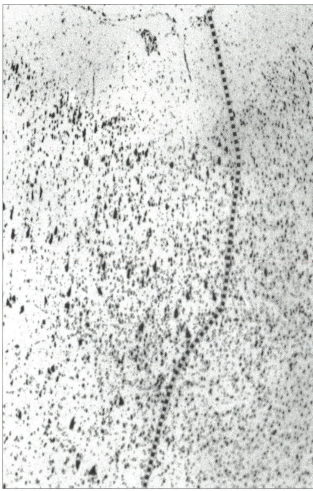

Fig. 12.15 Three examples of microdysgenesis in the cortex associated with generalized epilepsy. In each case, the normal cortex is shown on the right.

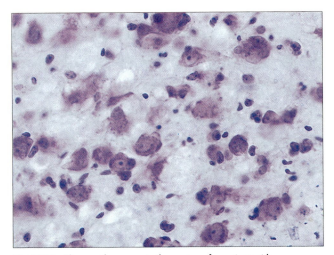

Fig. 12.16 Abnormal neurons in the cortex of a patient with generalized epilepsy (haematoxylin and eosin).

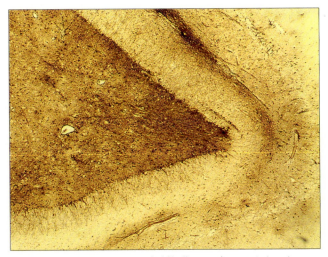

Fig. 12.17 Marked increase in glial fibrillary acidic protein (GFAP) immunoreactivity in the dentate gyrus.

Clinicopathological studies indicate that these kinds of lesions are very common in epilepsies that arise early in childhood and are resistant to treatment. This type of pathology is common in paediatric localization-related epileptic syndromes (e.g. temporal lobe epilepsy) and is often found after resection of the cortex, even when imaging studies have shown no overt abnormality.

Disordered cortical cytoarchitecture is the pathology thought to predispose to diverse types of epilepsy, including primary generalized epilepsy, West's syndrome, and temporal lobe epilepsy. The precise relationship between the extent and types of cortical abnormality and epilepsy is a matter of robust debate. This is, in part, due to the growing realization that variants of cortical architecture are comparatively common in 'normal' brains. Thus, some pathologists consider ectopic neurons as minor variations on the cytoarchitectural theme, whereas others interpret them as the morphological substrate of increased susceptibility to epilepsy. The threshold whereby the former becomes the latter remains to be defined.

Other Changes

Since the last century, both glial reactivity (Fig. 12.17) and dendritic degeneration have been related to the presence of epilepsy. Glial reactivity has been demonstrated experimentally to be a consequence of seizure activity. It is also possible that the formation of a glial scar in response to some pathological event could subsequently act to generate or induce a seizure focus. Dendritic degeneration is a non-specific finding, but it may be associated with membrane changes, including receptor hypersensitivity, that could contribute to epileptogenesis.

Another morphological change has been described relating to excitatory neurotransmission in the mossy fibre system in experimental epilepsy and in humans. This fibre system originates in the dentate granule cells of the hippocampus and usually terminates within the dendritic fields of the CA3 and CA4 principal neurons (the terminations being associated with kainate receptors). In adults with temporal lobe epilepsy, and apparently also in children with various types of generalized epilepsy, these fibres terminate abnormally in the inner molecular layer of the dentate gyrus, as a result of sprouting induced either by loss of other inputs or by abnormal neuronal discharges.

Ultrastructural Pathology

Seizures induce swelling of perineuronal astrocytic processes throughout the pyramidal layer of the hippocampus. Swollen mitochondria are seen in the neuron and in focal dendritic swellings. These appearances are similar to the excitotoxic changes caused by glutamate overactivity.

PHYSIOLOGY

Physiological Mechanisms

The physiological response of neurons to seizures have been extensively studied. The goal of such experimentation has been to describe:

- circumstances that give rise to the initial epileptic discharge (ictal or interictal);
- the causes and characterization of the transition from the interictal to the ictal state;
- physiological and synaptic mechanisms that propagate the spread of seizure discharge; and
- the processes that lead to the cessation of seizure activity.

At present, the complete details of these processes cannot be described with absolute certainty.

Although much is known about the physiological basis of the abnormal discharges accompanying seizure phenomena, the cellular mechanisms responsible for epileptogenesis remain conjectural. There may be a primary defect in the neuronal membrane that results in an instability of the resting membrane potential; possible underlying mechanisms include an abnormality of potassium conductance, a defect in the voltage-sensitive calcium channels, or a deficiency in the membrane ATPase linked to ion transport. There may be primary defects in the GABAergic inhibitory system or in the somatostatin-containing neurons that regulate it in the hippocampus, or in the sensitivity or arrangement of the receptors involved in excitatory neurotransmission.

Initiation and propagation of seizure activity

Interictal spikes (recorded with a focal or more general distribution by EEG) correspond at the cellular level to the synchronous occurrence in principal neurons of a paroxysmal depolarizing shift in the resting membrane potential. This is associated with a brief burst of action potentials and is followed by a phase of hyperpolarization. Such an event can be triggered by a synchronous volley in afferent fibres or by the spontaneous discharge of 'pacemaker' epileptic neurons. In experimental models in which the epileptic process has been dissected, it appears that:

- interictal discharges become frequent;
- the phase of hyperpolarization reduces and can disappear;
- the cycle of paroxysmal depolarization with burst firing occurs at ever decreasing intervals within neurons;
- these discharges are associated with increased extracellular potassium and decreased extracellular calcium;
- localized burst firing is initially associated with enhanced inhibitory activity in projection areas;
- with repetition, inhibitory activity fades and excitatory neurotransmission predominates; this causes synchronized burst firing in related cortical areas or deep brain nuclei, which in turn causes the spread of seizure activity;
- termination of seizure activity is associated with arrest of burst firing and replacement of the paroxysmal depolarizing shifts by sustained hyperpolarization, probably as a consequence of active intrinsic inhibitory processes.

NEUROCHEMICAL PATHOPHYSIOLOGY

It is clear that various neurotransmitters are intimately involved in the physiological processes described above. Two transmitters have been the focus of particular interest – GABA and somatostatin (Fig. 12.18).

These two transmitters are intimately related to each other in the cortex and in the hippocampus. Somatostatin is a neuropeptide that has excitatory effects, and GABA is an inhibitory transmitter. The two transmitters are co-localized within the same neuron in the cortex, and are found in separate neurons in the hippocampus. Increased excitability in neurons could arise from either:

- a direct loss of inhibitory (GABAergic) input; or
- a selective loss of the excitatory input (somatostatinergic) to the inhibitory system.

Both mechanisms may be operative in epileptogenesis. A selective loss of inhibitory terminals or cell bodies has been described in the epileptic focus created by aluminium in monkey cortex. Measurement of glutamic acid decarboxylase activity in focal epileptic tissue has suggested that GABA synthesis may be impaired in a minority of patients with focal seizures. A deficit in the GABA–benzodiazepine-receptor complex may be a predisposing or contributory cause of epilepsy. The number of benzodiazepine receptors in the midbrain appears to be reduced in two genetically determined epilepsy syndromes in rodents. A positron emission tomography study in humans with the C-labelled benzodiazepine receptor ligand Flumazenil has shown a decrease in the number of benzodiazepine receptors in the presumed epileptic focus in patients with partial epilepsy.

However, an immunocytochemical study in temporal lobectomy specimens found no evidence of a selective reduction in neurons containing glutamic acid decarboxylase (GABA) in the focus. In addition, experiments show that somatostatin neurons are selectively vulnerable to processes used to duplicate the pattern of epileptic damage in the hippocampus in animals.

It is possible that glutamate is also involved in the neurochemical pathology. Preliminary studies indicate increases in the density of glutamatergic binding sites, both in children with various types of generalized seizures and in adults with temporal lobe seizures. Electrophysiological studies provide evidence for hypersensitivity of N-methyl-D-aspartate (NMDA) receptors, both in the hippocampus of rats in which an epileptic tendency has been induced by repetitive electrical stimulation (kindling), and in the cortex of patients with focal epilepsy.

Glutamate and pathology

One consequence of seizure activity is the release of glutamate into the extracellular milieu. This can give rise to excitotoxic effects, because of the increased excitation induced by the glutamate. Some of the pathology found in the brains of patients with epilepsy is almost certainly due to the excitatory effects of glutamate.

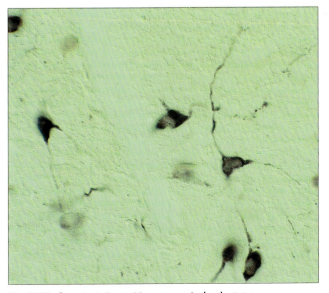

Fig. 12.18 Somatostatin-positive neurons in the dentate gyrus.

GENERALIZED AND PARTIAL EPILEPSY – PHYSIOLOGICAL DIFFERENCES

Research studies indicate at least two physiological characteristics that differentiate generalized and partial epilepsy:

- genetic models of generalized epilepsy are associated with abnormalities in inhibitory transmitter systems (increased inhibitory circuitry leads to inhibition of the normal inhibitory system);
- paroxysmal depolarization shift may not be the primary trigger for aberrant neuronal firing in generalized epilepsy.

Seizures – Electrophysiological Characteristics

Many seizure syndromes can be identified by the location of the initial seizure activity and the pattern of spread.

Neonatal seizures

Neonatal seizures may be manifest as various rhythmic movements or as postural spasms. They are widely thought to originate in the brain stem or midbrain without cortical involvement in the abnormal discharges. However, in some cases, slow abnormal discharges may be recorded from the cortex.

Absence seizures (3 Hz spike and wave)

Absence attacks are associated with:

- 3 Hz spike and wave patterns;
- symmetrical neocortical discharges; and
- simultaneous thalamic involvement.

Electrophysiological studies indicate that the seizures originate in the cortex and that activity spreads quickly via corticothalamic connections into the thalamus. Activity in the two cerebral hemispheres is co-ordinated by propagation of the seizure through the corpus callosum. The brain stem is not intimately involved in this circuit. This sequence of events is supported by the fact that absences can be triggered by unilateral electrical stimulation of the medial frontal cortex. This pattern of activity gives the physiological basis for the 3 per second spike and wave discharges.

Myoclonic syndromes

These syndromes can be categorized on the basis of their anatomical pattern of seizure activity:

- primary cortical (focal, multifocal, or generalized) with a rostrocaudal spread of activity;
- primary brain stem (reticular) with activity spreading both rostrally and caudally; and
- segmental or spinal.

Only the cortical form is believed to be a true form of epilepsy.

Common Anticonvulsants		
Drug	**Indications**	**Side effects**
Carbamazepine	partial and generalized tonic–clonic seizures	diplopia, dizziness, headache, nausea
Clobazam	adjunctive therapy in refractive epilepsy	sedation, depression, irritability
Clonazepam	myoclonic and generalized tonic–clonic seizures	sedation
Ethosuximide	absence seizures	nausea, vomiting, lethargy, ataxia, dizziness, psychosis
Phenobarbitone	partial and generalized tonic–clonic, clonic and tonic seizures	fatigue, depression; in children: insomnia, aggressive behaviour
Phenytoin	partial and generalized tonic–clonic seizures; status epilepticus	drowsiness, dysarthria, tremor, ataxia
Primidone	partial and generalized tonic–clonic seizures	nausea, vomiting, drowsiness, diplopia, nystagmus, ataxia, psychosis
Sodium valproate	primary generalized epilepsies; partial seizures; prophylaxis of febrile convulsions	tremor, weight gain, alopecia, peripheral oedema
Vigabatrin	adjunctive therapy in refractory partial epilepsy	fatigue, dizziness, irritability, depression, headache

Fig. 12.19 Drugs used in the treatment of epilepsy, their indications and important side-effects.

may secondarily g
prevalent cases of e

Aetiology

By and large, the
also give rise to p
exception: epilepsy

Clinical Present

Localization-relate
of clinical sympto
from the physiolog
restricted to specifi
of the brain region
the motor cortex m
muscles within a
sequential activati
seizures). Complex
in patients with s
system, or frontal l

Given the varyi
produce partial se
seizure activity, it
variable. Dramatic
ization-related epil
can disturb norm
complications aris
(Fig. 13.3). An int
epilepsies are the p

TREATMENT

Epilepsy can be controlled by a range of drugs (Fig. 12.19). Several clinical issues are of particular importance in achieving successful management of therapy:

- when to start therapy;
- appropriate therapeutic dose (with regard to side effects);
- non-compliance when seizures are controlled; and
- when to stop therapy.

These issues need to be dealt with on a case-by-case basis. They are heavily influenced by the age, occupation, and social status of the patient.

DIFFERENTIAL DIAGNOSIS

It is important to determine whether seizures are caused by acute symptomatic events (which do not necessarily require anti-epileptic drug treatment) or by spontaneous aberrant electrical activity (which indicates an epileptic disorder which can be treated with appropriate therapy) (Fig. 12.20).

Acute symptomatic seizures can be caused by a variety of factors, including raised body temperature in children under five, substance abuse, and metabolic disturbances. Diagnosis of a symptomatic seizure is helped by the fact that most occur in patients with an acute encephalopathy together with an associated confusional state or systemic disturbance. These features often last considerably longer than the period of seizure activity,

and this, together with the presence of other associated symptoms and signs, generally suffices to provide the correct diagnosis and to indicate treatment.

Syncope and pseudoseizures (non-epileptic attack disorder) are most frequently mistaken for epilepsy.

Syncope

Syncope, or vasovagal attack, results in cerebreal hypoperfusion and loss of consciousness. Several features characterize syncope:

- it is precipitated by postural hypotension (patients have just risen or are standing);
- onset tends to be gradual, with dizziness or loss of vision leading to unconsciousness;
- unconsciousness is accompanied by flaccidity, pallor, and slow pulse;
- EEG shows a slowing of activity;
- tonic–clonic muscle spasms are absent; and
- recovery is prompt with little or no retrograde amnesia.

These characteristics allow a distinction to be made between epilepsy and syncope.

Non-epileptic attack disorder (NEAD)

NEADs (and even pseudostatus epilepticus) are common, and it has been reported that as many as 20 per cent of patients referred for investigation of a suspected seizure disorder have NEAD. Such patients often have extensive (and expensive) histories of inconclusive investigations and treatment refractory seizures.

NEAD can arise as a result of neurological, cardiovascular, psychiatric, or emotional causes (Fig. 12.21). In many cases,

Simple partial		
Consciousness		
Age group		
Duration		
Symptoms		
Ictal EEG		
Special features		
Complex parti		
Consciousness		
Age group		
Duration		
Symptoms		
Ictal EEG		

Fig. 13.2 A classific

Differential Diagnosis of Epilepsy	
Syncope	**Psychogenic attacks**

reflex syncope
  postural
  'psychogenic'
  micturition syncope
  cough syncope
  valsalva
	pseudoseizures
	panic attacks
	hyperventilation

cardiac syncope
  dysrhythmias (heart block,
    tachycardias, etc)
  valvular disease (especially
    aortic stenosis)
  cardiomyopathies
  shunts
	Transient ischaemic attacks
	
	Migraine
	
	Narcolepsy
	
	Hypoglycaemia

perfusion failure
  hypovolaemia
  syndromes of autonomic failure	

Fig. 12.20 Differential diagnosis of epilepsy.

Non-Epileptic Attack Disorders	
Organic attack disorder	**Psychiatric disorder mistaken for epilepsy**

neurological
  cataplexy
  third ventricle cyst
  transient ischaemic attacks
  migraine (basilar)
  benign drop attacks
	hyperventilation attacks
	panic attacks
	anxiety with derealization/
	  depersonalization
	episodic dyscontrol syndrome

cardiovascular
  fainting
  Stokes–Adams attacks
  mitral valve prolapse
  atrial myxoma
  aortic stenosis
	Emotionally based attacks

other organic
  insulinoma (and other
    hypoglycaemias)
  phaeochromocytoma
	swoon – cut-off behaviour
	tantrum – immature displays
	  of emotion
	abreaction or symbolic attack
	deliberate simulation

Fig. 12.21 A classification of non-epileptic attack disorders (NEAD).

non-familial (

days 4–6 and

supervenes. T

τ activity.

Early myoclo

or massive n

suppression a

and slow wav

logical abnor

aemia has be

Infancy

West syndron

sion or delay

and a hypsar

poor respons

intellectual h

Benign myocl

show bouts o

generalized s

seizures and t

Severe myocl

lateral or bila

With time, t

which are ofte

seizures with

occur. Early l

polyspike-wav

later. Delay i

and seizures a

Childhood

Myoclonic ast

astatic seizur

generalized t

bilaterally sy

waves superi

rhythms. The

Lennox–Gast

diagnostic inc

atonic attacks

waking interi

Mental deve

trolled by dru

Childhood ab

ized by sudde

tonic, or autc

frequent and

seizures in 40

Auras may occur without the subsequent onset of more obvious seizure activity. This can occur in the early stages when the epilepsy is still evolving, or when seizures are only partially controlled by drugs. Patients quickly learn to equate their auras with seizure onset.

Localization-related Epilepsy and Age

Childhood

In many instances, the localization-related epilepsy syndromes of childhood are benign and remit in puberty. A family history of such seizures is sometimes found. Generally, intellectual functions are unimpaired and neurological deficits are rare.

Rolandic epilepsy (benign epilepsy with centrotemporal spikes)
This type of epilepsy is some three times commoner than generalized petit mal absence seizures. Onset is normally between the ages of three and 13. Seizures usually occur at night, after a few hours sleep, and are associated with sensory and motor symptoms (usually limited to the face and neck), which involve tonic, clonic, or tonic–clonic contractions of the face, lips, tongue, pharynx, and larynx with consequent anarthria and drooling. There may be unilateral paraesthesia. At night, seizures may become generalized. However, this type of seizure is not associated with secondary generalization and loss of consciousness if it occurs during the day. The loss of the capacity for speech, and the uncontrolled vocalization due to seizure activity, result in considerable distress for both the child and parents. In general, EEG investigations reveal a high-voltage lateralized centro-temporal spike focus.

The cause of the seizures is unknown, although genetic factors are implicated. Correct diagnosis of the syndrome obviates the need for extensive investigations and enables the introduction of anticonvulsant therapy. The syndrome is responsive to medication, which can usually be discontinued after several seizure-free years.

Benign epilepsy with occipital spikes   Occipital foci with spiking on eye closure give rise to seizures in which visual symptoms (flashing lights, loss of colour, etc) are the main features. These seizures result in severe postictal headache in many patients.

Kojewnikow's syndrome   There are two main types. In one type, patients with an identified rolandic lesion who also have a static neurological abnormality have partial motor seizures followed by well-localized myoclonic jerks. The EEG in these cases shows a focal abnormality.

In the other type, patients that were previously normal develop partial motor seizures followed rapidly by associated myoclonic jerks. Focal and diffuse spikes and/or spike-waves with additional background abnormalities are found on EEG. Neurological deficits and intellectual impairment are progressive.

Adolescence

The onset of partial epilepsy in adolescence is characterized by simple partial seizures with accompanying motor or sensory symptoms. There may be secondary generalization (which may be unilateral) and loss of consciousness. As a rule, there are neither neurological deficits nor loss of intellectual function. Between seizures, EEG is often normal or only mildly abnormal.

Adulthood

Localization-related seizures in adults are often the consequence of other types of brain pathology. Penetrating head trauma is a common cause of seizures in adult males (see Chapter 5) and infections of the meninges or CNS can result in scars, which can induce seizure activity. Substance abuse can be a cause of adult-onset fits in patients with no previous history or familial background of epilepsy. Tumours are a relatively minor cause of localization-related epilepsy in adults.

The clinical features of such conditions are dependent on the size of the lesion and its anatomical site. In this instance, the commonest type of localization-related epilepsy, temporal lobe epilepsy, is of particular interest (Fig. 13.4).

Temporal lobe epilepsy   Partial seizures generated by foci within the temporal lobe have been of particular interest to psychiatrists and neurologists because of the complexity of the psychological phenomena that can accompany them. These manifestations include complex visual hallucinations, paranoia, altered mood, aggressiveness, and a schizophrenia-like psychosis. If the underlying seizure activity is undetected then misdiagnosis of a psychiatric disorder is possible.

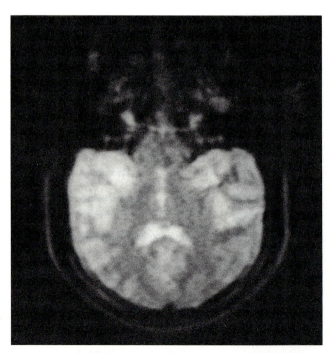

Fig. 13.4   T$_2$-weighted MRI scan showing a high intensity lesion in the right medial temporal lobe.

Patients display a significant degree of psychiatric morbidity and social problems. Surveys suggest that up to 50 per cent of men have experienced difficulties with employment, and interviews suggest that this is largely due to psychiatric difficulties – most commonly neurotic disorders and depression. Patients with temporal lobe epilepsy are more than twice as likely to experience such problems. Children also show hyperactivity and behavioural disorders. Fugues, twilight states, and postictal disorders can also lead to considerable problems in social adjustment.

Old age

Older patients are much more likely to have partial seizures than younger ones, and approximately 70 per cent of patients have partial seizures. It is thought that this difference is directly attributable to the increased levels of neurodegenerative disease and focal cerebral pathology in older people.

Cerebrovascular disease is one of the commonest types of pathology that leads to seizures. Although seizures are a common sequel to stroke, seizure activity is occasionally the presenting symptom of the underlying cerebrovascular disease (Fig. 13.5) (see Chapter 3). Primary neurodegenerative diseases, including Alzheimer's disease and tumours, are commonly associated with epilepsy. Some 10 per cent of patients aged 60 or over with a tumour (metastases or inoperable gliomas) suffer from seizures. Metabolic disturbances are also associated with seizure activity, though it is often difficult to disentangle the relative contributions of alcohol abuse, previous drug treatments, and poor nutrition.

The symptoms and signs associated with these seizures vary and are dependent on the localization of the seizure focus and the occurrence of secondary generalization. Motor, somatosensory, special sensory, autonomic, or psychiatric symptoms can be seen at the initial presentation.

Diagnosis

Obtaining a clear-cut diagnosis of a localization-related epileptic disorder in older patients can be difficult for the following reasons:

* difficulties in obtaining an adequate or complete history;
* presence of concurrent vascular or cerebrovascular disease;
* possible presence of primary neurodegenerative disease; and
* side effects of ongoing drug therapy.

EEG and imaging procedures sometimes fail to give a clear diagnostic picture because of age-related brain atrophy, coincident cerebrovascular lesions, and alterations in cerebral perfusion. Increasing frequency of fits, difficulty in controlling fits, and marked changes in cognitive or psychiatric state are indications that additional investigations are required to exclude the possibility of other concurrent disease.

Imaging

MRI studies reveal evidence of high-intensity lesions in the medial temporal lobe of the majority of patients with temporal lobe epilepsy. Morphometric studies of hippocampal size have shown accompanying volume loss. PET reveals hypofunction in the area of the seizure focus interictally in most patients; SPECT does so too, but it is less sensitive than PET. While functional imaging techniques are not consistent enough to be diagnostic, they can help to localize the seizure focus before surgery.

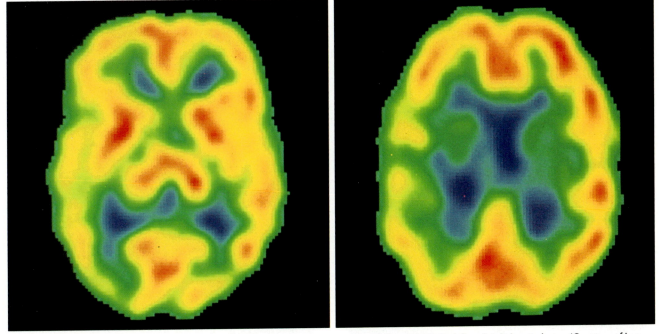

Fig. 13.5 A scan of blood flow using Tc99m HMPAS SPECT, through the basal ganglia (left) and through the cortex (right) in a patient with multi-infarct dementia and seizures. The scan shows several large areas of reduced flow in both the left and right hemispheres. (Courtesy of Len Holman MD, Boston, Massachusetts.)

Neuropathology

The neuropathology of partial epilepsy is essentially the same as that described for generalized epilepsies. Any type of brain lesion can result in a seizure focus. The two main types of pathology associated with temporal lobe epilepsy are Ammon's horn sclerosis and microdysgenesis. Both types of pathology occur more often in men than women.

Differential diagnosis

Diagnostic difficulties arise from the more subtle symptomatology exhibited by patients, particularly those with temporal lobe epilepsy. The possibility of another concurrent neuropsychiatric disorder or psychological disturbance should always be explored, particularly in older patients.

Treatment

Drug therapy is analogous to that used to treat generalized epilepsy. The guidelines for determining a therapeutic programme are essentially the same whatever the patient's age. Several variables will require particular attention:

• starting treatment;
• drug dosage; and
• likelihood of stopping drug therapy.

Given the increased risks of injury following a fit (e.g. broken limbs from a fall) and the possibility of extensive postical periods, there is a temptation to begin therapy after a single well-documented tonic–clonic seizure that was clearly unrelated to drugs, alcohol, or pyrexia. This should be balanced against the compliance problems inevitably experienced by patients already taking other medications and the likely side effects, both those of the anticonvulsant of choice and those arising from polypharmacy. Such decisions can only be made on a case-by-case basis.

Management of seizure activity in elderly patients is of considerable importance. Osteoporosis is common, and falls after a fit can result in extensive fractures. The loss of social confidence and anxiety caused by the sudden onset of seizure activity and the confusion experienced postictally can lead to considerable disruption in social functioning and can place considerable burdens on other family members.

Surgery

Localization-related epilepsy is by definition focal; if the lesion can be adequately localized, it is possible to remove the lesion surgically. Such an approach has been used successfully to treat patients with refractory temporal lobe epilepsy (Figs 13.6 and 13.7). Studies from centres in the USA, UK, and Europe suggest

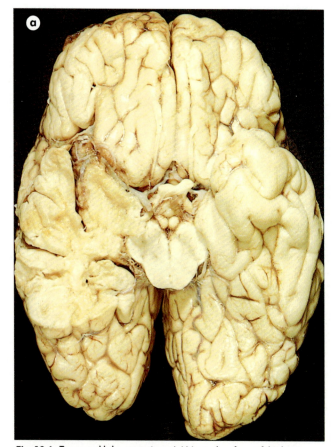

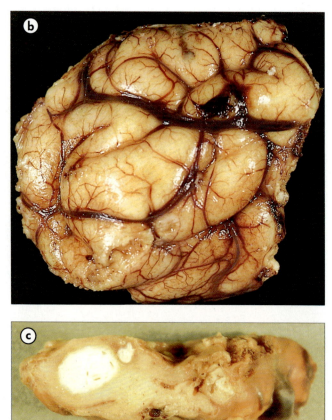

Fig. 13.6 Temporal lobe resections. (a) Ventral surface of the brain, showing extent of temporal lobe resection; (b) a specimen from a resected anterior temporal lobe; (c) calcified lesion found in a resected portion of the temporal lobe. (Courtesy of Dr CJ Bruton, London.)

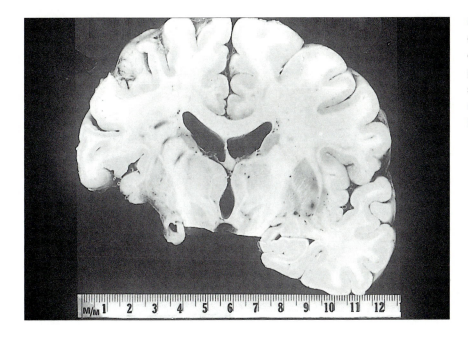

Fig. 13.7 Coronal slice of brain, showing extent of resection of the temporal lobe in a patient who continued to have seizures post-operatively. The surgery was not successful because the hippocampus was not removed. (Courtesy of Dr CJ Bruton, London.)

that up to 60 per cent of patients remain free of seizures after surgical resection of parts of the temporal lobe.

Physiology

Localization-related seizures are characterized by several physiological phenomena (Fig. 13.8):
- initiation by neurons firing rapid bursts of action potentials;
- synchronization of bursts in groups of neurons; and
- spread of seizure activity along anatomical pathways.

Initiation – paroxysmal depolarization shift

The neurons within a focus have characteristic patterns of discharge activity with interspike intervals as short as 2 ms. This burst pattern of discharge is generated by an abnormal, abrupt depolarization of neuronal membranes – paroxysmal depolarization shift.

The generation of rapid bursts of action potentials is a property of many neurons. This ability is conferred by the presence of voltage-dependant calcium channels in neuronal membranes. These channels have relatively slow kinetics so that, once activated by a depolarizing stimulus, they sustain the depolarization for tens of milliseconds. This extended depolarization can drive rapid bursts of fast action potentials, which are mediated by voltage-dependant sodium channels. These prolonged calcium-dependant bursts are terminated after hyperpolarization due to potassium channels being activated by influx of calcium. The ion channels thus mediate calcium influx and potassium efflux, and provide the basis for the rhythmic firing of neurons; this rate is largely determined by the kinetics of the after-hyperpolarizations. Detailed experiments have shown that the burst discharges in neurons are regulated by voltage-dependant sodium and potassium conductance in the cell body, and by calcium conductances in one or more dendritic compartments.

These discharge mechanisms are important in the establishment of an epileptic focus, and particular neurons that demonstrate these phenomena (e.g. Hippocampal CA2 and CA3 neurons, layer 4 cortical neurons) are thought to be involved in seizure initiation in the human brain. However, although the burst activity of neurons may facilitate seizure initiation, other mechanisms must be involved in the synchronization of activity between neurons and in the propagation of the seizure activity through the brain.

Synchronization One such mechanism is thought to involve strong recurrent excitatory connections that provide a neural substrate for positive feedback using glutamate as an excitatory transmitter acting on NMDA and AMPA receptors. Two properties seem to be required for the synchronization of burst activity in pyramidal cells: connections between the cells must be divergent; and connections must allow a single cell to drive its post-synaptic targets.

Other synchronizing mechanisms have been identified; these include electrical field interactions, which may regulate the fine dynamics of the bursts, and alterations in the extracellular ion concentration (especially potassium), which are related to spreading depression and spreading excitation.

Synaptic plasticity may also be involved in the development or 'ripening' of a focus. Persistent electrical stimulation can serve to strengthen existing synaptic contacts and to induce the formation of new contacts or even a degree of neuronal re-wiring. It is thought that the NMDA receptor is intimately involved in these kinds of changes and that future therapy may be targeted on these processes.

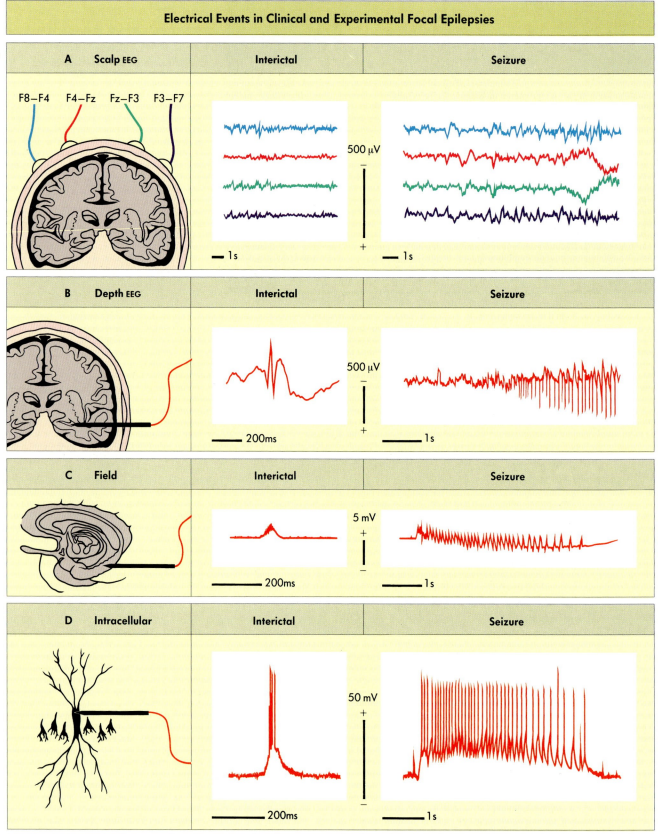

Fig. 13.8 (a) Conventional EEG recordings from a patient's scalp, showing the contrast between an interictal spike and the much more prolonged seizure discharge. The signals are small and noisy because of the volume of tissue between the source of the currents and the electrodes; (b) intracranial recordings from another patient with a mesial temporal epileptic focus. These signals are larger and less noisy because the electrodes are much closer to the source of the signal; (c) *in vitro* recordings from rat brain slices which had received an injection of 6 ng tetanus toxin into the hippocampus ten days earlier. These field potentials are analogous to the depth recordings obtained in (b), but a wider bandwidth is used than is typical in clinical work; (d) an intracellular recording from the same rat brain as in (c). (Courtesy of Dr J Jefferys, London.)

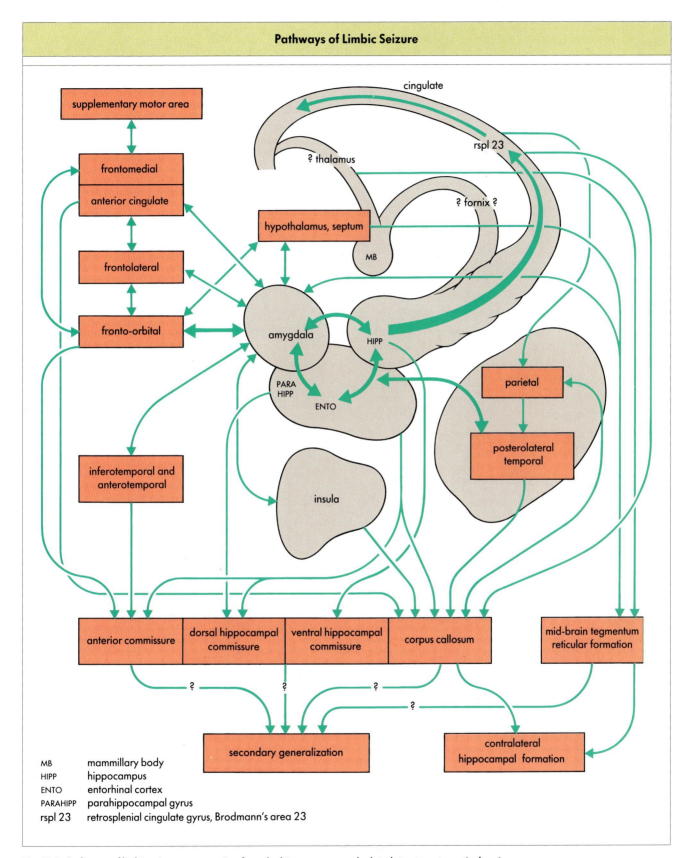

Fig. 13.9 Pathways of limbic seizure propagation from the hippocampus and related structures to cortical regions.

Kindling

This is the phenomenon whereby mild repetitive stimulation of brain areas leads to a permanent reduction in seizure threshold. In this way, a stimulus which does not cause seizure activity on first presentation can eventually precipitate seizure activity. The processes are analogous to learning and probably involve synaptic plasticity and the NMDA receptor. This phenomenon is of some clinical significance and could be involved, for example, in the gradual emergence of epilepsy after head trauma.

Spread of seizure activity

Focal motor seizures usually originate in or near the primary motor cortex but may involve the secondary motor area on the medial aspect of the frontal lobe. Anatomical connections between cortical areas (horizontal fibres in layer 6) mediate the spread of seizure activity.

Jacksonian march is thought to be due to a strictly localized seizure propagating at a speed of some 5 mm.s^{-1}. Activation of intrinsic GABAergic neurons may limit local cortical (homotopic) spread of seizure activity by creating an 'inhibitory surround'. Clinical signs of seizure activity are thought to reflect activation of basal ganglia, thalamic, and brain stem nuclei. Changes in the pattern of cortical discharge may underlie the transition from clonic to tonic activity.

Typical temporal lobe (complex partial) seizures start in the medial portion of one temporal lobe, although other limbic regions or cortical areas projecting to limbic regions can also be involved. Several anatomically defined types of seizure have been described using depth electrodes – e.g. hippocampal or mediobasal limbic, amygdalar, lateral posterior temporal, and opercular. These types correlate with different types of symptoms. However, the spread of seizure activity involves a set of common structures (Fig. 13.9) and patients tend to show similar clinical signs. The circuit within which seizure activity becomes established can be disrupted by surgical removal of the amygdala and hippocampus (amygdalo-hippocampectomy) or by resection of the anterior temporal lobe (see Fig. 13.6). This is not necessarily the case when the original focus is extratemporal.

SUMMARY

Generalized seizures

(i)   Generalized seizures are characterized by simultaneous discharges in all cortical areas from the seizure onset.

(ii) Generalized seizures are characterized by the absence of an aura and loss of consciousness.

(iii) Generalized seizures account for about 30 per cent of epilepsy.

(iv) Genetic lesions are often associated with the occurrence of primary generalized epilepsy.

(v)   Abnormalities in the organization of inhibitory transmitter systems may be a physiological characteristic.

Partial seizures

(vi)   Partial seizures are characterized by a focus of seizure activity in a specific brain area.

(vii) Partial seizures are the most common type of epilepsy.

(viii) Prodromata and auras remain consistent in a given patient and can be used to localize a focus and warn of an attack.

(ix)   A wide variety of neurological and psychiatric signs and symptoms occurs.

(x)   The incidence of partial epilepsy rises sharply after 60 years of age.

(xi)   Temporal lobe epilepsy is common and associated with psychiatric symptoms.

(xii) Any type of pathology can give rise to an epileptic focus.

(xiii) Temporal lobe epilepsy is a common sequel to fetal anoxia or febrile convulsion, which cause Ammon's horn sclerosis.

(xiv) Partial epilepsy is characterized physiologically by the presence of a paroxysmal depolarization shift.

(xv)   Synaptic plasticity and the glutamate neurotransmitter system are involved in the development of a focus and the propagation of seizure activity.

(xvi) Surgical removal of a seizure focus often succeeds in ending seizure activity.

(xvii) Differential diagnosis includes psychosis and primary degenerative dementias.

SECTION 4

Psychoses

Psychosis is a clinical description of a person's mental state. It describes mental states characterized by gross distortions of thought, delusions, hallucinations, and disturbed or inappropriate emotion.

The diagnosis is phenomenological, based on observation of the patient's behaviour and analysis of the patient's own descriptions of his or her mental state. As can be expected, this category of disease covers a wide spectrum of disordered thought and behaviour and many types of syndromes. Historically, the psychoses have been divided into two broad groups: organic (e.g. Alzheimer's disease, epileptic psychoses), and functional (e.g. schizophrenia, manic depression).

The historical basis of this division was simple, and rested on the presence of a readily identifiable brain pathology or a well-documented electrophysiological or metabolic disturbance in the organic psychoses. Advances in imaging techniques have improved our ability to detect subtle pathology, and improvements in neuropathological technique have allowed us to detect pathology where none was previously suspected; therefore, the concept and practice of assigning syndromes like schizophrenia to the category of functional psychoses is obsolete.

Psychoses (in particular schizophrenia and mood disorder) provide the core of the psychiatrist's caseload. The spectrum of clinical presentation is varied and covers the manifestations of disordered mental processes from childhood to old age. A large number of psychotic syndromes have been described (Fig. 2), although the aetiological validity of many of these remains suspect.

Diagnosis   Disturbances in mental state are common and part of our existential heritage. The expression of such disturbances is deemed appropriate if it falls within the cultural norms of a given society (e.g. depression and grieving after bereavement, aggression in competition, jealousy in love, religious ecstasy and visions). However, in all societies there comes a point when the behaviour that results from a disturbance in mental state is deemed inappropriate and is no longer tolerated. The dividing line can be difficult to determine in some circumstances (e.g. when does grief become a morbid form of depression?) and simple in other circumstances (e.g. a person who believes himself or herself to be an alien from Mars). Diagnosis of psychosis is only justified after an extensive interview with the patient to establish exactly the mental state and to place this state in the context of the patient's cultural norms.

Wherever possible, investigations should be made to determine whether additional factors, such as substance abuse or concurrent systemic or central nervous system disease or disorder, is causing or contributing to the disturbed mental state.

It is generally useful as a prognostic guide to subdivide psychosis further into acute and chronic psychosis. Acute psychotic reactions last for hours or days and are usually associated with precipitating factors (e.g. pyrexia, psychogenic drugs, side effects of therapy, nervous system disease, stress) or with substance abuse. Acute psychotic reactions have a good prognosis. Chronic psychosis tends not to be closely related to precipitating factors or continues long past the advent of such influences. Chronic psychotic states can have a poor prognosis. The two largest categories of chronic psychosis are schizophrenia and mood disorder.

14 Schizophrenia

INTRODUCTION

The story of Dr Jekyll and Mr Hyde encapsulates what too many lay people understand by the term schizophrenia. Such a powerful and seductive literary image has also encouraged the use of the term 'schizophrenic' as an everyday word to describe people or even organizations that have changing opinions or that demonstrate an inconstant approach to policy. This is a matter of regret, not because of the abuse of a technical term, but for its trivialization of one of the most serious psychiatric disorders in adult psychiatry.

Descriptions of patients affected by delusions and hallucinations have been traced back to ancient writings, but the modern concept of schizophrenia dates from the work of Bleuler and Kraeplin in the 1900s. The concept was based on the phenomenology associated with the illness and, as invariably occurs in such situations, the subjective interpretation of phenomenology has led to considerable dispute and confusion. This is not the place to dissect the milestones in the evolution of the concept (see recommended reading), and in truth it seems reasonable to state that the syndrome of schizophrenia as we know it today came into existence in the 1970s with the development of operationally defined criteria to aid diagnosis.

Despite this uncertain start, the use of such criteria has greatly improved diagnostic reliability and confirmed that schizophrenia is present worldwide. Schizophrenia is a disease of early adulthood which affects some 0.5–1 per cent of the population. In the USA, it is estimated that 30–50 per cent of all psychiatric beds are occupied by schizophrenics. Since the disease strikes in early adulthood and can last for decades, the economic and social costs are huge.

A significant proportion of patients spontaneously remit, and drug therapy (using dopamine-receptor antagonists) has significantly improved the treatment of other patients. However, a large proportion of patients show no response and continue with a chronic course. Recent studies have begun to show the presence of abnormal brain structure in the brains of patients with schizophrenia and to demonstrate that, far from being a 'functional psychosis', schizophrenia is probably a consequence of incomplete brain development.

Definition

Schizophrenia is characterized by a fundamental disturbance of personality, a characteristic distortion of thinking, bizarre delusions, altered perceptions, inappropriate emotional responses and possibly a degree of autism. These symptoms are experienced in a setting of clear consciousness and (generally) undiminished intellectual capacity (World Health Organization). Explicit diagnostic criteria based on phenomenological characteristics are contained in the DSM-IIIR.

The types of symptom referred to above are neatly encapsulated in Schneider's first rank symptoms (Fig. 14.1).

EPIDEMIOLOGY

Adults have a 0.5–1 per cent lifetime risk of developing schizophrenia and the incidence is some 15–20 new cases per 100 000 of the population. A large WHO study has demonstrated that the risk is relatively constant across the world and that the symptoms of the syndrome are very similar in each country. There are few exceptions to this pattern of homogeneity, although a high prevalence of schizophrenia has been reported in Croatia and the west of Ireland.

The disease can occur any time between early teens to late seventies, though the vast majority of cases show an onset between 15 and 45 (Fig. 14.2). In European studies, average peak incidence in men is at 27, three years earlier than that seen in women (see Fig. 14.2), although both sexes are affected equally. Studies in other countries using more rigid diagnostic criteria have reported earlier ages of onset.

Schneider's First Rank Symptoms
Auditory hallucinations of specific type
Audible thoughts: voices repeating or anticipating the patient's thoughts out loud Two or more voices discussing the patient in the third person Voices commenting on the patient's thoughts or behaviour
Thought disorder of specific type
Thought withdrawal by some external agency Thought insertion by some external agency Thought broadcasting so that thoughts are conveyed to others
Feelings, impulses, or acts experienced as under external control
Primary delusion – an unshakeable belief arising in an unaccountable manner from a commonplace event

Fig. 14.1 Schneider's first rank symptoms of schizophrenia.

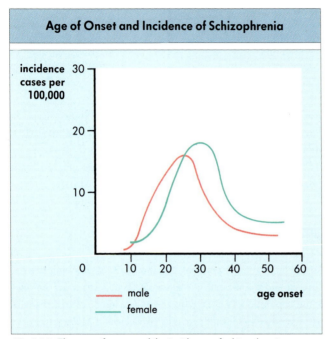

Age of Onset and Incidence of Schizophrenia

incidence cases per 100,000

— male
— female

age onset

Fig. 14.2   The age of onset and the incidence of schizophrenia.

Increased prevalence of schizophrenia has been demonstrated in people from lower socioeconomic backgrounds (social classes 4 and 5). Rates are also higher in inner city areas. This has been interpreted by some investigators to mean that poverty, limited education and associated handicaps, or the stress of modern life predispose to schizophrenic illness. However, studies also demonstrate that the social class of the parents of schizophrenics does not differ appreciably from that of the control population. The association between schizophrenic illness and low socio-economic status has been interpreted to reflect 'downward drift'. According to this explanation, the patients' psychiatric disorder interferes with education and work performance, so that the patients find it difficult to complete advanced schooling or function effectively in demanding positions of responsibility. As a result, their socioeconomic status, which is defined by income, educational achievement, and employment, is inevitably reduced. This example of the difficulty in interpreting epidemiological research in schizophrenia gives but a flavour of the often bitter disputes that erupt periodically in the field.

AETIOLOGY

The cause of schizophrenia is not known. However several factors have been the subject of speculation in the development of aetiological hypotheses:

- genetics – schizophrenia is often familial and monozygotic twins develop the disease concordantly much more frequently than do dizygotic twins;
- season of birth – winter months show an excess of births;
- viral pandemics – reported excess of patients with schizophrenia born three to six months after influenza pandemics;

- fetal, birth or perinatal infection or trauma;
- neurological or neuropsychiatric conditions can give rise to schizophrenia-like symptoms;
- abnormal development – psychological surveys, and imaging and neuropathological studies suggest a failure in brain development.

Genetics

Family studies have clearly demonstrated increased risks for developing schizophrenia in the relatives of patients. The risk increases with genetic proximity (Fig. 14.3). Several factors from these studies are worthy of comment:

- parents are often unaffected and thus have a lower risk than siblings;
- if one of the parents has schizophrenia, it is most likely to be the mother;
- risk in offspring is greatly increased if both parents have schizophrenia; and
- symptoms vary greatly within families.

Schizophrenia greatly reduces the probability of a patient marrying and producing offspring; thus parents of affected children could be unaffected carriers or they may produce offspring before the onset of their illness. This latter point is also relevant to the fact that the affected parent is more likely to be female. The average age of onset is later in women than in men and it could also be argued that social mores allow more latitude for women in the equation between marriageability and socioeconomic success.

The variability of symptoms may result from the phenotypic spectrum of the disorder.

Genetic Risk of Schizophrenia

Monozygotic twin affected	50 per cent
Dizygotic twin affected	15 per cent
Sibling affected	10 per cent
One parent affected	15 per cent
Both parents affected	35 per cent
Second-degree relative affected	2–3 per cent
No affected relative	1 per cent

Fig. 14.3 Life expectancy of schizophrenia in relatives of patients with the disease.

Studies on the concordance for schizophrenia in monozygotic and dizygotic twins show concordance rates of about 50 per cent in monozygotic twins. This is about three times the rate seen in dizygotic twins, who have rates comparable to that of full siblings (10 per cent). These data support the case for a genetic component in schizophrenia. This concept is also consistent with the results obtained from the study of the adopted children of parents with schizophrenia. Such offspring manifest the same high risks of schizophrenia, despite their being brought up by their normal non-biological parents.

Viral pandemics

Several studies in Europe and the USA have shown that patients with schizophrenia have an excess of births (some 5 per cent) during the late winter and early spring months of the year. Though most schizophrenics are not born during these months, the data suggest that something associated with such births predisposes to schizophrenic illness. This observation has been tied together with studies that show that peaks of excess births can be related to viral pandemics, particularly influenza, that occurred during the third to sixth months of gestation.

Such studies are difficult to conduct and even more awkward to analyse statistically. One recent study, which used data from the clinical records of mothers, found no influenza effect. Studies on other types of neurological defects (e.g. Down's syndrome) have also demonstrated a similar season of birth effect. It might be concluded, therefore, that the effect of season of birth and viral pandemics on the subsequent development of schizophrenia is likely to be small.

Fetal, birth, or perinatal trauma or infection

Several studies have suggested that patients with schizophrenia show an increased incidence of fetal distress or adverse events during or shortly after birth. These findings, however, have been disputed. The whole issue is clouded by the problem of retrospectively gathering data decades after the events occurred. In the UK Perinatal Mortality Survey, which had access to detailed information gathered contemporaneously with the birth, no increased incidence of adverse fetal, birth, or perinatal events was found. The question remains open. However, it would be reasonable to assume that such events do not give rise to a large number of patients with schizophrenia later in life. Such a view can be buttressed by considering that a common cause of fetal or birth injury is anoxia and subsequent Ammon's horn sclerosis (see Chapter 12). Studies have shown that although such a lesion carries a very high degree of risk for the subsequent development of temporal lobe epilepsy, these lesions are not associated with the development of schizophrenia. An alternative perspective of adverse perinatal events is the possibility that they are the result, not the cause, of abnormal brain development.

Neurological disorders

There is a substantial literature documenting the existence of schizophrenia-like psychoses in a variety of disorders from temporal lobe epilepsy to metachromatic leucodystrophy to cortical Lewy body disease. It has often been suggested that cases of schizophrenia might be due to undiagnosed neurological disorders. Although this undoubtedly occurs, exhaustive studies of large series of patients suffering from schizophrenia indicate that the incidence of underlying diagnosable organic disease was less than 5 per cent.

Abnormal development

A substantial body of evidence suggests that schizophrenia is an abnormality of brain development. Psychological studies of children at risk, prospective cohort studies, imaging studies, and neuropathological investigations support this contention (see page 14.15).

What Causes Schizophrenia?

Consideration of the literature allows us to calculate tentatively what percentage of cases of schizophrenia are caused by the factors discussed above:
- genetic – 80 per cent;
- neurological disorder – less than 5 per cent;
- fetal/birth/perinatal events – less than 3 per cent;
- season of birth and viral pandemics – less than 5 per cent; and
- others – 5 per cent.

Clinical Course

Descriptions of the typical course of schizophrenia are difficult to frame. There are two main reasons for this:
- schizophrenia can last for decades and there is a relative paucity of well-documented follow-up studies (Bleuler's work being a magnificent exception); and
- schizophrenia often has a fluctuating course and can remit, never to occur again.

Therefore, the typical descriptions of schizophrenia are often those pertaining to chronic unremitting sufferers and these may represent a minority of patients. On first presentation, it is difficult to define the course of a patient's illness since there are as yet no reliable imaging or laboratory investigations that can be used to assign patients objectively to prognostic categories. Several surveys indicate that patients who receive a firm diagnosis of schizophrenia will, eventually, be found to fall into three (admittedly broad) categories:
- 20 per cent have a small number of psychotic episodes followed by a return to their premorbid level of function (good prognosis);
- 60 per cent have an episodic course characterized by psychotic episodes, which may be precipitated by negative life events or adverse social circumstances; deterioration in personality and inadequate social function are present; and
- 20 per cent have a disorder marked by personality deterioration together with severely impaired social function and integration (poor prognosis).

Chronic schizophrenia occurs in somewhat less than 1 per cent of the population, but because of its early onset, chronicity, and associated disability, it is one of the most important psychiatric illnesses. The distinction between good and poor prognosis forms of schizophrenia is often not made in epidemiologic surveys, nor is the possibility raised that some of the good prognosis cases may in fact be other disorders, though available evidence suggests that the good prognosis cases are more common than the poor prognosis ones. The combined prevalence of both good and poor prognosis disorders is probably between 1 and 2 per cent of the population.

CLINICAL FEATURES

Presentation and Diagnosis

The clinical course of schizophrenia often spans decades. Once the syndrome is established, the characteristic symptoms are those of:
- delusions;
- delusions of control;
- hallucinations (auditory and sensory, less often visual));
- thought disorder (insertion, broadcast, echo, withdrawal, repeated aloud);
- flattening of and/or incongruity of affect; and
- speech disorder (poverty of content, incoherence, neologisms).

The first rank symptoms of Schneider provide a useful first approximation of a diagnosis of schizophrenia. More formal diagnosis requires that the patient's history and symptoms fulfils one of the recognized sets of operationalized criteria. Such criteria have been shown to be valid and reliable for diagnosis in different centres and countries.

Onset and Course

The peak age of initial diagnosis is in the mid twenties (see Fig. 14.2). The late teens and early twenties are the time when psychiatric symptoms become manifest. Strange behaviour, social withdrawal, and delusions/hallucinations are noted at this time. The symptoms are often glossed over or viewed as difficulties of adolescence or of growing up. The symptoms may be brief and vague at first and their significance is not appreciated by the patient's family. In patients who live alone, symptoms can persist and develop over a considerable period of time. Eventually, the symptoms and resulting behaviour changes disrupt normal social functioning. Psychiatric consultation is often the result of this disruption (e.g. loss of employment, antisocial activity, examination failure, family strife).

As a consequence of this pattern of presentation, patients are frequently interviewed while in an agitated, anxious or aggressive state. A considerable degree of skill is required when dealing both with patients and relatives in order to obtain the full history required for accurate diagnosis and for the eliciting of important prognostic information (such as mode of onset).

In the 80 per cent of patients who experience multiple psychotic episodes, the illness generally has a fluctuating course. One or more psychiatric hospitalizations commonly occur. Neuroleptic therapy and current medical policy dictates that most patients have a pattern of acute admission, carefully monitored drug therapy, return to the community and, after varying intervals, subsequent readmission. Such a pattern has been graphically described as a 'revolving door' admission pattern. Even when therapy is successful and symptoms are controlled, patients often lead disordered lives. They have great difficulty in forming satisfactory personal relationships; as a result they fail to find partners and to marry. They also have poor job histories and seldom achieve positions of responsibility. Their position is often one of neighbourhood eccentrics or hermit-like denizens of inner cities, undertaking sporadic unskilled work or being supported by welfare. It is probable that many of the homeless people in large cities are affected by schizophrenia.

In a proportion of cases (10–20 per cent), symptoms are refractory to neuroleptic therapy and patients become almost permanent residents in specialized hospitals.

As patients age, and with increasing lengths of illness, various studies have noted a relative loss of positive symptoms (hallucinations, delusions) and an increase in negative symptoms (affective flattening, speech disorder). This has been interpreted by some as evidence that schizophrenia is a progressive (in a neurodegenerative sense) disorder. However, it has been pointed out that normal ageing is associated with significant changes in personality, and that age could modify the expression of the symptoms in patients with schizophrenia. In addition, neuropathological studies do not support the view of schizophrenia as a degenerative condition.

Neurological signs

Numerous studies have described the presence of soft neurological signs in patients with schizophrenia. These are exemplified by minor changes in measurements of reflex responsiveness, electrodermal reactivity, or EEG (P300 wave) and minor defects in perception or attention. Such studies have no utility in an everyday clinical setting but do serve to demonstrate an organic involvement of the brain in the syndrome of schizophrenia.

Prognostic indicators

Many of the difficulties in the clinical management of patients with schizophrenia arise from the lack of definitive prognostic indicators. When patients are admitted for the first time, it is difficult to predict which ones will suffer a few episodes and then reattain their premorbid state and which ones will have a chronic relapsing course with drug-refractory symptoms. As a result of this, therapy is difficult to tailor to the individual and neuroleptics are prescribed both to patients who will not require them and those for whom they will prove ineffective. Given the known side effects of neuroleptics, this implies that a large proportion of patients are exposed to undesirable risks.

A number of interrelated factors provide a guide to prognosis:

- onset;
- positive and negative symptoms;
- response to treatment;
- social circumstances; and
- aetiology.

Onset Age and the nature of the onset are closely associated as prognostic factors. The earlier the age of onset (i.e. 15–20 as opposed to 30–35) the poorer the prognosis. Patients with an early age of onset generally have an insidious onset.

A slow insidious onset indicates a worse prognosis than an abrupt onset. The mode of onset is a useful prognostic indicator.

Insidious onset A skilled clinical interview often reveals that a patient had personality abnormalities, such as excessive shyness, social awkwardness, withdrawal from personal relationships, and inability to form close relationships (the so-called schizoid personality), before their first psychotic episode. Often, these traits will have been present for years and date from early adolescence and will have been the subject of comment and concern to the patient's family for months or years before the appearance of frank psychotic symptoms. Studies have also shown that schizophrenics have greater difficulties in achieving developmental milestones and expected levels of academic achievement and that they have lower scores on intelligence tests than do their siblings and other controls in childhood and adolescence. Such work indicates that antisocial and delinquent behaviour throughout childhood may be an early manifestation of the illness. The long history implied by an insidious onset is an indicator of a poor prognosis.

Abrupt onset Such cases are characterized by the relatively sudden appearance of aberrant behaviour. Such behaviour may be a response to the sudden occurrence of hallucinations and delusions and is generally accompanied by considerable fear and anxiety. This is often expressed as phases of acute excitement with restlessness and agitation, and leads to considerable difficulty in communicating with the patient. Such states also tend to resolve quickly. Although the symptoms experienced by the patient may be indistinguishable from those found in the operational criteria, the nosological status of abrupt-onset states that resolve over a few days or weeks has been the subject of much discussion. A diagnosis of schizophrenia requires that symptoms be present for an extended period of time. Psychotic episodes with an abrupt onset that resolve quickly have also been labelled as *bouffées délirantes* or schizophreniform psychoses. Such states are also a common result of alcohol or drug abuse.

Positive and negative symptoms Positive symptoms are especially associated with an abrupt onset, whereas cases with an insidious onset tend to show more negative symptoms (Fig. 14.4). Negative symptoms become more prominent the longer the patient has been ill. While not part of the diagnostic criteria,

Positive and Negative Symptoms	
Positive symptoms	**Negative symptoms**
Delusions	Thought disorder
Hallucinations	Language disorders
	Affective flattening or incongruity

Fig. 14.4 Positive and negative symptoms in schizophrenia.

cognitive deficits – especially memory dysfunction and executive-type cognitive disabilities – are frequently associated with the illness. The more prominent the cognitive deficits, the worse the outcome tends to be.

Response to treatment Neuroleptics have a much greater therapeutic effect on positive symptoms than on negative ones. Thus, patients with mainly positive symptoms are more likely to benefit from drug therapy and be able to cope in the community after discharge from hospital. Recent advances in pharmaco-therapy have produced the 'atypical neuroleptics' like Clozapine which may be more effective against certain negative symptoms.

Social circumstances Negative life events, such as divorce, family difficulties, and unemployment, significantly affect relapse rate. The progressive breakdown in the social structure of the patient's life makes non-compliance with drug therapy and failure to attend clinics increasingly likely. The nature of the ill-ness dictates that effective management of the condition is only achieved with regular contact between physician and patient in a stable social setting.

Aetiology A family history is one of the only aetiological factors that can be established with some confidence. Early age of onset, insidious onset, and chronicity have all been associated with a family history of schizophrenia.

Subtypes of schizophrenia Careful description and document-ation of the phenomenology of symptoms in schizophrenia has resulted in the syndromal delineation of several subtypes (Fig. 14.5). It should be emphasized that, although these subtypes have clinical utility as an aid to categorizing and managing patients, they do not claim to reflect the consequences of different aetiological factors.

Suicide

Suicide accounts in large part for the raised mortality rate associated with schizophrenia. Almost 10 per cent of patients commit suicide during the course of their illness. The risk is particularly great in young males and during the first years of the illness. Suicide in patients with schizophrenia is often achieved by using bizarre means.

Subtypes of Schizophrenia

Catatonic schizophrenia

Clinical picture dominated by catatonic signs (catatonic stupor, catatonic negativism, catatonic rigidity, catatonic excitement, or catatonic posturing)

Paranoid

Clinical picture marked by both:
- preoccupation with one or more systematized delusions or with frequent auditory hallucinations related to a single theme
- none of the following: incoherence, marked loosening of associations, flat or grossly inappropriate affect, catatonic behaviour, grossly disorganized behaviour

Hebephrenic

The following criteria are met:
- incoherence or marked loosening of associations
- flat or inappropriate affect
- grossly bizarre or disorganized behaviour
- the criteria for catatonic subtype are not met

Undifferentiated

Clinical picture marked by:
- prominent delusions, hallucinations, incoherence, or grossly disorganized behaviour
- the criteria for catatonic, paranoid, or disorganized subtypes are not met

Residual

Clinical picture marked by the following:
- absence of prominent delusions, hallucinations, incoherence, marked loosening of associations, or grossly disorganized behaviour
- continuing evidence of the disturbance, as indicated by two or more of the following: flat or inappropriate affect, poverty of speech, social isolation or withdrawal, poor grooming and hygiene, peculiar behaviour.

Fig. 14.5 Subtypes of schizophrenia, adapted from the Proposed Criteria for the *DSM-IV* Subtypes of Schizophrenia.

Chemical Structures of the Four Major Groups of Antipsychotic Drugs used to treat Schizophrenia

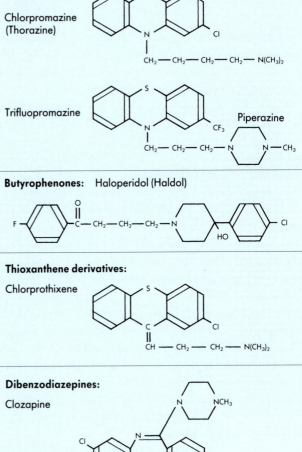

Fig. 14.6 Chemical structures of the four major groups of antipsychotic drugs used in the treatment of schizophrenia.

TREATMENT AND ANTIPSYCHOTIC DRUGS

Treatment of psychotic symptoms with drugs was discovered serendipitously in the 1950s. The first such drug was reserpine and this was quickly followed by the class of drugs now known as the typical antipsychotics (Fig. 14.6):
- phenothiazines (e.g. chlorpromazine);
- butyrophenones (e.g. haloperidol); and
- thioxanthenes (e.g. chlorprothixene).

These drugs have been augmented by the recent addition of the atypical antipsychotics, the dibenzodiazepines (e.g. clozapine).

Antipsychotics were originally used to tranquilize patients. Extensive clinical studies showed that, when administered over

a period of weeks, the tranquilizing effects were supplemented by a marked diminution of positive psychotic symptoms. Negative symptoms were not improved by treatment with typical neuroleptics, although recent data indicate that some of these symptoms can be ameliorated by the atypical neuroleptics.

All of these drugs act on the dopaminergic system by a direct antagonistic effect at the various receptor sites (Fig. 14.7). The different receptor sites are found in different brain areas, have different binding kinetics, and activate a variety of second messenger systems (Fig. 14.8).

Antipsychotics show a range of affinity for dopamine receptors and this is related to their clinical efficacy (Fig. 14.9). Antipsychotics are known to affect other neurotransmitter and neuro-

The Four Main Dopaminergic Tracts in the Brain

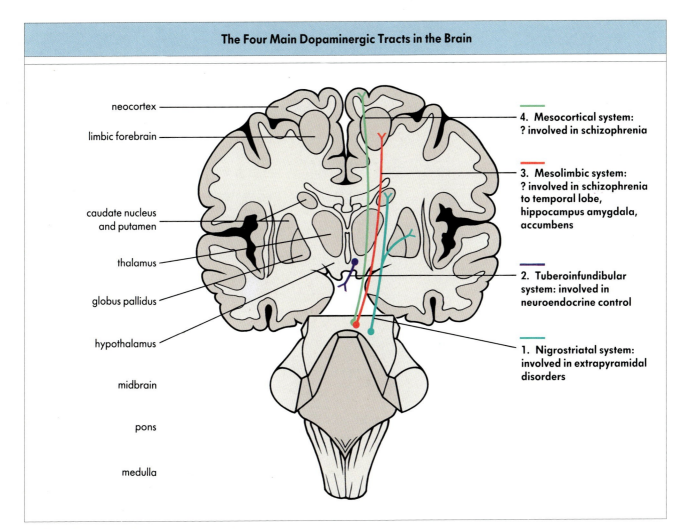

neocortex

limbic forebrain

caudate nucleus
and putamen

thalamus

globus pallidus

hypothalamus

midbrain

pons

medulla

4. **Mesocortical system:**
? involved in schizophrenia

3. **Mesolimbic system:**
? involved in schizophrenia
to temporal lobe,
hippocampus amygdala,
accumbens

2. **Tuberoinfundibular
system:** involved in
neuroendocrine control

1. **Nigrostriatal system:**
involved in extrapyramidal
disorders

Fig. 14.7 The four main dopaminergic tracts in the brain.

peptide systems. Although their interaction with the dopamine system has been intensively studied, the fact that binding to central dopamine receptors occurs within minutes, yet the antipsychotic effects develop over weeks, suggests that other systems are involved in the antipsychotic effect.

Antipsychotic side effects

Treatment with antipsychotics is often long term, and this inevitably results in side effects in some patients (Fig. 14.10). The most prominent side effects are extrapyramidal, and include torsion dystonia, rigidity, tremor, and chronic tardive dyskinesia.

IMAGING

CT and MRI

The advent of *in vivo* imaging techniques has dramatically altered our clinical paradigm of schizophrenia. CT studies have demonstrated ventricular enlargement in the brains of patients with chronic schizophrenia (Fig. 14.11). MRI studies have replicated this finding and also documented the presence of a diffuse reduction of cortical grey matter. This reduction, although affecting many cortical areas, appears to be concentrated on the area of the temporal lobes. Carefully controlled studies on monozygotic twins discordant for schizophrenia have demonstrated 15 per cent losses of temporal lobe grey matter and increases in the size of the lateral ventricle (Fig. 14.12).

Many studies have tried to correlate the changes seen on scans with clinical symptoms and/or aetiological factors. Clear and consistent correlations with specific clinical symptoms have yet to emerge, although there is a trend for large ventricles to be associated with early age of onset and poor premorbid functioning. Meta-analysis of the pooled data from many CT studies indicates that the phenomenon of larger ventricles is unimodal. This is a finding of some considerable significance, since it suggests that the phenomenon of brain abnormality in schizophrenia is a unitary one and, by extrapolation, that the various syndromal manifestations of phenomenology are but reflections of a common pathological process.

Postsynaptic Dopamine Receptor Family

	D$_1$ and D$_5$	D$_{2a}$	D$_{2b}$	D$_3$ and D$_4$
Molecular structure	seven membrane-spanning regions	seven membrane-spanning regions	seven membrane-spanning regions	seven membrane-spanning regions
Effect on c-AMP	increases	decreases	increases phospho-inositide turnover	—
Effective neuroleptics (antagonists)				
Typical				
phenothiazines	potent	potent	—	—
thioxanthenes	potent	potent	—	—
butyrophenones	weak	potent	—	—
Atypical				
clozapine	inactive	weak	weak	potent

Fig. 14.8 Some characteristics of dopamine receptors and the antagonist effects of various neuroleptics on each other.

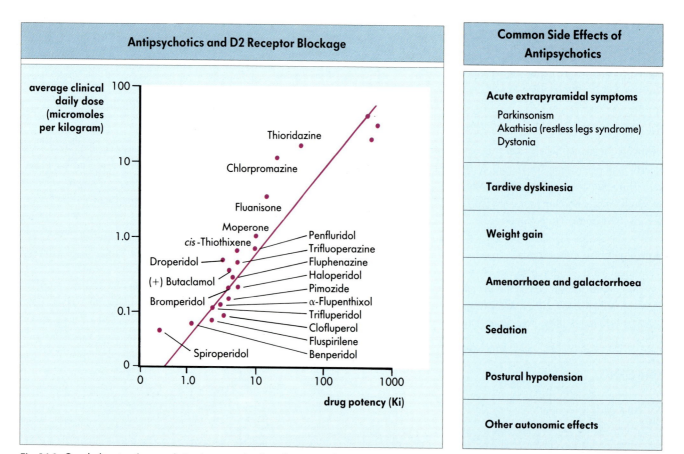

Fig. 14.9 Graph showing the correlation between the clinical potency of various antipsychotic drugs and the drugs' ability to block dopamine D2 receptors.

Common Side Effects of Antipsychotics

Acute extrapyramidal symptoms
Parkinsonism
Akathisia (restless legs syndrome)
Dystonia

Tardive dyskinesia

Weight gain

Amenorrhoea and galactorrhoea

Sedation

Postural hypotension

Other autonomic effects

Fig. 14.10 Common side effects of drugs used in the treatment of schizophrenia.

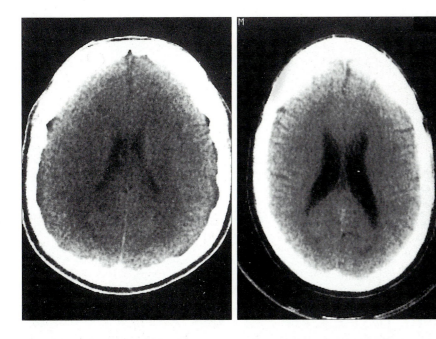

Fig. 14.11 CT scans showing enlargement of the lateral cerebral ventricles in a chronic schizophrenic (right), compared to a normal control (left).

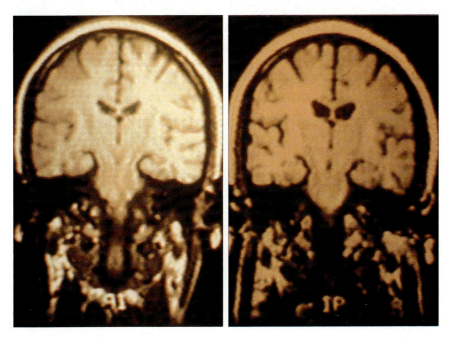

Fig. 14.12 MRI scans through the bodies of the lateral ventricles in a pair of monozygotic twins who are discordant for schizophrenia. Note the increase in the CSF spaces in the schizophrenic twin (right) compared to the unaffected twin (left).

Despite the increased sensitivity of MRI for detecting minor pathological damage (e.g. periventricular hyperintensities, white matter damage) there is little evidence from either CT or MRI studies of increased amounts of other pathological damage in the brain in schizophrenia.

PET and SPECT

PET studies show the presence of relative hypometabolism and reduced blood flow (rCBF) in the dorsolateral prefrontal cortex of patients who are given psychological tasks (e.g. the Wisconsin Card Sort) that activate this brain region (Fig. 14.13). The result is in striking contrast to those obtained when patients are required to perform reasoning tasks that do not activate the prefrontal cortex; these show no abnormalities in cerebral blood flow. A similar result is seen when comparing discordant monozygotic twins (Fig. 14.14).

The findings of hypofrontality appear to be independent of neuroleptic treatment and to be present in untreated patients on their first admission. Preliminary reports indicate that one effect of neuroleptic treatment is to diminish the degree of hypofrontality.

Some PET and SPECT studies have also demonstrated bilateral hypermetabolism in the temporal lobes of patients with schizophrenia, though hypometabolism has also been reported.

Attempts to demonstrate increased numbers of dopamine receptors using specific ligands and PET scans have not produced conclusive information.

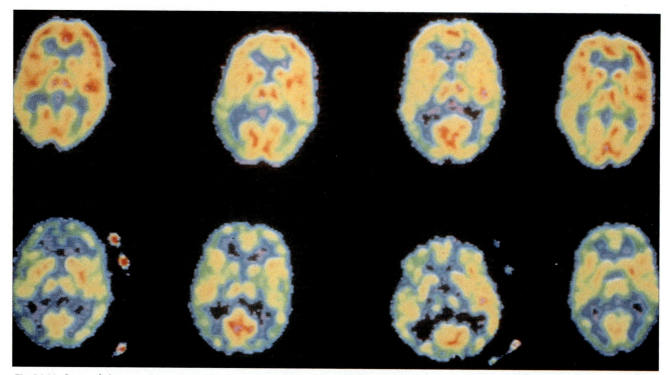

Fig. 14.13 Scans of glucose utilization with F18 deoxyglucose and PET scanned through the level of the basal ganglia in four normal subjects (upper row) and in four subjects with schizophrenia (bottom row). There is reduced glucose utilization, particularly in the frontal regions, in the schizophrenic patients. (Courtesy of Monte Buchsbaum, MD, University of California, Irvine.)

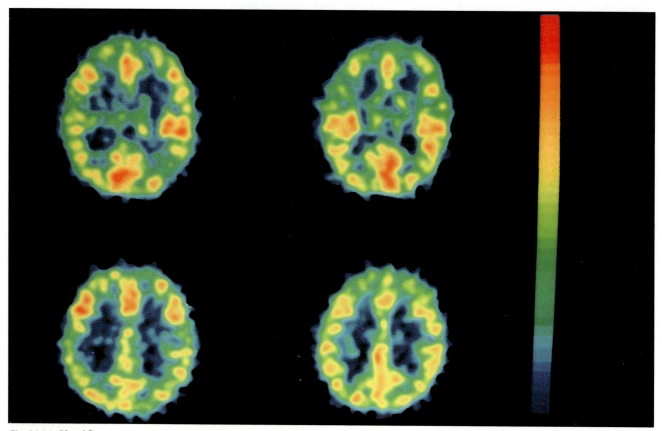

Fig. 14.14 Blood flow (measured using oxygen 15 water and PET) during the performance of the Wisconsin Card Sorting Task (a task that activates prefrontal cortex in normal subjects) in a schizophrenic twin (right column) and an unaffected twin (left column). The arrows indicate the relatively focused failure of activation in the affected twin compared with the unaffected twin. This indicates a behaviour-specific failure of an anatomically focused function.

PHYSIOLOGY AND PATHOLOGY

Neurophysiology

EEG studies have shown inconclusive results, although variable degrees of abnormal temporal lobe activity are a recurring theme. Motivational problems and the complications due to neuroleptic treatment have confused the interpretation of many other neurophysiological studies. However, abnormalities in the control of eye movements during tracking appear to be a relatively robust phenomena and have been proposed as a schizophrenia trait marker in large families.

Gross pathology

Ventricular enlargement in the brain of patients with chronic schizophrenia can be visible to the naked eye (Fig. 14.15). Brain weight reductions of some 5 per cent and a reduced (fixed) brain length of 0.8 cm have been observed bilaterally in men and women in some, but not all, studies. Otherwise, brains appear normal and do not display marked structural aberrations, and sulcogyral patterns are within normal limits. No other gross

pathological phenomena has been consistently associated with schizophrenia. However, it should be remembered that a diagnosis of schizophrenia offers no immunity from a supervening disease process and that patients examined in post-mortem studies are often in their sixth, seventh, or eighth decade. This fact may account for the sporadic case reports that link schizophrenia to various types of pathology.

Quantitative assessment of various brain structures demonstrates volume reductions and reduced cross-sectional areas of particular brain regions (Fig. 14.16):

- the entorhinal cortex;
- the hippocampus;
- the temporal lobe grey matter; and
- the central grey matter.

There is diffuse reduction in cortical volume; this particularly affects the medial temporal lobe (Fig. 14.17).

Microscopic Pathology

In most respects, the brains of patients with schizophrenia appear to differ little from those of controls of a similar age. The data from imaging studies suggests a relatively diffuse process, perhaps more focused on the temporal lobe, and the data from carefully controlled neuropathological studies are consistent with this. Neuronal loss has been described in the insula, entorhinal cortex, and prefrontal cortex. Quantitative studies indicate reductions of approximately 20 per cent in neuronal number of the anterior hippocampus and entorhinal cortex, with smaller reductions in particular cortical layers of the cingulate (layer 5) and prefrontal (layer 6) cortex. In addition, changes in the cytoarchitectural arrangement of neurons in entorhinal cortex, hippocampus, and insula have been observed.

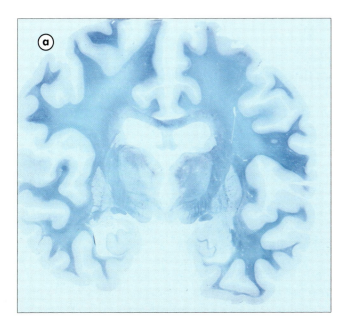

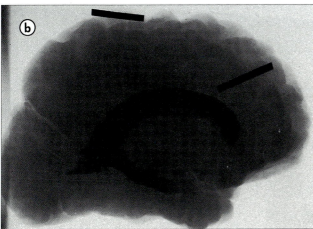

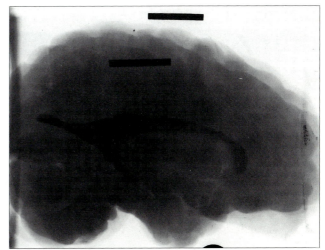

Fig. 14.15 (a) Lateral ventricular enlargement in a 53-year-old woman with schizophrenia (myelin stain). (Courtesy of Dr P Falkai, Dusseldorf.) (b) Radiographs of post-mortem brains in which radio-opaque dye has been injected into the ventricular system, showing the larger ventricles in the schizophrenic (right) compared to the normal control. (Courtesy of Dr CJ Bruton, London.)

Structural Abnormalities in the Brain in Schizophrenia

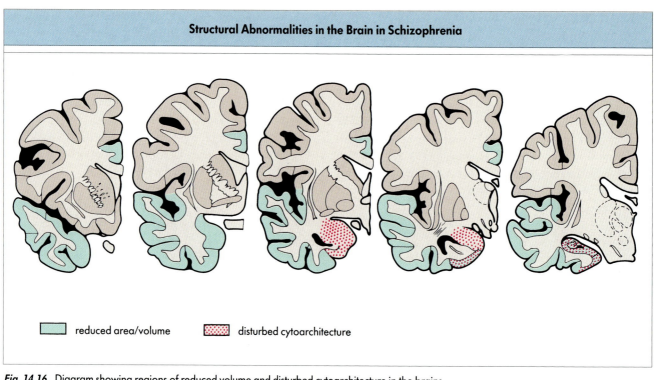

reduced area/volume   disturbed cytoarchitecture

Fig. 14.16 Diagram showing regions of reduced volume and disturbed cytoarchitecture in the brains of patients with schizophrenia.

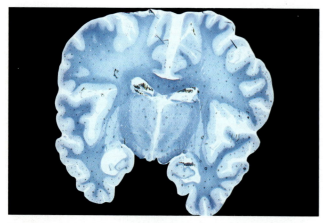

Fig. 14.17 Coronal section from the brain of a 49-year-old woman with schizophrenia, showing marked decrease in the size of the hippocampus and marked increase in the size of the temporal horn. (Courtesy of Dr P Falkai, Dusseldorf.)

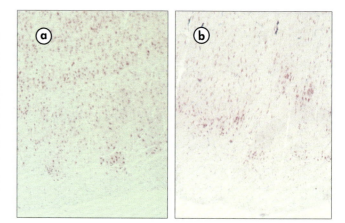

Fig. 14.18 Section from the entorhinal cortex in (a) a normal control, showing well-developed laminae and clusters of layer 2 neurons, and (b) a schizophrenic patient, showing marked loss and disturbance in organization of layer 2 entorhinal neurons.

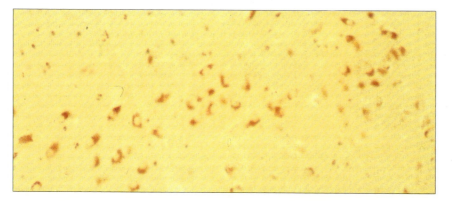

Fig. 14.19 Layer 2 entorhinal neurons immunostained for nitric oxide synthase.

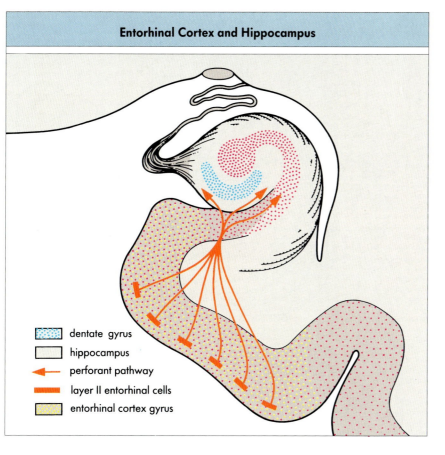

Entorhinal Cortex and Hippocampus

dentate gyrus
hippocampus
perforant pathway
layer II entorhinal cells
entorhinal cortex gyrus

Fig. 14.20 Neuronal connections between the entorhinal cortex and the hippocampus.

Entorhinal cortex and layer 2 neurons   One interesting finding that has been reported by several groups is a disturbance in the organization of and loss of layer 2 (pre-α) neurons. These modified pyramidal neurons are of considerable interest functionally because:

- they are modified pyramidal cells organized into unique clusters (Fig. 14.18);
- they contain large amounts of the enzyme nitric oxide synthase (Fig. 14.19);
- their projections form part of the 'perforant pathway' (Fig. 14.20); and
- they receive inputs from almost all areas of association cortex (Fig. 14.21).

The degree of disorganization is variable and difficult to quantify. Cytoarchitectural disturbances in this region could lead to a disturbance in the functioning of synaptically connected distant brain regions (e.g. dorsolateral prefrontal cortex, cingulate cortex, hippocampus) and result in considerable compromise and distortion of the input and integration of information from many sensory modalities.

Absence of gliosis   The presence of larger ventricles in the brains of patients with schizophrenia suggests, by analogy to Alzheimer's disease, a neurodegenerative condition. Exhaustive studies have failed to reveal neuropathological evidence of neurodegenerative change and, in particular, reveal a marked absence of the reactive or activated glial cells (gliosis) that characterize most known neurodegenerative processes.

Schizophrenia: a neurodevelopmental pathological process

Thus, the pattern of pathological differences found in the brains of patients with schizophrenia may be characteristic:

- slightly larger ventricles;
- slightly reduced brain weight and length;
- disorganization of cortical neurons and reduced neuronal number in the medial temporal lobe;
- reduced neuronal number in other cortical areas; and
- absence of gliosis or neurodegenerative change.

These changes fit the pattern expected in a disorder of brain development. Neuropathological studies indicate that similar abnormalities of brain structure can be demonstrated in all subtypes of schizophrenia. This is consistent with the data derived from imaging studies.

Neurochemistry

The symptoms of schizophrenia can be ameliorated and treated by neuroleptic therapy. This fact has led to extensive investigations aimed at finding a culpable neurochemical.

Most neuroleptics block dopamine receptors (D2 subtype) and drugs that increase dopamine levels in the brain (e.g. L-DOPA, amphetamine, cocaine) can cause a psychotic state that resembles paranoid schizophrenia. These observations led to the dopamine hypothesis of schizophrenia: that excess of dopaminergic transmission (particularly in the mesolimbic pathway) causes schizophrenia.

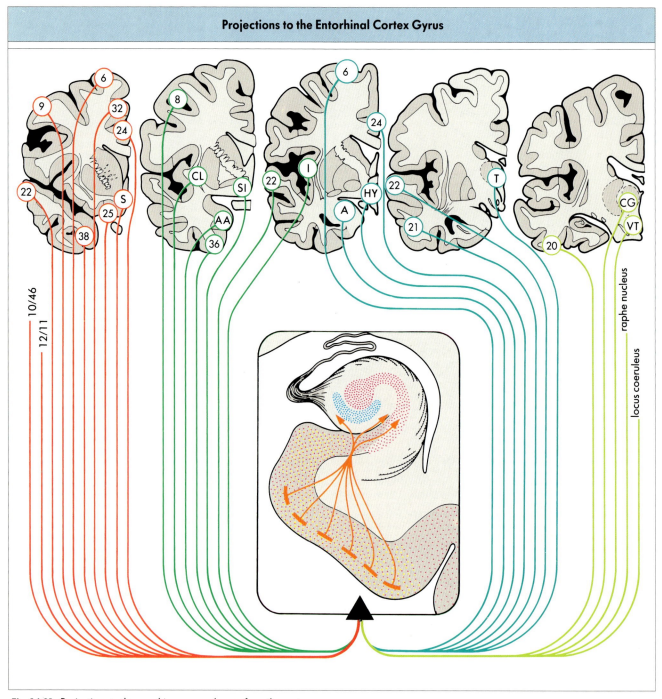

Fig. 14.21 Projections to the parahippocampal gyrus from the cortex.

Although an attractive and simple hypothesis, this has received little support in the way of undisputed experimental data. In schizophrenia, CNS levels of dopamine are unaltered, D2 receptor numbers appear unchanged, dopamine metabolites are unaltered, and the synthesizing enzymes of the dopamine system appear unaffected.

Pharmacokinetic studies indicate that CNS dopamine receptors are blocked by neuroleptics within 20 minutes of administration. Yet clinical efficacy reaches its maximum over days or weeks.

This suggests that the blockade of the dopamine system gradually affects other systems in the brain to produce a therapeutic effect.

Other transmitter systems that have been implicated in schizophrenia include noradrenaline, glutamate, and several neuropeptides. Interestingly, both glutamate and cholecystokinin octapeptide are present within layer 2 neurons in the entorhinal cortex and both are thought to have a role in cortical development. A direct dopaminergic innervation of these neurons has also been reported in the human brain.

A specific deficit in a single transmitter system seems unlikely in schizophrenia. However, the powerful therapeutic effect of neuroleptics indicate that a small number of transmitters, perhaps in particular brain areas, are critical for the generation of psychotic symptoms.

Molecular biology

The evidence of genetic factors in schizophrenia has prompted many linkage studies. To date, no definitive evidence of linkage to any marker has been demonstrated: studies that show evidence of weak linkage to such markers as the pseudo-autosomal region of the X chromosome and chromosome 5 are best regarded as tentative. Such studies are in their infancy, and improved statistical methods for dealing with incomplete penetrance, availability of specific probes for target genes, and improved sequencing technology should provide more definitive data in the near future.

Laterality

The association between left hemisphere temporal lobe lesions (e.g. epilepsy) and increased risk of a schizophreniform psychosis, relative left hemisphere hypometabolism in schizophrenia, presence of speech disorders and other neuropsychological left-hemisphere deficits have given rise to the view that schizophrenia is a disorder of the left hemisphere. This has been supported by reports of greater left-sided ventricular enlargement and left-sided pathology.

The concept that schizophrenia arises as a consequence of damage limited to the left side of the brain is incorrect. Many scanning and pathological studies indicate damage in both hemispheres. However, studies also indicate that structural changes are often greater on the left. This seeming paradox may be explainable by the fact that the human brain has a lateralized pattern of development (Fig. 14.22).

Schizophrenia as a disorder of brain development

Work over the past 20 years has changed our view on the pathological processes that underlie schizophrenia. These can be summarized (Fig. 14.23) as:

- schizophrenia is probably caused by or influenced by a genetic disorder, perhaps of brain development;
- abnormal brain development affects the whole brain but is particularly marked in the medial temporal lobe;

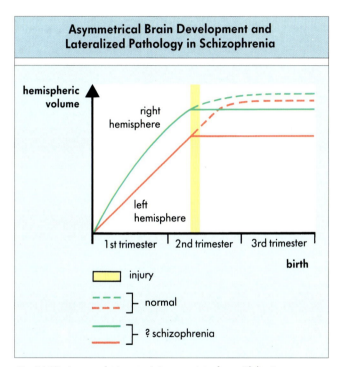

Fig. 14.22 A second-trimester injury can interfere with brain development and lead to pronounced left hemisphere pathology.

Fig. 14.23 Possible factors in the development of schizophrenia, showing the time of life during which they are operative.

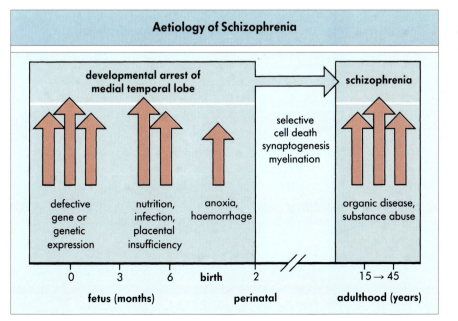

- left hemisphere is affected more than the right, perhaps because of lateralized pattern of normal brain development;
- disarray in layer 2 neurons alters connectivity between entorhinal cortex and hippocampus and leads to aberrant functional connectivity between hippocampus and frontal cortex;
- abnormalities in intellectual development could be present from early childhood;
- psychotic symptoms emerge at a particular stage of postnatal brain development (between 15–25 years of age); and
- syndromal subtypes of schizophrenia are phenotypic manifestations of a single underlying pathological process which varies in degree but not in kind.

DIFFERENTIAL DIAGNOSIS

The clinical phenomena of schizophrenia have been described and the various criteria for making the diagnosis have been outlined. However, the diagnosis often cannot be made simply on positive findings of schizophrenia, but must include an absence of features more characteristic of other syndromes. The conditions to be considered in the differential diagnosis include the following:

- substance abuse;
- other psychiatric disorder;
- paranoid states;
- other neuropsychiatric disease; and
- cultural differences.

Substance abuse

Many drugs (e.g. amphetamine, LSD, cocaine, phencyclidine, and cannabis) can produce an acute psychosis that mimics schizophrenia (Fig. 14.24). Of these, amphetamine psychosis and phencyclidine psychosis are the most difficult to distinguish, as the symptoms can be identical with those of paranoid schizophrenia. The other hallucinogens tend to cause visual rather than auditory hallucinations and produce a 'psychedelic' experience. Cannabis may produce an 'amotivational syndrome'. Debate continues over whether individuals who develop drug psychoses are constitutionally predisposed. Alcoholic hallucinosis may also be mistaken for schizophrenia, and once again there is dispute over whether this arises in those who have a genetic predisposition to schizophrenia.

Other psychiatric disorder

The boundaries between schizophrenia and affective disorder are vague. One should be particularly aware of the intensification of affect that may be an early symptom of schizophrenia, and of the occasional occurrence of first-rank symptoms and of over-inclusive thinking in manics. Even when the greatest care is taken, patients diagnosed on their initial hospitalization as schizophrenic will sometimes need to be reclassified as having affective disorder, and *vice versa*.

It may at times be difficult to differentiate between schizoid personality and schizophrenia, and obsessional neurosis may also be wrongly diagnosed as schizophrenia. A careful history should demonstrate that even the most persistent or bizarre obsessional thought does not have the quality of absolute certainty of a delusion.

Paranoid states

The exact classification of paranoid states has been a matter of controversy for years, and some authorities regard the differences between paranoid personality, paranoia, and paranoid schizophrenia as merely a matter of degree. Paranoia is a relatively rare condition characterized by an intricate, complex, and logically elaborated delusional system without hallucinations. The delusions are systematized, firmly knit, and more or less isolated so that the rest of the personality remains intact. Those with paranoid personality and generally rigid and inflexible, suspicious, and morbidly sensitive. They often have a dominant personality, and their suspiciousness relating to their *idée fixe* leads to difficulties in maintaining personal relationships. Paranoia is rare before 30 years of age and is usually associated with social isolationism. However, sometimes a paranoiac may consider his abilities unique and seek to demonstrate this by joining particular social or political organizations.

Erotomania (de Clerambault's syndrome) is characterized by a delusional belief that the patient (usually female) is loved by another person. This person, usually of a relatively higher socioeconomic status who may only have had a fleeting contact with the patient, is thought to indicate their love by various indirect means that only the patient knows and understands. As a result, the other person is pestered by unwelcome letters, visits, and telephone calls from the patient. Erotomania can persist for many years without a disintegration of the personality. However, some patients experience a slow deterioration reminiscent of chronic schizophrenia.

Morbid jealousy is characterized by delusions of marital infidelity and a search for evidence of adultery. Spouses may be followed, or have their mail intercepted or their underwear repeatedly examined for seminal stains. Accusations of affairs can develop into violent attacks which occasionally end with the homicide of the partner and/or the suspected lover. Morbid jealousy is a symptom which may occur in paranoid states, schizophrenia, alcoholism, or depression psychosis.

In *folie à deux*, the delusional idea of one person is seemingly transferred to another so that both come to share the psychopathology. This type of condition is usually confined to persons living together, such as a husband and wife or a brother and sister. The personality in the person to whom the delusion is transferred is typically passive and dependent. The second person usually recovers within a few months if separated from the patient that first develops the delusion.

Other neuropsychiatric disease

Imaging, EEG, and neuropsychological evaluation together will enable a reliable distinction between schizophrenia and many other neuropsychiatric disorders to be made. Care is required in

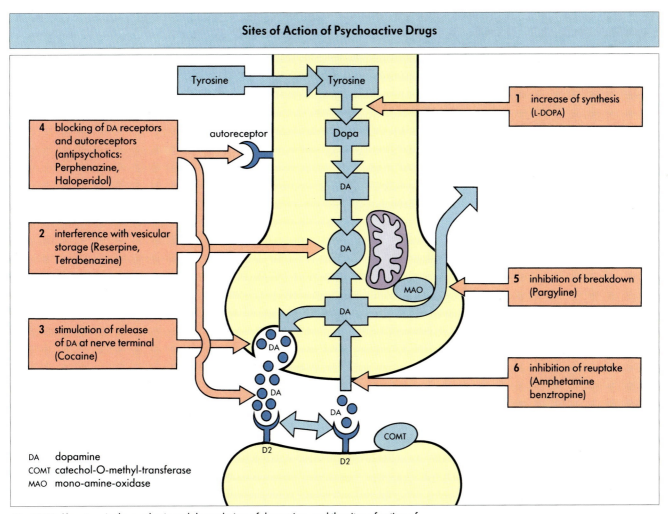

Fig. 14.24 Key steps in the synthesis and degradation of dopamine, and the sites of action of various psychoactive drugs.

dealing with patients who have temporal lobe epilepsy (see Chapter 13) or suspected puerperal psychosis.

Cultural differences

Migrant populations tend to be at increased risk of receiving the diagnosis of schizophrenia. Part of this may be a consequence of psychiatrists considering unfamiliar beliefs (e.g. believing in possession, spells, or evil spirits) as delusions. Similar considerations may apply to subcultural groups in Western society such as spiritualists.

Features of everyday adolescent crises – exultation, preoccupation with abstract ideas, new beliefs and intolerance of the ideas of others, unpredictability, introspection and social withdrawal, and extreme shyness commonly occur in schizophrenia. Deriving a firm diagnosis is even more difficult when a young patient subscribes to the beliefs of a cultural subgroup whose practices differ from those of the clinician. Schizophrenia is a

serious mental disorder, and so care and time are required before diagnosing the syndrome in a difficult or rebellious adolescent.

SUMMARY

(i) Schizophrenia is a major category of psychosis characterized by gross disturbance in mental state, hallucinations, delusions, thought disorder, and inappropriate affect.

(ii) The prevalence of schizophrenia is similar world-wide, and represents a lifetime risk of approximately 1 per cent.

(iii) Schizophrenia is caused in part by genetic factors, although environmental events such as fetal infection, birth trauma, perinatal damage and adult neuropsychiatric disorder, may be involved in some cases.

(iv) Peak age of onset is in the third decade of life.

(v)   Onset of symptoms is followed by remission, a fluctuating course, or chronic illness (in 20 per cent, 60 per cent and 20 per cent of patients respectively).

(vi) Acute onset, response to medication, and adequate social circumstances are related to good prognosis.

(vii) Insidious or early onset, poor response to medication, negative symptoms and poor social circumstances are related to poor prognosis.

(viii) Antipsychotics block dopamine receptors.

(ix) CT and MRI scans indicate larger ventricles and diffuse loss of cortical grey matter, especially affecting the temporal lobe.

(x)   PET and SPECT scans may show hypometabolism in the prefrontal cortex, especially during cognitive activation.

(xi) Pathology is characterized by developmental abnormalities, most clearly affecting the medial temporal lobe.

(xii) Differential diagnosis includes substance abuse, other psychiatric conditions, and other neuropsychiatric disorder.

15 Mood Disorders

INTRODUCTION

During his pioneering studies on the phenomenology of psychoses, Emil Kraeplin championed the careful distinction between:

- disturbance of a patient's intellectual and cognitive abilities (disorders of thought) – like schizophrenia; and
- disturbances of the emotion and mood (disorders of affect) – like depression and mania.

The major mood disorders are a varied group of conditions whose common clinical expression is a sustained disturbance of emotion and mood. Patients that suffer from these disorders show extreme states of mood which can vary from euphoria to despair. The three mood states which are most commonly involved are:

- euphoria, which when sustained becomes mania;
- depression; and
- anxiety.

As a result of altered mood, these patients also have changes in their sleep patterns, appetite, cognitive ability, sexual behaviour, and psychomotor function.

Disturbances in mood are increasingly being described in childhood; however, mood disorder typically strikes in early adulthood and middle age, and women are more affected than men. The major mood disorders are subdivided into:

- depressive disorder (depression only);
- manic disorder (manic–depressive disorder); and
- anxiety-related disorders.

There is evidence of a substantial genetic contribution to the aetiology of these disorders. Drug therapy is very successful in treating many patients. Although anxiety disorders are not considered part of the mood disorder spectrum in some nosologies, they will be considered here because they overlap phenomenologically in a number of respects.

Definition

Mood disorders are the result of sustained and inappropriate moods of depression, mania, or anxiety.

EPIDEMIOLOGY

Estimates of the prevalence of primary mood disorder vary considerably depending on the sampling procedure. Studies of isolated populations in Iceland and Denmark indicated that the lifetime risk for primary mood disorder is 5 per cent for men and 9 per cent for women. Studies performed at the National Institute of Mental Health (USA) tend to confirm these findings; they report a prevalence of bipolar and unipolar disorders of about 5 per cent in the general population. These figures indicate that some 8 000 000 people in the USA have mood disorder at any one time with a resultant huge social and economic cost (some $60 billion in 1990).

The average age of onset is about 30 for depressive disorders, and 20 for manic disorder. However, onset can occur at any age, though onset of a primary depressive disorder is relatively rare in patients over 60. Primary mood disorder is commoner in women than men (ratio approximately 3:2). This distinction is most marked in depressive disorder; men and women have an almost equal risk of suffering manic disorder.

Episodes of illness typically last for six to 24 months if untreated and 70 per cent of patients with depressive mood disorder will experience a second and possibly subsequent episodes.

Primary mood disorder is the most frequent cause of psychiatric admission. Together, depression – primary and secondary – are the commonest diagnoses in psychiatry. The diagnosis of depressive mood disorder accounts for almost 90 per cent of diagnoses of mood disorder.

AETIOLOGY

Genetic factors are the best identified causes. An increased risk of mood disorder has been shown to occur in the relatives of patients with a mood disorder:

- lifetime risk to relatives of depressive disorder, 20 per cent;
- lifetime risk to relatives of manic disorder, 24 per cent; and
- lifetime risk in general population, 6 per cent.

Family, twin and adoption studies show a picture of the importance of genetic background similar to that seen in schizophrenia. However, no clear pattern of heritability has been described and the presence of a single gene responsible for mood disorder is considered unlikely. Molecular biological studies have not uncovered reliable linkage to any single marker.

Relationships between socioeconomic factors and mood disorder have been proposed. However, other than the common sense supposition that increased rates of stress or negative life events may predispose to mood disorder, little of substance has been uncovered.

DIAGNOSIS AND CLINICAL COURSE

Mood disorder is diagnosed (Fig. 15.1) according to operationalized criteria (DSM III-R) which assign to patients diagnoses of:

- depressive disorder (also called unipolar disorder);
- manic (manic–depressive) disorder (also known as bipolar disorder); and
- anxiety states.

These are syndromal diagnoses and exact demarcation between the various types of mood disorder is often difficult.

Depressive, manic and manic–depressive disorders and anxiety states have different natural histories and differential responses to drug therapy.

Diagnostic Criteria for Major Depressive Episode

a. At least five of the following symptoms have been present during the same two-week period and represent a change from previous functioning; at least one of the symptoms is either (1) depressed mood, or (2) loss of interest or pleasure.

1. depressed mood most of the day, nearly every day
2. markedly diminished interest or pleasure in all, or almost all, activities most of the day, nearly every day
3. significant weight loss or weight gain when not dieting, or decrease or increase in appetite nearly every day
4. insomnia or hypersomnia nearly every day
5. psychomotor agitation or retardation nearly every day, observable by others
6. fatigue or loss of energy nearly every day
7. feelings of worthlessness or excessive or inappropriate guilt (which may be delusional) nearly every day
8. diminished ability to think or concentrate, or indecisiveness, nearly every day
9. recurrent thoughts of death, recurrent suicidal ideation without a specific plan, or a suicide attempt or a specific plan for committing suicide.

b.
(1) It cannot be established that an organic factor initiated and maintained the disturbance.
(2) The disturbance is not a normal reaction to the death of a loved one.

c. At no time during the disturbance have there been delusions or hallucinations for as long as two weeks in the absence of prominent mood symptoms (i.e. before the mood symptoms developed or after they have remitted).

d. Not superimposed on Schizophrenia, Schizophreniform Disorder, Delusional Disorder, or Psychotic Disorder, No Other Specified Diagnosis.

Fig. 15.1 Diagnostic criteria for a major depressive episode, adapted from DSM-III-R.

Depressive Disorder

Onset of symptoms usually occurs in adulthood (average age 30) and episodes can last for six to 24 months if untreated. In the past, considerable attention was paid to distinguishing reactive depression (i.e. where a precipitating event is identified) and endogenous depression (i.e. where no such event is identified). The usefulness of such a distinction is doubtful, since the symptoms, course, and treatment of the two are essentially the same. The presenting symptoms are:

- feelings of worthlessness, guilt, doom, despair, or ideas of self-harm;
- anorexia with weight loss;
- insomnia or early morning awakening;
- loss of energy, general tiredness, or fatigue;
- agitation or psychomotor retardation; and
- loss of interest in usual activities, including sex.

It is also common for depressed patients to complain of pains, tachycardia, breathing difficulties, gastrointestinal dysfunction, headache, or other somatic disturbances.

Sadness or despondency characterize the dysphoric mood experienced by patients with depressive illness. Patients also describe themselves as feeling hopeless, irritable, fearful, worried, or simply discouraged. Sometimes, patients present with an apparent unipolar disorder complaining of insomnia and anorexia whilst reporting minimal feelings of dysphoria. In extreme cases, patients may even weep profusely whilst maintaining that they do not feel sad.

Patients with depressive disorder often have low expectations of recovery and are concerned about their loss of emotional stability and have fears of 'losing their mind'. This type of pessimistic outlook is in itself a diagnostic indicator, since patients with conventional somatic illnesses seldom give up all hope of improvement, even when seriously ill.

Agitation is marked in some patients; these patients pace to and fro, wring their hands, bemoan their fate, and try to get reassurance from anyone who will listen. Psychomotor retardation can also be prominent, and slowing of thought and motor behaviour occurs. Speech is an effort and simple tasks can take a long time. Psychomotor retardation can be so severe that a patient becomes mute or even stuporous.

Depressive disorder can also be associated with paranoid symptoms including exaggerated ideas of reference associated with notions of worthlessness and hypochondriacal or nihilistic delusions. Hallucinations (often accusatory voices or visions of dead relatives) associated with guilt occur. Delusions and hallucinations occurring in primary mood disorder are usually 'mood congruent' (i.e. their content is consistent with the person's dominant mood).

Depressed patients may or may not mention events that they consider important in producing their illness. Occasionally, the precipitating event is trivial and may be difficult to relate to the catastrophic change in the patient's mental state. Detailed interviews often reveal that some symptoms began before the so-called precipitating event. It is probable that some patients who begin to feel depressed need to identify a precipitating event and do so retrospectively.

Precipitating events include employment problems, death of relatives, moving or leaving home, and difficulties with personal relationships. Pregnancy and childbirth appear as frequent precipitating factors for women: in one series, 37 per cent of female manic depressives and 17 per cent of female depressives had their first episode of depression during pregnancy or in the post-partum period.

Changes in social habits often accompany depressive illness, e.g. uncharacteristic episodes of heavy drinking in a middle-aged person with no previous history of alcoholism may indicate the onset of depression. Sometimes the converse (i.e. a person drinking less than normal) is also seen.

Many depressive episodes are inextricably bound up with anxiety states. Drug therapy is often particularly effective in such cases. Approximately 70 per cent of patients that suffer a depressive episode will experience another.

Depression in children

Children can have episodes of depression that resemble depression in adulthood:

- crying;
- social withdrawal;
- hypersensitivity to environmental events; and
- behavioural problems.

It is not certain whether such episodes are an early manifestation of primary mood disorder. There are at least two important differences between childhood and adult depression:

- childhood depression is more common in boys; adult depression is more common in women; and
- the sleep of depressed children does not differ from that of age-matched normal children; depressed adults differ from normal adults in taking longer to fall asleep, awakening more often throughout the night, and experiencing greater early-morning wakefulness.

Mania

The characteristic features of mania (also known as bipolar disorder) are:

- euphoria;
- hyperactivity; and
- flight of ideas (Fig. 15.2).

Not all manic patients are euphoric; in some the predominant feature is one of irritability or agitation. Flight of ideas is a rapid digression from one idea to another. Characteristically, these flights of ideas are understandable and follow a logical sequence, although some connections between ideas may be tenuous. These flights are generally expressed in pressured speech (i.e. speech in which a great deal is said in a short period of time). The exposition of the ideas may be accompanied by rhyming, punning, and amusing associations. The tenuous logic of the flights of

Diagnostic Criteria for Manic Episode
a. A distinct period of abnormally and persistently elevated, expansive, or irritable mood.
b. During the period of mood disturbance, at least three of the following symptoms have persisted (four if the mood is only irritable) and have been present to a significant degree 1. inflated self-esteem or grandiosity 2. decreased need for sleep 3. more talkative than usual or pressure to keep talking 4. flight of ideas or subjective experience that thoughts are racing 5. distractibility 6. increase in goal-directed activity or psychomotor agitation 7. excessive involvement in pleasurable activities which have a high potential for painful consequences (unrestrained buying sprees, sexual indiscretions, foolish business investments).
c. Mood disturbance sufficiently severe to cause marked impairment in occupational functioning or in usual social activities or relationships with others, or to necessitate hospitalization to prevent harm to self or others.
d. At no time during the disturbance have there been delusions or hallucinations for as long as two weeks in the absence of prominent mood symptoms.
e. Not superimposed on Schizophrenia, Schizophreniform Disorder, Delusional Disorder, or Psychotic Disorder, No Other Specified Diagnosis.
f. It cannot be established that an organic factor initiated and maintained the disturbance.

Fig. 15.2 Diagnostic criteria for a manic episode, adapted from DSM-III-R.

ideas is in marked contrast to the incoherence and tangentiality of speech found in patients with schizophrenia.

Manic patients are often amusing and may engage the physician in humorous behaviours. It has often been said that when so amused, a diagnosis of mania or hypomania (mild mania) should be considered.

Psychotic syndromes also occur:

- persecutory and grandiose delusions;
- hallucinations; and
- ideas of reference.

These are usually mood-congruent and take the form of grandiose ideas about the patient's position in the universe or inflated assessments of the patient's abilities. Patients can exhibit depression and mania simultaneously, crying whilst describing a grandiose scheme, for example.

Compared to patients with depressive disorder, bipolar patients tend to have:

- an earlier age of onset (late 20s);
- cyclical depressions;
- a higher frequency of post-partum onset;
- a greater tendency for suicide attempts;
- more likelihood of being delusional;
- more likelihood of having psychomotor retardation at some stage; and
- more likelihood of having a family history of the disorder.

Studies indicate that manic patients that have had depression respond better to lithium than do depressives. Most manic patients will experience episodes of depression.

Anxiety States

There is a considerable debate as to the exact status of anxiety states, since many of their clinical features are seen in depression and mania. One of the important manifestations of anxiety disorder is the occurrence of fear manifested by:

- high levels of arousal;
- heightened responsiveness;
- sweating, increased pulse, increased blood pressure; and
- ideas of flight or escape and planning of avoidance strategies.

A degree of anxiety is useful as it can heighten responses to environmental stimuli, but sustained high levels of anxiety can be deleterious. Many anxiety syndromes have been described but the two most important are panic attacks and generalized anxiety.

Panic attacks

These are brief (typically 15–30 minutes) periods of terror or fear that arise unexpectedly and have no clear cause. The attacks are characterized by a sense of fear and an intense activity of the sympathetic nervous system, shortage of breath, dizziness, trembling in limbs, and increased pulse rate.

Attacks usually emerge in the late 20s and occur several times a week over a period of months to years. Some 60 per cent of patients also suffer from depression, and depression occurs more commonly in their relatives than the normal population. It has been suggested that panic attacks are a form of depression. This is supported by the observation that tricyclic antidepressants and monoamine oxidase inhibitors are effective treatments.

An interesting feature of panic attacks is their ready precipitation in some patients following an intravenous infusion of sodium lactate or inhalation of carbon dioxide. Antidepressants block this effect.

Generalized anxiety state

The main symptom is excessive worry or anxiety lasting for months. Other symptoms include:

- motor tension;
- autonomic hyperactivity; and
- heightened vigilance.

As mentioned previously, this type of disorder is often related to previous episodes of depression. These states are best treated by benzodiazepines, which suggest a role of GABA in the pathophysiology of the disease.

Suicide

There is a clear association between depression and suicide. Between 50 and 70 per cent of suicide victims can be found retrospectively to have had symptoms characteristic of depression. Some 10–15 per cent of patients with a diagnosis of depression eventually commit suicide. Attempted suicide is even more common. Although most people who commit suicide have made previous suicide attempts, only a small percentage of attempters eventually kill themselves. Typically, no more than 4 per cent are dead by suicide within five years after an attempt. The more medically serious the attempt, the more likely it is that a person will subsequently die by suicide.

Severity of symptoms is not clearly associated with increased suicide risk. An increased risk is associated with age greater than 40, with being male, with alcoholism, and with threatening to commit suicide.

PHYSIOLOGY

There is a confused literature on the changes of various physiological responses in depression. In the light of the varied clinical expression this is, perhaps, not unduly surprising.

Depression in adults is associated with a reduction in slow-wave sleep (stages 3 and 4), shortened rapid eye movement latency, and increased REM density. As previously noted, sleep studies of depressed children demonstrate none of these differences.

IMAGING

PET Studies

PET studies have demonstrated that depressive and manic patients show different metabolism rates and different patterns of cerebral activity. Depressed patients show a reduction of glucose metabolism in structures above the tentorium (Fig. 15.3), whereas manic patients have higher values. The clinical significance of this finding is uncertain.

Psychological studies suggest that right hemisphere deficits are more prominent in mood disorder. PET studies, however, have suggested that left hemisphere activity, especially in the frontal lobes, is more likely to be abnormal. Depressed patients may show impairment in abstract thinking (using the Halstead–Reitan Category Test), and impairment in short-term memory which improves as symptoms dissipate. However, long-term memory is not affected. Memory impairment with depression is occasionally so profound as to prompt a diagnosis of dementia, the so-called pseudodementia. However, memory returns to normal after recovery from the depression.

CT and MRI

Recent studies have demonstrated the presence of slight structural abnormalities in the brains of patients with depression. The changes include enlarged ventricles and slight reductions in cortical mass. However, because such non-specific findings have not been reported in young first-episode patients and appear to increase with time after the first episode, these changes may be epiphenomena. Further studies are required.

Recently, a series of studies of primarily elderly patients with depressive disorders has reported increased prevalence of high-intensity white matter lesions on MRI scan (Fig. 15.4). These studies have raised the possibility that such pathology, even if of a non-specific aetiology (e.g. cerebrovascular disease), increases the risk of depression in elderly persons.

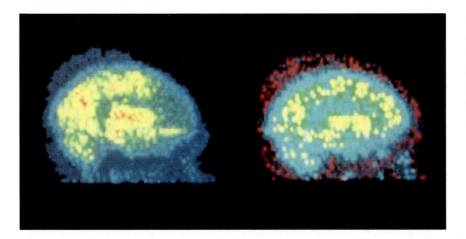

Fig. 15.3 PET scans of glucose utilization, using F18-deoxyglucose as a tracer, in a depressed subject. It shows frontal hypometabolism (left) which improves after treatment with antidepressant medication (right).   (Courtesy of Lewis Baxter MD, UCLA School of Medicine, Los Angeles.)

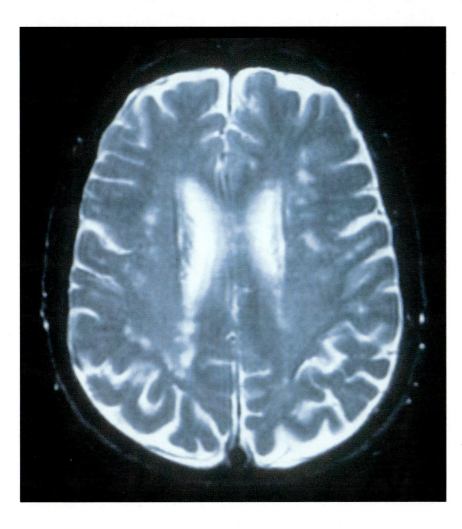

Fig. 15.4 MRI scan showing high-intensity white-matter lesions in a patient with a first episode of late-life depression.

NEUROCHEMISTRY

Antidepressants affect the function of the serotonergic, the noradrenergic, and (in many instances) the dopaminergic transmitter systems (Fig. 15.5). Both tricyclic antidepressant and monoamine oxidase inhibitors affect the uptake and/or accumulation of these neurotransmitters, and may lead to changes in the dynamics of both pre- and post-synaptic receptors.

The exact mechanisms by which this takes place are not certain. However, research evidence suggests that depression may be due to changes in one of several transmitter systems. Since these systems interact, the totality and the dynamics of the neurochemical changes induced by antidepressants, and how this alleviates depression, remain to be defined.

Neuroendocrine function

Hypothalamic function is often disturbed in mood disorders. The clearest example of this is hypersecretion of cortisol from adrenal cortex caused by increased adrenocorticotropin secretion from the pituitary; this occurs in about 60 per cent of patients. Release of adrenocorticotropin is controlled by corticotropin-releasing hormone in the hypothalamus. Normally, cortisol secretion peaks at about 8.00 am and is lower in the early morning and in the evening (Fig. 15.6). Excess secretion in depressed patients occurs during the afternoon and evening, resulting in a loss of this normal diurnal pattern. This change in secretion pattern may relate to sleep disorders and is not seen in other psychiatric illnesses.

The hypersecretion of cortisol is sometimes resistant to normal feedback mechanisms. This can be tested for by administration of the synthetic corticosteroid dexamethasone, which acts to suppress adrenocorticotropin. The dexamethasone suppression test (DST) is only fairly sensitive for affective disorder: about 50 per cent of patients with depression have a positive result (i.e. resist suppression of blood cortisol levels following a dose of dexamethasone). The specificity of the test is higher: only about 10 per cent of normal control subjects are non-suppressors. Specificity drops to less than 70 per cent when other conditions are considered, however; these include dementia, schizophrenia, alcohol abuse, and anorexia.

The American Psychiatric Association takes the view that a positive DST does not predict a good response to antidepressants and that a negative test is not an indication for withholding antidepressant treatment. It has been suggested that the DST could be useful in determining the cases in which antidepressant treatment should be discontinued. The use of the DST in clinical practice is still controversial.

NEUROPATHOLOGY

Assessment of the nature of the changes in brain structure that might be present in affective disorder is in its infancy. A limited number of studies have reported the presence of large ventricles, and some have indicated that this effect may be more apparent in the temporal horn in the right cerebral hemisphere. However, the literature describing the pathological features of depression is remarkable for its paucity rather than its reliability, and thus it demands a cautious interpretation.

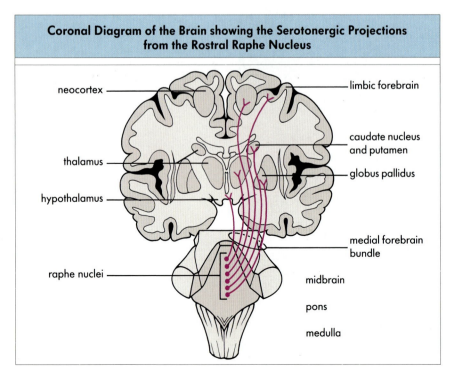

Coronal Diagram of the Brain showing the Serotonergic Projections from the Rostral Raphe Nucleus

neocortex

limbic forebrain

caudate nucleus and putamen

globus pallidus

thalamus

hypothalamus

medial forebrain bundle

raphe nuclei

midbrain

pons

medulla

Fig. 15.5 Coronal diagram of the brain, showing the serotonergic projections from the rostral raphe nuclei.

TREATMENT

There are three main medical treatments for affective disorder:

- electroconvulsive therapy;
- antidepressants; and
- lithium.

Electroconvulsive Therapy

This therapy involves the induction of a generalized brain seizure under general anaesthesia. On average, six to eight seizures given at two-day intervals over several weeks produce a marked therapeutic effect in some 90 per cent of patients, particularly in older patients with marked psychomotor retardation. The mechanism of action is unknown, but is often associated with changes in aminergic transmitter systems. This therapy is useful for patients with cardiovascular disease, as these patients may not tolerate some antidepressant drugs, owing to their cardiovascular side effects.

Despite its proven efficacy and its lack of side effects (e.g. no observable memory deficits six months after treatment) electroconvulsive therapy has entered the canons of modern demonology. Its use is often decried and is a frequent subject of public vilification and hostility. This situation is unfortunate in the light of its therapeutic usefulness.

Antidepressants

There are three classes of antidepressants (Fig. 15.7):

- monoamine oxidase inhibitors;
- tricyclic compounds; and
- serotonin-uptake blockers.

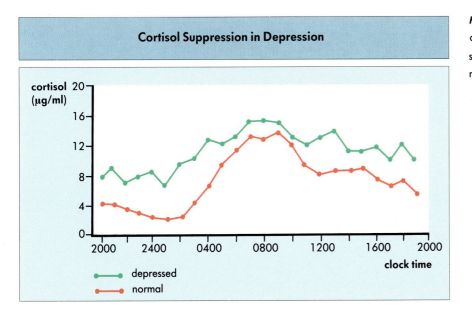

Cortisol Suppression in Depression

Fig. 15.6 Mean hourly plasma cortisol concentrations over a 24-hour period in a series of depressed patients, compared with normal subjects.

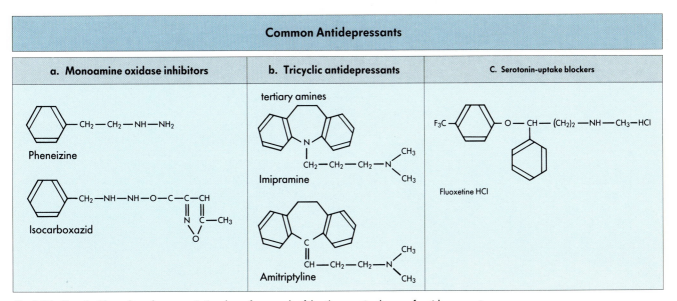

Fig. 15.7 Chemical formulae of representative drugs from each of the three main classes of antidepressants.

Monoamine oxidase inhibitors   Monoamine oxidase inhibitors increase the concentration of serotonin, noradrenaline and, to a lesser degree, dopamine in the brain by blocking the degradation of these transmitters by monoamine oxidase (Fig. 15.8).

Tricyclic antidepressants   Tricyclic antidepressants block the reactive uptake of serotonin, noradrenaline and dopamine, thereby increasing the amount and prolonging the active period of these transmitters in the synaptic cleft (see Fig. 15.9).

Serotonin-uptake blockers   These are highly selective for serotonin and act by causing a delayed decrease in the sensitivity of an inhibitory presynaptic autoreceptor. This causes an increased release of serotonin (see Fig. 15.9). The net effect is improvement in the efficiency of serotonergic transmission.

Once depressive symptoms have remitted, there may be a period in which the patient is at an increased risk of recurrence. There is no practical method of determining the length of this period and so it is common practice to continue medication for at least six months after the remission of acute symptoms.

Lithium

Lithium salts are highly effective in the treatment of mania and manic depression. Lithium acts by blocking the enzyme inositol-1-phosphatase, which causes a build-up of inositol phosphate (IP3) and subsequently affects calcium metabolism. The net effect of lithium is to damp down excess neuronal activity by reducing the responsiveness of neurons whose transmitter receptors are coupled to the IP3 pathway (Fig. 15.10).

DIFFERENTIAL DIAGNOSIS

The diagnosis and classification of mood disorders remains controversial. DSM-III-R does not distinguish between 'primary' and 'secondary' mood disorder. This distinction may be important since, although the symptoms of primary and secondary mood disorder are similar, the two conditions have different prognostic and therapeutic implications.

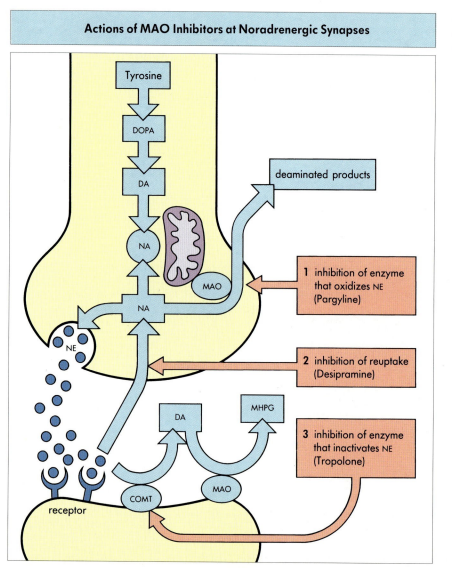

Actions of MAO Inhibitors at Noradrenergic Synapses

Fig. 15.8 Mechanisms of action of monoamine oxidase inhibitors at noradrenergic synapses.

Primary mood disorder, which occurs in the absence of a pre-existing psychiatric disorder or a chronic debilitating medical illness, consists of discrete episodes interspersed with periods of normality. In secondary mood disorder, there is a pre-existing illness which is often chronic, and the patient is not well between episodes of depression.

Depressions that are symptomatically indistinguishable from primary mood disorder occur commonly in obsessive compulsive disorder, phobic disorder, panic disorder, somatization disorder, alcoholism, drug dependence, and antisocial personality. In fact, almost all psychiatric disorders, including schizophrenia and brain syndromes, are associated with an increased risk of secondary depression (secondary mania is much less common).

Treatment plans will be heavily influenced by a diagnosis of secondary mood disorder, as both the pre-existing illness and the depressive syndrome must be treated.

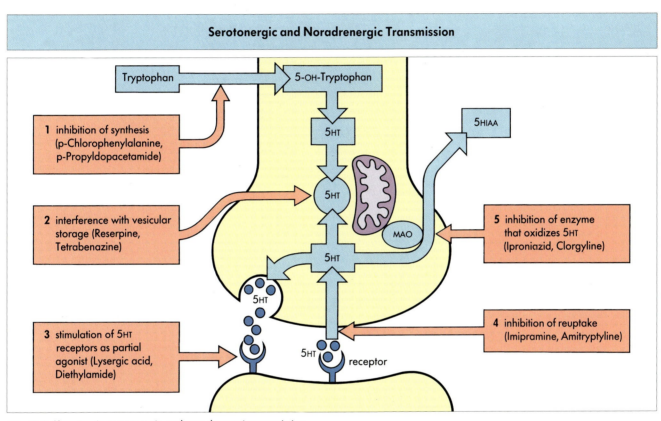

Fig. 15.9 Key steps in serotonergic and noradrenergic transmission.

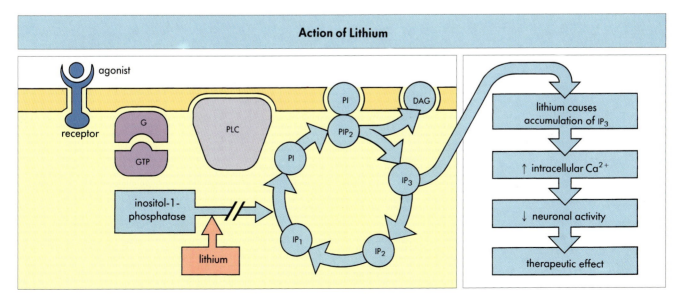

Fig. 15.10 Lithium affects the phosphoinositide second-messenger system, by blocking the action of the enzyme inositol-1-phosphate, which causes the accumulation of IP3 in the cytoplasm.

The following points are useful in the differential diagnosis of a primary mood disorder:

- mood-congruent psychotic features (schizophrenia has mood-incongruent psychotic features);
- acute depression of recent onset (in dementia it is often insidious);
- memory and insight usually preserved; depressed patients often communicate a sense of distress and complain of their symptoms (dementia has shallow emotions and patients tend not to complain); and
- no deficits of higher cortical function (these deficits – e.g. aphasia – are seen in dementia).

SUMMARY

(i)   Mood disorders are sustained disorders of mood.

(ii)   The three main categories of mood disorder are depression, mania, and anxiety.

(iii) Depression affects more women than men and has a peak onset of around 35 years of age.

(iv)   More than one episode is experienced by 60 per cent of patients.

(v)   Presenting symptoms include tiredness, sleep disturbance, guilt, low self-esteem, and irritability.

(vi)   Mania affects men and women equally and has a peak onset around 25 years of age.

(vii) Presenting symptoms include grandiose delusions, amusing flights of ideas, and hyperactivity.

(viii) Between 10 and 15 per cent of patients commit suicide.

(ix)   Treatments include electroconvulsive therapy, tricyclic antidepressants, and serotonin-uptake blockers.

(x)   Alterations in serotonin and noradrenaline are a likely cause of symptoms.

(xi)   Structural abnormalities and disturbed cerebral perfusion may be found in the brain.

(xii) Differential diagnosis includes secondary mood disorders, schizophrenia, and dementia.

Suggested Further Reading

Dementia

Copeland JRM, Kelleher MJ, Kellett JM *et al.* A semistructured clinical interview for the assessment of diagnosis and mental state in the elderly. The Geriatric Mental State Schedule 1. Development and reliability. *Psychol Med* 1976; **6**: 439–449.

Gurland B, Kuriansky J, Sharpe L, Simon R, Stiller P, Birkett P. The comprehensive assessment and referral evaluation (CARE). Rationale, development and reliability. *Int J Aging Hum Dev* 1977; **8(1)**: 9–42.

La Rue A. *Aging and neuropsychological assessment.* New York: Plenum Publishing Corporation, 1992. (Puente AE, Reynolds CR, eds. *Critical Issues in Neuropsychology*).

Rapp PR, Amaral DG. Individual differences in the cognitive and neurobiological consequences of normal aging. *Trends Neurosci* 1992; **15**: 340–345.

Robins LN, Heelzer JE, Crougham J, Ratcliffe KS. National Institute of Mental Health Diagnostic Interview Schedule: its history, characteristics and validity. *Arch Gen Psychiatry* 1981; **38**: 381–389.

Roth M, Kuppert FA, Tym E, Mountjoy CO, *et al.* Camdex: *The Cambridge Examination for Mental Disorders of the Elderly.* Cambridge: Cambridge University Press, 1988.

Roth M, Tym E, Mountjoy CO, *et al.* CAMDEX: a standardized instrument of the diagnosis of mental disorder in the elderly with special reference to the early detection of dementia. *Br J Psychiatry*; in press.

Sjögren T, Sjögren H, Lindgren AGH. Morbus Alzheimer and morbus Pick. A genetic clinical and patho-anatomical study. *Acta Psychiatr Neurol Scand (suppl)* 1952; **82**: 1–152.

Slater E, Roth M. *Clinical Psychiatry.* 3rd edn. London: Baillière Tindall, 1987.

Wing JK, Cooper JE, Sartorius N. *The Measurement and classification of psychiatric symptoms.* Cambridge: Cambridge University Press, 1974.

Alzheimer's disease

Burns A. Clinical diagnosis of Alzheimer's disease. *Dementia* 1991; **2**: 186–194.

Hardy J, Allsop D. Amyloid deposition as the central event in the aetiology of Alzheimer's disease. *Trends Pharmacol Sci* 1991; **12**: 383–388.

Lantos PL. Ageing and dementias. In: *Systemic Pathology.* 3rd edn. Edinburgh: Churchill Livingstone, 1990.

Mirra SS, Heyman A, McKeel D, *et al.* The consortium to establish a registry for Alzheimer's disease (CERAD). *Neurology* 1991; **41**: 479–486.

Orrell MW, Sahakian BJ. Dementia of frontal lobe type [Editorial]. *Psychol Med* 1991; **21**: 553–556.

Roberts GW, Lofthouse R, Allsop D, *et al.* CNS amyloid proteins in neurodegenerative diseases. *Neurology* 1988; **38**: 1534–1540.

Cerebrovascular dementia

Adams JH. Head Injury. In: Adams JH, Duchen LW, eds. *Greenfield's Neuropathology.* 5th edn. London: Edward Arnold, 1992.

Bouma GJ, Muizelaar JP, Stringer WA, Choi SC, Fatouros P, Young HF. Ultra-early evaluation of regional cerebral blood flow in severely head-injured patients using xenon-enhanced computerized tomography. *J Neurosurg* 1992; **77**: 360–368.

Garcia JH. The evolution of brain infarcts. *J Neuropathol Exp Neurol* 1992; **51**: 387–393.

Garcia JH, Brown GG. Vascular dementia: neuropathologic alterations and metabolic brain changes. *J Neurol Sci* 1992; **109**: 121–131.

McGonigal G, McQuade CA, Thomas BM, Whalley LJ. Survival in presenile Alzheimer's and multi-infarct dementias. *Neuroepidemilogy* 1992; **11**: 121–126.

Nussbaum M, Treves TA, Korczyn AD. Evaluation of the Hachinski ischemic scale in a prospective study. *Dementia* 1992; **3**: 10–14.

Pulsinelli W. Pathophysiology of acute ischaemic stroke. *Lancet* 1992; **339**: 533–536.

Rothwell NJ. Functions and mechanisms of interleukin 1 in the brain. *Trends Pharmacol Sci* 1991; **12**: 430.

Siesjö BK. Pathophysiology and treatment of focal cerebral ischemia. Part I: Pathophysiology. *J Neurosurg* 1992; **77**: 169–184.

Siesjö BK. Pathophysiology and treatment of focal cerebral ischemia. Part II: Mechanisms of damage and treatment. *J Neurosurg* 1992; **77**: 337–354.

Dementia with cortical Lewy bodies

Hansen L, Salmon D, Galasko D. The Lewy body variant of Alzheimer's disease: a clinical and pathologic entity. *Neurology* 1990; **40**: 1–7.

Head trauma

Adams JH. Head Injury. In: Adams JH, Duchen LW, eds. *Greenfield's Neuropathology*. 5th edn. London: Edward Arnold, 1992.

AIDS dementia

Budka H, Wiley CA, Kleihues J, *et al*. HIV-associated disease of the nervous system: review of nomenclature and proposal for neuropathology-based terminology. *Brain Pathol* 1991; **1**: 143–212.

Maj M. Organic mental disorders in HIV-1 infection. *AIDS* 1990; **4**: 831–834.

Masliah E, Ge N, Morey M, De Teresa R, Terry RD, Wiley CA. Cortical dendritic pathology in human immunodeficiency virus encephalitis. *Lab Invest* 1992; **66**: 285–291.

Miller D, Riccio M. Non-organic psychiatric and psychosocial syndromes associated with HIV-1 infection and disease. *AIDS* 1990; **4**: 381–388.

Royce RA, Luckmann RS, Fusaro RE, Winkelstein W Jr. The natural history of HIV-1 infection: staging classifications of disease. *AIDS* 1991; **5**: 355–364.

Shapshak P, Yoshioka M, Sun NCJ, *et al*. HIV-1 in postmortem brain tissue from patients with AIDS: a comparison of different detection techniques. *AIDS* 1992; **6**: 915–923.

Prion disease

Brown P, Preece MA, Will RG. 'Friendly fire' in medicine: hormones, homografts, and Creutzfeldt–Jakob disease. *Lancet* 1992; **340**: 24–27.

Harrison P, Roberts GW. Life, Jim, but not as we know it. *Br J Psychiatry* 1991; **158**: 457–470.

Mayer RJ, Landon M, Laszlo L, Lennox G, Lowe J. Protein processing in lysosomes: the new therapeutic target in neurodegenerative disease. *Lancet* 1992; **340**: 156–159.

Prusiner SB. Molecular biology of prion diseases. *Science* 1991; **252**: 1515–1522.

Prusiner SB, McKinley MP. *Prions*. San Diego: Academic Press, 1987.

Parkinson's disease

Johnson WG, Hodge SE, Duvoisiin R. Twin studies and the genetics of Parkinson's disease – a reappraisal. *Movement Disorders* 1990; **5 (3)**: 187–194.

Maraganore DM, Harding AE, Marsden CD. A clinical and genetic study of familial Parkinson's disease. *Movement Disorders* 1990; **6**: 205–211.

Forno LS. Pathology of Parkinson's disease: the importance of the substantia nigra and Lewy bodies. In: *Parkinson's Disease* (Stern G, ed). London: Chapman and Hall, 1990.

Gibb WRG. Neuropathology in movement disorders

Epilepsy

Brodie MJ. Status epilepticus in adults. *Lancet* 1990; **336**: 551–555.

Chadwick D. Diagnosis of epilepsy. *Lancet* 1990; **336**: 291–296.

Gram L. Epileptic seizures and syndromes. *Lancet* 1990; **336**: 161–164.

Gross RA. A brief history of epilepsy and its therapy in the western hemisphere. *Epilepsy Res* 1992; **12**: 65–74.

Jefferys JGR. Basic mechanisms of focal epilepsies. *Exp Physiol* 1990; **75**: 127–162.

Manford M, Hart YM, Sander JWAS, Shorvon SD. The National General Practice Study of Epilepsy. *Arch Neurol* 1992; **49**: 801–808.

Meldrum BS. Anatomy, physiology, and pathology of epilepsy. *Lancet* 1990; **336**: 231–234.

Meldrum BS, Bruton CJ. Epilepsy. In: Adams JH, Duchen LW, eds. *Greenfield's Neuropathology*. 5th edn. London: Edward Arnold, 1992.

Porter RJ. New antiepileptic agents: strategies for drug development. *Lancet* 1990; **336**: 423–424.

Shorvon SD. Epidemiology, classification, natural history, and genetics of epilepsy. *Lancet* 1990; **336**: 93–96.

Schizophrenia

Arnold SE, Hyman BT, Van Hoesen GW, Damasiol AR. Some cytoarchitectural abnormalities of the entorhinal cortex in schizophrenia. *Arch Gen Psychiatry* 1992; **48**: 625–632.

Bleuler E. *Dementia praecox or the group of schizophrenias*. (Zinkin J, translator.) New York: International Universities Press, 1950.

Ciaranello RD, Ciaranello AL. Genetics of major psychiatric disorders. *Annu Rev Med* 1991; **42**: 151–158.

Daniel DG, Goldberg TE, Gibbons RD, Weinberger DR. Lack of a bimodal distribution of ventricular size in schizophrenia: a Gaussian mixture analysis of 1056 cases and controls. *Biol Psychiatry* 1991; **30**: 887–903.

Kendell RE, Brockington IF, Leff LP. Prognostic implications of six alternative definitions of schizophrenia. *Arch Gen Psychiatry* 1979; **35**: 25–31.

Kraepelin E. *Dementia praecox and paraphrenia.* (Barclay RM, translator.) New York: RE Drieger, 1971.

Mednick SA, Machon RA, Huttunen MO, Bonett D. Adult schizophrenia following prenatal exposure to an influenza epidemic. *Arch Gen Psychiatry* 1988; **45**: 189–192.

O'Callaghan E. Sham P, Takei N, *et al.* Schizophrenia after prenatal exposure to 1957 influenza epidemic. *Lancet* 1991; **337**: 1248–1250.

Overall JE, Gorham DR. The brief psychiatric rating scale. *Psychol Rep* 1962; **10**: 799–812.

Pulver AE, Stewart W, Carpenter WT; *et al.* Risk factors in schizophrenia. *Br J Psychiatry* 1983; **143**: 389–396.

Reynolds GP. Developments in the drug treatment of schizophrenia. *Trends Pharmacol Sci* 1992; **13**: 116–121.

Schneider K. *Klinische Psychopathologie.* 5th edn. (Hamilton MW, translator.) New York: Grune and Stratton, 1959.

Spitzer RL, Williams JBW, Gibbon M, First MB. The structured clinical interview for *DSM-III-R* (SCID). I: History, rationale, and description. *Arch Gen Psychiatry* 1992; **49**: 624–629.

Stevens JR. Abnormal reinnervation as a basis of schizophrenia: a hypothesis. *Arch Gen Psychiatry* 1992; **49**: 238–243.

Suddath RL, Cristison GW, Torrey EF, Casanova MF, Weinberger DR. Cerebral anatomical abnormalities in monozygotic twins discordant for schizophrenia. *N Engl J Med* 1990; **12**: 789–794.

Weinberger DR. Implications of normal brain development for the pathogenesis of schizophrenia. *Arch Gen Psychiatry* 1987; **44**: 660–669.

Weinberger DR, Berman KF, Suddath R, Torrey EF. Evidence of dysfunction of a prefrontal–limbic network in schizophrenia: a magnetic resonance imaging and regional cerebral blood flow study of discordant monozygotic twins. *Am J Psychiatry* 1992; **149**: 890–897.

Wing JK, Cooper JE, Sartorius N. *The description and classification of psychiatric symptoms: an instruction manual for the PSE and Catego systems.* Cambridge: Cambridge University Press, 1974.

Mood disorders

Ciaranello RD, Ciaranello AL. Genetics of major psychiatric disorders. *Annu Rev Med* 1991; **42**: 151–158.

Kandal ER, Schwartz JK, Jessell TM. *Principles of neural science.* 2nd edn. New York: Elsevier Science Publishing Co, 1991.

Kendell RE, Zealley AK. *Companion to Psychiatric studies.* 3rd edn. Edinburgh: Churchill Livingstone, 1983.

Styron W. *Darkness visible: a memoir of madness.* New York: Random House; 1990.

Priest RG, Baldwin D. *Depression and Anxiety.* London: Martin Dunitz Ltd; 1992.

Index